RENEWALS 4

DATE DUE

D0350821

NOV - 8			
GAYLORD			PRINTED IN U.S.A.

Illness and
Shamanistic Curing
in Zinacantan

Illness and Shamanistic Curing in Zinacantan

An Ethnomedical Analysis

HORACIO FABREGA, JR. AND
DANIEL B. SILVER

Stanford University Press
Stanford, California
1973

Stanford University Press
Stanford, California
© 1973 by the Board of Trustees of the
Leland Stanford Junior University
Printed in the United States of America
ISBN 0-8047-0844-4
LC 73-80621

To Joan and Sybil

Preface

THIS STUDY RECORDS our efforts to understand how Zinacantecos construe illness and how they organize themselves socially to obtain medical care. Our original intention was to do a community-wide sociological and psychological study of the various occupational types in Zinacantan, with special reference to the *h'iloletik*, a body of shamanistic curers who control almost all medical practice and much of the religious ritual in the community. The scope and focus of the study, however, changed in response to our own developing interests and the limitations of field conditions. The breadth of information needed and the analytic requirements of studying diverse occupational types were extensive; and, although it has become easier every year to procure informants in Zinacantan, we still lacked the census data and range of contacts necessary for a truly representative sampling. These factors, then, together with our special interests, led to a reduction in the scope of the study and prompted us to focus more intensively on one occupational group, the h'iloletik.

Preliminary research in Zinacantan by members of the Harvard Chiapas Project, as well as the investigations of those working in other Mayan communities, had filled in some of the general outlines of the comprehensive picture of health, illness, and medical care that we sought. Large areas demanded closer analysis, however. This is reflected in the emphases of our fieldwork and in the present report, both of which are devoted to ethnographic description and to more analytical topics involving medical concerns.

The first six months of Daniel Silver's field stay (1963–64) were devoted primarily to studying Tzotzil, observing curing ceremonies, and evaluating the suitability of various testing materials. During this time, and throughout the year, he lived in San Cristóbal de las Casas, working with Zinacanteco informants there. Since most of the township of Zinacantan is readily accessible by trail and road from San Cristóbal, there was no problem of isolation involved in this procedure. There were regular short stays in hamlets and in Hteklum, the ceremonial center of Zinacantan, for the purpose of observing curing ceremonies and organized fiestas. In the course of the year, about a dozen major curing ceremonies were observed, as well as several public ceremonies. The remainder of the year was devoted to more systematic investigation. At various times two to four literate informants were employed to write texts in Tzotzil and Spanish on various aspects of Zinacanteco medical belief, and the information contained in these was analyzed and condensed. A voluminous questionnaire on medical beliefs was developed and administered to eleven informants as an exploratory exercise. Finally, during this period an economic census of about 400 households was compiled in interviews with three informants.

In 1967 both authors worked in Chiapas from June to August. During part of this time we administered the projective test and collected social background data on a group of healing practitioners and nonpractitioners. Horacio Fabrega was also involved in fieldwork in the Mayan community of Tenejapa, where he examined medical beliefs and interpretations. We were able to confer frequently, and attempted to consolidate our impressions about health, illness, and medical practice in the region.

Last, Fabrega returned to Chiapas in April–June 1969. This time in the field was devoted to administering to a large group of informants a questionnaire dealing with attributes of illness; the questionnaire items had resulted from Silver's earlier work. During this time we were also able to evaluate the medical judgments of Zinacantecos by eliciting responses to photographs of persons who showed obvious signs of disease. Further aspects related to the processual characteristics of medical care in Zinacantan were also investigated. Fabrega has since continued work in the Chiapas area, and impressions gained from these subsequent studies have been offered where appropriate.

We have tried to fit this report into the pattern of material available elsewhere, so as to minimize duplication of effort. The reader, for example, will find only brief mention of the *cargo* system (F. Cancian,

1965), or of Zinacantan's saints (Early, 1965). Evon Vogt's survey monograph fills in many of the gaps and provides a general description of the community of Zinacantan (Vogt, 1969).

The phonemes of Tzotzil are discussed in Weathers (1947, 1950) and in L. Colby (1960). They include a phonemic glottal stop and both glottalized and unglottalized forms of t, p, ts, ch, and k. We have indicated the phonemic stop by a single quote symbol ('); glottalized consonants are followed by a prime sign (').

Acknowledgments

OUR FIELDWORK WAS DONE, and this book written, both within the general framework of the Harvard Chiapas Project and with the assistance of research grants from the Public Health Service. Work with the Harvard Project was supported by a research training fellowship (No. 5 FL-MH-15, 710-02) and a research grant (No. MH-08349-01) from the National Institute of Mental Health, United States Public Health Service. Further assistance was obtained from NIMH through research grants No. MH-14131-01 and No. MH-16000-01, and through a general research support grant administered through the College of Human Medicine, Michigan State University. We are grateful to NIMH for its generosity, and to many members of its staff for assistance. Preparation of the manuscript was aided by support from the International Studies Program, Michigan State University; and we would like to express our thanks to John Hunter, Director of the Latin American Studies Center, for this help.

We have drawn heavily on the work of others, both published and unpublished, for general background on Zinacanteco culture and for specific data on curing practices to compare with our own observations. We are grateful to all members of the Harvard Project, past and present, for their generous assistance, both in personal discussion and in the field notes they have left in the Project files. None of them, however, should be held responsible for the data or conclusions herein, for which we are solely responsible.

We are deeply grateful to Professor Evon Z. Vogt, not only for unfailingly useful advice and supervision but for innumerable instances of extraordinary kindness and generosity. He has consistently provided us with support and guidance. The extent to which we have depended on his ideas and insights will be clear throughout this book.

Assistance and helpful comments, both in the field and since, were also received from Drs. Frank Cancian and Robert Laughlin and from George Collier. Our stay in San Cristóbal benefited from the friendship and assistance of Sra. Gertrudes Duby de Blom and Sr. Jose Rubio V. Ben Orlove offered help in obtaining data in the field; and we also benefited from conversations with and suggestions by Peter K. Manning. Finally, our work would have been impossible without the efforts of our informants Domingo de la Torre Pérez and Anselmo Pérez Okotz, or without the loyal friendship of Mariano Pérez Pérez of Pat'osil.

Miss Carole Ann Wallace deserves special acknowledgment and recognition. She performed most of the statistical analyses that we have used throughout the book, a number of which required developing special computer programs. In addition, she was responsible for scoring the inkblot protocols that served as the basis of the study reported in Chapter 5, and for coding the medical judgments analyzed in Chapter 7. Finally, she helped to organize the preparation of the book, supervised the typing, and was responsible for proofreading the manuscript. Joan Fabrega offered some support in this capacity, and we wish to acknowledge her help.

Miss Sherrilyn Boatman typed the early drafts for the book, as well as the final manuscript. It is a pleasure to express our appreciation to her for her patient and very skillful secretarial assistance.

Parts of Chapter 1 of this study appeared in *Yale Journal of Biology and Medicine* 43 (1971): 385-404. The material in Chapter 5 appeared in *Behavioral Science* 15 (1970): 471-86. The material in Chapter 7 appeared in *Southwestern Journal of Anthropology* 26 (1970): 305-14. And the material in Chapter 9 appeared in *Milbank Memorial Fund Quarterly* 48 (1970): 391-412. We thank the publishers of these journals for permission to modify and expand these articles for the present work. Our Figure 1 is modified from Jane F. Collier, *Law and Social Change in Zinacantan* (Stanford University Press, 1973), p. xiv. The map in Figure 5 is modified from Evon Vogt, *Zinacantan* (Harvard University Press, 1969), pp. 376-77, by permission of the Belknap Press of Harvard University Press.

H.F.
D.B.S.

Contents

Tables

Figures

Chapter one

Introduction

THE MEMBERS of all human groups have always had to contend with problems that interfere with their ability to carry out the daily tasks of living. Some of these problems stem from physical and/or social changes in their environment and affect the lives of the group members collectively. Other problems are of a more individualistic and personal nature. More or less regularly, people are observed "not feeling well," withdrawing from organized and productive work, changing in their manner of carrying out vital life functions, and seeking rest and comfort, often with help from their immediate comembers. All these are hallmarks of what we have come to call illness and disease. All groups, furthermore, have available to them as part of their inherited and learned cultural traditions a set of explanations about the causes of illness, and tied to these explanations are ways of eliminating or treating the illness. The sum total of a group's way of defining illness, of explaining its sources and occurrences, and of dealing with its burdens may be termed the group's system of medical care.

Several different approaches have been used to study illness and medical care in a group. When the groups studied are those of Western nations, a frequent approach is one that we have come to call epidemiological. The epidemiological approach is designed to make explicit the level and distribution of disease in a human community; it depends on applying the accumulated knowledge of Western biological science and medicine, and it is an integral feature of public health disciplines, which are concerned with maintaining a high level of health in the community. The focus of epidemiological studies, "disease," signifies a biomedical category or entity that is indicated and diagnosed by specialized examinations and tests. In recent years, social scientists and physicians have been interested in studying additional factors that are not, strictly speaking, epidemiological, although they are related to the level and distribution of disease in this biological sense—for example, general medical orientations and reasons for any delay in seeking medical care, social consequences devolving from the labeling of oneself as "sick" or "patient," and actual evaluations of the medical care that is administered. Implicit in these latter studies is the belief that static profiles of how much disease is found in a community offer only one rather limited medical view of the community. The way in which disease is experienced, defined, and handled by members of the community as well as by medical practitioners is felt to offer a more dynamic if not more dramatic picture of medical problems. Specifically, these studies inform us in a more realistic fashion about the burden and consequences of disease in the community.

When investigators have studied medical issues in isolated and nonliterate groups, rather different approaches and aims have been pursued. If the analytic unit is disease as defined biomedically, we might term the approach ecological: that is, the biological characteristics of persons living in isolated groups are examined with the intent of gaining knowledge about how they are affected by characteristics of the ecosystem. The immediate aim of these studies is to gain information on immunological, physiological, and genetic factors that contribute to good health and to disease. In the process, the investigators have sometimes uncovered unusual infectious diseases that have yielded insights regarding the biology of man. In addition to describing human biophysical traits that may have a direct bearing on health and disease, ecological studies also examine broader questions that are central to the fields of population genetics and cultural ecology. It is reasoned that man as a biological creature was formed in communities analogous to those that today we term "primitive," "isolated," or "nonliterate." Consequently, the biological defenses that protect against disease and that may have allowed for the survival of man need to be carefully examined *in situ* in order to understand the growth and movements of populations. Thus an ultimate aim of "ecological" studies is to clarify evolutionary questions and to derive an understanding of the characteristics that are unique to man as well as those that he shares with other primates.

There are practical payoffs associated with this line of investigation.

For example, some contemporary medical problems, the so-called chronic diseases, are believed to be in part consequences of the control that man has gained over his environment, a control that now enables him to live longer under conditions less "natural" than those to which he is biologically accustomed. Hence ecological studies, insofar as they clarify the basic biophysical features of man, may also indirectly clarify the causes of degenerative diseases. In brief, by explicating the biology of man as seen in his more natural and isolated "primitive" settings, and by studying the characteristics of these settings that influence genetic equipment and physiological functions, we may better understand the medical problems that are associated with other modes of social organization. In this sense, then, epidemiological and ecological studies complement each other.

A third way to conduct a community study of illness and medical care can be identified, which we may term ethnomedical. In this instance, medical problems are examined with a view to the form and meaning given these problems by members of the community. Epidemiological studies, of course, can also interpret disease-related issues along the highly specific lines determined by a group's culture. Disease specified biomedically, in fact, is precisely how members of Western cultures, especially social planners and medical practitioners, have come to conceptualize and explain deviations in bodily wellbeing; biomedical terms have wide currency even among laymen, and are often used by them when they speak and think about their medical difficulties. Special theoretical problems are created by this application of an impersonal and technologically based language to the highly personal, private, and socially consequential matters that are invariably associated with any instance of illness and disease (see Fabrega, 1972). Suffice it to say here that many competing and conflicting views exist at present.

Ethnomedical studies, especially when they are conducted among non-Western groups uninfluenced by biomedicine, bring into sharp relief the alternative or "nonbiomedical" meanings and implications of illness, disease, and medical care. Such studies base their definitions on a community's own beliefs about illness and on the various practices that have been established to cure illness. Altogether different definitions of disease and strategies for coping with its effects thus stand out dramatically. The ethnomedical approach is the one classically associated with the discipline of anthropology; and it is by nature broad, synthetic, and comparative, resting on a framework that emphasizes holism, process, and change. In ethnomedical studies the investigator tries to analyze problems of illness and medical care in relation to other cultural activities of the group. The perception of illness, in effect, is one more example of the way behavior is structured and organized by underlying cultural rules. And an analysis of medical treatment may allow access to beliefs regarding religious and malevolent agencies, giving the anthropologist some idea of the ultimate values that the culture holds sacred. Indeed, the members of a cultural group often display both their actual personal relationships and their views of those relationships most dramatically during illness and other uncontrollable calamities.

A long-range goal of ethnomedical studies, shared by anthropological studies in general, is to analyze how sociocultural units function and change. Illness and disease are so problematic to members of a group that in continually being forced to cope with these occurrences they strive to develop new and better ways of resolving the problem. Changing strategies for dealing with disease often initiate and always reflect other complex changes that can be observed in a sociocultural group, giving the anthropologist a rich area for the development and testing of theory. The approach followed here is basically ethnomedical, and for this reason we will discuss earlier studies in this general area later on.

It should be clear, then, that our primary concern is with medical issues as these are interpreted by the Maya Indians of Zinacantan. For this reason, no physiological or immunological data will be presented; for we, like the Zinacantecos, must not regard disease as a strictly biomedical category or fact. Instead, we work in a cultural framework, viewing the term "disease" entirely as a product of the behavioral and sociopsychological experiences and culturally specific concepts that have significance in Zinacantan; and we prefer to use the term "illness" to refer to this sociopsychological entity.

Even though we will not concern ourselves with disease in the strictly biomedical sense, this study does take up indirectly and by implication some of the questions we have described as epidemiological and ecological. For example, we have attempted to uncover perceptions about the social and physiological components of illness in Zinacantan and interpret them in biomedical terms. Also, using the biomedical point of reference regarding disease entities, we have attempted to examine the Zinacanteco ways of evaluating and explaining illness. Lastly, we have addressed ourselves to what can be termed the "objective" factors associated with the decision to seek medical care. Implicitly, we have used the biomedical frame of reference to analyze Zinacantecan medical forms and experiences, and this comparative orientation has obviously influenced our choice of questions and methods of procedure. But in addition to describing and analyzing the problems of illness and medical care comparatively, we have also attempted to meet the requirements for good descriptive ethnography: for example, we have described in detail the ritual practices associated with public and private ceremonies in Zinacantan, and have also dealt with the diverse nonmedical occupational patterns of male Zinacanteco healers.

By way of summary, let us emphasize that a particular medical problem—that is, an occurrence of illness—must be examined in terms of the setting in which it occurs. Necessarily, the native conceptions that give the problem its meaning should be described in great detail; and whenever possible the biological correlates or implications of the illness and the way in which it is handled should be brought into focus. The process of medical care should be seen as a series of social events that reflect cultural rules and have potential biological implications for the cultural group. The basic units of analysis—what we may term "disease" and "medical care"—should thus be given multiple referents. The definition of these terms, in other words, must fall within three logically independent but complementary frameworks: the biomedical, the phenomenological, and the behavioral.

Ethnomedicine as a Special Field of Study

An examination of the literature in ethnomedicine (Fabrega, 1972) reveals that illness episodes are usually analyzed in one of three ways. First, they may be treated as indicating a point of stress and dysfunction in the sociocultural unit. The dysfunction may be viewed as determined by psychocultural factors; or it may be considered stochastic in the sense that it represents an obtrusion of "natural" forces that have no fixed reference in the culture. At any rate, the illness is then supposed to provide an opportunity for specific institutions and other culturally patterned processes to adjust or control the situation. Second, because illness is suffused with heightened emotion and concern, the analyst may examine it in terms of how religious and other "supernatural" ideas come to be expressed in symbolic actions, rituals, and practices that exercise powerful influences on the behavior of the sick one and his family. This paradigm is not exclusive of the "functional" approach; but it is analytically distinct, since the main effort of the ethnographer in this case appears to be devoted to processional and symbolic issues. Finally, an illness may be analyzed as an instance of the way sociocultural patterns "shape" both the expression of disability itself and the general aspects of illness and medical care (regardless of whether the medical occurrence is psychoculturally determined or stochastic, as in the first approach). In all three of these cases, anthropologists seem to be motivated by an interest that is above all descriptive.

Regardless of the approach taken by a given anthropological writer, it usually happens that his description of an illness episode is not differentiated in a way that allows others to build on their own impressions and insights gained in the field. The episode is treated either as part of an abstract biomedical category (e.g. pneumonia) that has no currency in the cultural group and glosses varied experiences and perceptions of the subjects or as a generic cultural type (e.g., Susto or Piblobtok) largely devoid of situational richness. Even the cultural formalization creates the illusion that all illnesses in a culture are similarly patterned and have the cultural significance that the ethnographer attributes to the one he examines. Illness episodes may obviously vary in their modes of onset and resolution, and in their social and temporal locations; and they obviously occur in individuals (or family units) characterized by particular histories. What is not altogether clear is what transpires situationally before and after clearly distinct illness/treatment episodes. That is, in ethnomedical studies one gains only a faint picture of the sequence of events leading to a request for medical care and continuing through the curing ceremonies and their aftermath. We feel that the complete social context of illness and medical care should be explicated if the description is to be useful in more than a limited context.

In the general domain of ethnomedicine it is possible to identify several areas that should be studied and clarified if we are to develop a culturally relevant picture of illness and medical care.

The Context and Constituents of Medical Judgments

In general, the "healing" that persons in a given culture experience from what have come to be called "folk" curing rituals and ceremonies is viewed by anthropologists as a consequence of primary psychosocial changes in identity and feeling. Essentially, the patient's self-conception and his value to himself and to his immediate group are enhanced by the ceremony, which depends on the manipulative and persuasive actions of the healer and occurs in a setting of heightened emotion. One may acknowledge that some benefits of ceremonial cures do depend on the pharmacological effects of the herbs or potions used; but the folk healer's use of these agents is usually sanctioned by supernatural revelation, and not by articulated explanations that relate the physical ingredients of the medicines to specific bodily processes.

Processes of many kinds no doubt underlie any occurrence of illness, and we must certainly include among them the physiological, the biochemical, and the sociopsychological. Evidently the "persuasion" associated with folk healing also has physiological and biochemical consequences for the individual, and both are adaptive and health-promoting. (See Frank, 1961.) All processes of the human mind and body are clearly implicated during an illness episode, though the centrality and importance of each process may vary. We must assume that some illness episodes are associated with underlying biomedical changes of kinds that are relatively refractory to psychosocial influences. Episodes of this type, which will most likely not be resolved or "cured" by folk healing, would appear to endanger the reputations of folk medical practitioners, who stand to lose if patients under their care die.

In other words, in nonliterate groups, matters of illness, disease, and death are interconnected with diverse personal, interpersonal, and sociostructural matters that are not only complex but also imbued with significance far beyond purely naturalistic happenings. Cosmic and supernatural factors of great concern to the individual and his group are at stake. Furthermore, the practitioner who is consulted does not draw on a public and systematically articulated body of medical knowledge that assigns the bases or causes of illness to impersonal agencies. Consequently, since he himself takes on part of the significance of and responsibility for the illness, he is placed in a very vulnerable and dangerous position.

Given these considerations, if one assumes that successful folk healing results from changes brought about primarily by psychosocial factors, then the professional success of folk healers would seem to depend on at least two related factors. First, there are the practitioner's interpersonal skills, which are in part reflected by his ability to emotionally arouse others and especially by his ability to influence and manipulate their behavior in line with particular decisions related to the treatment he administers. These skills can be regarded as stemming from persuasive or "charismatic" personality attributes (Romano, 1965). Second, a practitioner, in order to be successful, would seem to depend on what could be termed his "clinical judgment." The patients of successful practitioners "should" more often improve than not, which suggests that these practitioners might possibly select and treat only those persons whose underlying medical problem is likely to remit or improve. Success in making this essentially prognostic judgment appears to require some general appreciation of degrees of bodily functioning, a general understanding of illness behaviors, and an intuitive knowledge of the relationship between both of these. One would thus assume that practitioners, when compared to nonpractitioners, are more sensitive to the physical attributes and manifestations of illness that relate to prognosis.

Earlier studies of folk or primitive medicine have not dealt with this particular aspect of a healer's behavior. That is, the nature of the understanding that folk practitioners have of medical problems, even though we acknowledge that this understanding is culturally organized, has never been empirically investigated by means of testing materials that depict the physical manifestations or components of disease. In fact, the orientations and activities of folk practitioners have been investigated in a manner almost wholly independent of how the sick person is ill and what the outcomes of the illness reflect and mean. To the extent that a critical evaluation of the practitioner's knowledge and judgment is disregarded, the literature suggests that medical practice in primitive settings is constituted of decisions and actions based purely on ideology, and that folk practitioners are relatively insensitive to the dimensions of illness that reflect biological functioning. There exists, in other words, a need to clarify the extent to which this particular dimension of illness does affect the medical judgments of practitioners generally and their judgment of severity or prognosis specifically. A greater knowledge of this aspect of ethnomedicine will lead to greater understanding not only of the way illness is patterned, but also of the way illness is handled in primitive settings, the social significance associated with illness, and the role of the practitioner.

How Folk Medical Knowledge Is Distributed in a Culture

In ethnomedical studies, various exotic and unusual features or symptoms of illness that may or may not be intraculturally significant are very often given more attention by anthropologists than the rather basic question of what bodily and/or behavioral elements comprise the general model of illness in a culture. In other words, preoccupied with describing these so-called culture-bound syndromes or with rendering equivalent Western diagnoses of them, the ethnographer completely overlooks the cultural framework of illness referents that actually provides the basis for judgment-making in the group he is studying. Furthermore, the ethnographer interested in describing these syndromes and explaining their sources and mechanisms invariably reflects a psychiatric bias. That is, he assumes that since the unusual manifestations he sees are social and behavioral, they must be purely psychologic, and thereby he abandons his search for other bodily and physiological manifestations that might be present.

Although certain culturally differentiated illnesses have been described with some fidelity, the issue of how distinct and invariant their content may be within the culture has been largely overlooked. Investigators have simply not addressed themselves to the issue of uniformity. As a result, we know a good deal about the general and the exotic ways in which culture can shape illness manifestations; yet the underlying and related issues of how illness is modeled in a culture and how distinctly this model and its component parts appear in the minds of representative members of the culture have not been carefully explored. It is important that we evaluate empirically the degree of clarity and specificity with which native subjects construe illness, and this must be done by determining the extent to which they differentiate between various symptoms and signs, and how they regard the clustering of these signs in syndromes. Even if this biological dimension is disregarded, we must still specify the way in which purely native beliefs about illness are organized and patterned. In brief, researchers conducting even purely intracultural analyses of illness should strive to document how knowledge about illness (including its various types, their components, and their presumed sources and implications) is shared by members of the group.

Along the same lines, it is necessary to evaluate the extent to which native conceptions of illness are specific or special to folk medical practitioners as such. Past studies have not made altogether clear whether the folk healer validates his social position by commanding and using a special body of medically relevant information. Largely by implication, it is known that nonpractitioners who are comembers of the healer's cultural group have some understanding of the various native illness

terms and can often list the symptoms, general implications, and customary treatments of specific "folk illnesses." In this sense, knowledge of
health and illness can be said to be generally shared within the culture.
It is possible, however, that if precise attention were given to the kind
of understanding that different groups have of medical phenomena,
practitioners would be found to differ from nonpractitioners.

We would suggest that when a group of practitioners is compared
with a group of nonpractitioners in terms of their responses to inquiries
about given features of illness (e.g. cause or prognosis), several possibilities may result: (a) certain response options may be selected in differing proportions; (b) there may be differences in a group's response
variability when illness terms are considered singly; (c) there may be
differences in the response consistency that the subjects of one group
manifest across native illness terms; (d) the groups may differ in some,
none, or all of these dimensions. These possibilities should be evaluated
for any specific culture if we are to elicit a true ethnography of the native medical system. Furthermore, since the knowledge base of a people
influences its behavior, the concerns reviewed here bear directly on the
process of medical care, and hence on the study of how people adjust to
social and environmental constraints.

We can draw attention to the importance of the issues discussed in
this and the preceding section by emphasizing once again the unique-
ness of the field of ethnomedicine and the rich potential that it offers to
the anthropologist who works in the particular sector of medical beliefs
and theories of illness. For example, investigators in psychosomatic medicine have come to appreciate that illness and disease must be approached
in an integrated fashion—that there is a unity in the way men respond
to stress, and that bodily, psychological, and behavioral manifestations
must be examined together. In the last analysis, a group's theory of illness represents its formal basis for medical judgments and expectations,
and these, in turn, determine how individuals respond to and express
that which they regard as illness: the theory, in short, actually shapes
the patterning of illness itself.

Ethnomedical studies, therefore, particularly when conducted in non-
Western settings, offer the anthropologist an opportunity to examine altogether novel patterns of illness expression, and to see how culture, in
the form of perception categories and behavioral prescriptions, can
affect and shape even matters that are predominantly "physiological."

Ethnomedicine in this sense can contribute information of relevance to both psychosomatic medicine and social science. However, we must take more than an individualistic and purely relativistic view of the issues involved. Once having uncovered the basic cultural ingredients of illness and disease, our aim should be to determine what pattern, if any, inheres in the way a group's medical knowledge is distributed among its members, and what relation this system of knowledge bears to alternative ones (e.g., the biomedical system). In this context, the healer's view of illness must be compared with that of his comembers if we are to more clearly understand the bases for his power and jurisdiction in matters of social control—and ultimately to determine the functional roots of his role in the culture. Such investigations can not only contribute the basic information needed to develop what we could term a social frame of reference for illness and medical care—a sociomedical theory, as it were —but would also allow anthropologists of various theoretical persuasions the opportunity to examine and test in the medical sphere their own propositions about cultural maintenance and change. From this expanded perspective, then, we see that ethnomedicine offers both medical and anthropological researchers ample opportunity to uncover important information of a potentially theoretical nature.

The Personality of the Medical Practitioner

Although not considering their work as necessarily ethnomedical in focus, anthropologists who work in the field of culture and personality have addressed themselves to problems that are, from our standpoint, medical. This was implied when we mentioned that earlier studies of folk illness have concentrated on unusual behavioral manifestations and interpreted them psychologically—that is, as "unusual" forms of mental illness shaped by distinctive cultural patterns. If one views the requirements of ethnomedicine as necessitating an extensive and thorough probing of all facets of a group's orientation to illness and medical care, then it is clear that ethnomedicine as an investigative field also encompasses the motivations and personality of the medical practitioner himself.

The actual behavior of native healers, medicine men, and shamans has long intrigued travelers and missionaries; and, as we have indicated, it has received considerable attention from behavioral scientists. Psychiatric anthropology, in particular, has approached the relationship between culture and mental illness by using as a paradigm the adaptation of the shaman to his role. A persistent question has been whether shamans are socially deviant persons with an underlying psychotic personality whose pathology is somehow protected and concealed by the behavioral requirements of their role. Silverman (1967) has reviewed the literature pertaining to this general topic. He elaborates on the ideas of Devereaux (1956) and Wallace (1961); and, using psychiatric knowledge about the syndrome of schizophrenia, he develops a five-stage cognitive model to explain and compare shamanism with the schizophrenia process. Largely on the basis of anecdotal information, these investigators have assumed that significant psychological changes and modifications take place as shamans come to choose and adopt their role in the culture, and have then gone on to elaborate formally the sequence of changes taking place. Largely in response to these formulations, Handelman (1968) has stressed the need for psychological data in this general area. He emphasizes the importance of distinguishing role behavior from behavior directly traceable to personality dynamics. In other words, shamanistic behavior may not reflect dynamic psychological notions, but rather conscious and creative role playing.

Initially, impressionistic and scattered observations served to link shamans with psychopathology. Single case studies or life histories of shamans, often used in the structural-functional analysis of sociocultural units, also provided a profile of personality dynamics and functioning. But the picture that emerges from some of these studies is hardly pathological (Handelman, 1967). Moreover, case studies unfortunately cannot answer the question of whether shamans as a group tend to demonstrate psychopathology. In order to answer this question in any one culture as a whole, more extensive and controlled psychological studies are needed, and very few fieldworkers dealing with the problem have attempted a broad approach. A notable exception is the work of Boyer (Boyer, 1962, 1964; Boyer et al., 1964, 1967), who studied the personality configuration of Mescalero Apache Indians, using a sample that included shamans, pseudoshamans, and normals. His initial psychoanalytic impressions, which he felt were validated by subsequent Rorschach analyses, were that Apache shamans are not persons who have disguised serious psychological illness. On the contrary, judging by "their greater capacity to test reality and their ability to use regression in the service of the ego," they are healthier than their societal comembers.

These studies of Boyer et al. are the only ones in the literature that probe in a controlled fashion the psychological status or adjustment of folk healers, and many others like them are badly needed. But at this stage, Boyer's conclusions must be regarded as tentative. The details of his psychoanalytic observations and interpretations have not been published. In addition, information derived from psychoanalysis is difficult to measure and quantify reliably; hence it often cannot be used to conduct controlled comparisons of groups on discrete personality dimensions. Similarly, not enough data on the social characteristics and experiences of the Apache subjects have been reported, and the comparability of the groups cannot be established on this dimension either. One cannot determine in what fashion or to what extent the reported "personality" differences are caused by differences in the subjects' social backgrounds (e.g. acculturative exposures).

A related problem is that Boyer and his colleagues have not integrated their analysis of the projective material with a knowledge of the role behavior of their subjects. It is quite possible that psychological data now evaluated purely from the standpoint of the health/pathology continuum could be better interpreted from a perspective that also accounted for the unique learning experiences of the subjects. For example, group differences on particular Rorschach measures, rather than exclusively reflecting greater "health" in the psychodynamic sense, may in part result from unique learning experiences involved in the performance of the shamanistic role.

In sum, the conclusions of Boyer et al. regarding the greater adjustment or health of Apache shamans appear to rest entirely on psychological grounds. Information derived from analyzing the projective material has not been explicitly linked with information bearing on social adjustment. Because of this, problems that may result from the cross-cultural invalidity of the projective test used cannot be excluded.

The literature in ethnomedicine, then, demonstrates a need for the controlled evaluation of personality characteristics of shamanistic medical practitioners. And in this evaluation other, nonshaman members of the same cultural group should be used for comparative purposes. Finally, analyses of personality characteristics should be combined with information about the social adjustment of shamans and the distinguishing features of their work in the cultural unit.

The Social Characteristics of Shamans

Besides information on the personality features of shamans, we need more material on the actual role of the shaman. We should know the standard ways in which shamans are selected, the requirements or characteristics of the apprenticeship period, if one exists, and the predominant patterns of exercising the entitlements of the position of shaman. Is the treatment of medical problems the principal means of livelihood for shamans? In addition to diagnosing and curing, what other duties and responsibilities are attached to the position of shaman? What prestige or social ranking do shamans enjoy in the community? Are different types of practitioners recognized, and is there a way of describing their competence as practitioners? These are a few of the questions that we feel need to be asked and satisfactorily answered in order to understand the shamanistic role in a culturally appropriate manner. Not only will such information provide the ethnographic background needed for an understanding of cultural dynamics, but it will also allow us to develop a detailed picture of the context of medical care and practice in a nonliterate community.

It should be realized that in a group's plans, directives, and institutions for medical care we have a set of distinct social and cultural forms that are manipulated by persons whose roles in the culture are potentially far-reaching and critical for understanding how social life is organized. Ethnomedical studies, if they are going to do justice to the wide-ranging social implications that attach to the performance of these roles, will have to describe in depth the many characteristics of the persons who fill them.

The Dynamics of Medical Practice

Considerable attention has been given in this brief discussion of ethnomedicine to studies dealing with the shaman. The clarification of this area relates centrally to current concerns in the fields of transcultural psychiatry and psychological anthropology. An additional purpose in studying the folk practitioner, as we have indicated, is to allow for a more rational understanding of the role of his behavior in medical care. To recapitulate, delineating the nature of the medical knowledge and judgments of the practitioner should make explicit not only the relevance of different types of symbolic categories in medical transactions, but also the ultimate sources of his power and control over a host of social processes in which he is involved; and clarifying the influence of personality factors and social patterns of functioning should lead to a better understanding of why and how he applies these categories. This information should be supplemented by analyses of the actual process of medical care.

Although there is now an extensive literature on various facets of medicine in preliterate settings, we have surprisingly little information dealing with the processes and dynamics of concrete medical practice in these settings. An example of this is the lack of attention given to the various stages of the practitioner-patient relationship that mediates the delivery of medical care. As we have remarked, the implicit model that most investigators rely on could be termed time-limited and socio-psychological. That is, the modification of social and psychological factors assumed to relate to health status is regarded as central to the eventual healing that takes place. Factors promoting this healing or treatment, however, are believed to be set in motion during a sharply demarcated time interval.

Such a model does not consider the many influences and events that antedate and follow any curing ceremony. These events involve the particular healer and patient, as well as other key persons and health-focused relationships; they are related to the unique sociocultural patterns that structure medical practice in the setting, and they directly affect the nature of any healing or treatment that may take place. Issues of this type have been examined in our own society, but a comprehensive understanding of medical practice requires that related phenomena be studied in other settings.

Our lack of information regarding the details of practitioner-patient interactions in nonliterate settings beclouds the manner in which various specifiable biological and behavioral processes are handled in these settings. It is quite likely, for example, that patients with what we could term "Western" diseases having different underlying pathological processes are viewed and treated differently by the practitioner. In other words, the formal properties and what is termed the "natural history" of a given "Western" disease that a patient develops—if there is such a thing as a "natural" history of a disease—probably affect directly the type of healing relationship that ensues. It was mentioned earlier that social scientists have largely ignored the influence of these properties of diseases when studying folk medical practice. Frake (1961), for example, draws attention to the importance of various formal characteristics of skin lesions in classifying illnesses among the Subanun but goes no further. Although he uncovers many linguistic correlates of diagnostic situations, he discounts the influence that perceptions and interpretations of the physical characteristics of the lesions may have on the social features of the practitioner-client relationship.

An analysis of native treatment practices in terms of type of pathophysiological process would provide a deeper understanding of how this system functions. Furthermore, by focusing exclusively on the cultural and behavioral levels, a careful analysis of the events of medical care should yield insights about social organization. A native medical system, in other words, must be assumed a priori to possess unique characteristics that reflect both facts of social science and facts of human biology. Viewing the process of medical care as a complex of informational and socially relevant exchanges that have effects on and implications for various system levels would link the ethnographic tradition of anthropology with that of cultural ecology in a way that should enrich the field of medicine. Although there exists a large body of traditional epidemiological data dealing with the geographic distribution of diseases, there is at present little information describing in detail a native system of definition and treatment or a given cultural group's way of handling the manifestations of the disease. Consequently, in most nonliterate cultures that have been studied it is not possible to evaluate the extent of the actual social problems created by a disease or its potential influence in the culture.

Focus and Organization of the Book

Our discussion so far should have made clear the frame of reference that we bring to our investigation of illness and curing in Zinacantan, Mexico. We see in a group's orientation to illness and medical care a culturally determined system that has a variety of important functions for the members of the group and for the group itself. Illness and disease episodes are endemic in social groups, and by definition they interfere with everyday affairs and continually pose challenges and threats to the group members. Consequently, a successful culture must develop effective ways of coping with illness. This "coping" must be viewed broadly. It includes, above all, a language for describing what we can term a set of illness forms, which are indicated by social, behavioral, and biological changes of diverse sorts. The "language of illness" necessarily reflects and embodies a theory explaining the causes of illness, the reasons for its presence in the world, the manner in which illnesses come and go, and the implications that they carry for the individual and the group.

Perhaps the most salient aspects of a cultural group's way of coping with the burdens posed by illness and disease are those personified by the individual practitioners whose function it is to control and eliminate these maladies. Treatment practices have certainly attracted the attention of anthropologists, as have the psychological characteristics of folk practitioners and shamans. However, the curers, their attitudes, and their ways of coping with illness are only part of the group's system of medical care. Medical matters in nonliterate societies ramify into and exemplify actions and functions that one could also term economic and religious. Furthermore, just as illness and the pursuit of medical care embody complex and diverse problems, so also do medical practitioners serve diverse functions in the group. In order to obtain a rational understanding of illness and medical care, then, one must also examine a great many aspects of the life situation of the people generally, and of the sick person and practitioner specifically. In brief, one is forced to conceptualize and handle illness and medical care as social phenomena that are marked in a culturally distinct manner but have various sources and extensions in the culture as a whole.

In addition to tracing the interconnections of matters we would wish to call illness or medical care, we must also determine their total patterning in the culture. This entails a careful probing of how members of the group define illness, how they agree and disagree about causes and treatment, and whether practitioners differ in any special way in their understanding of these matters. The principal rituals and ceremonies, too, as well as all the other activities that take place during treatment, must be explicated richly if one is to obtain a balanced ethnography of the group's orientation toward illness.

Our aim is to describe and analyze how the Maya Indians of Zinacantan orient themselves toward medical problems, and how they organize themselves to seek relief from the many problems associated with illness. In line with this basic ethnomedical goal, we have attempted to examine many aspects of this native medical system that we feel to have been passed over in similar studies of other cultures.

In Chapter 2, the salient characteristics of the community of Zinacantan that bear on medical matters are reviewed. In Chapter 3, we describe the different types of medical practitioners found in Zinacantan. How-

ever, we concentrate on the *h'iloletik*, or shamans, since they are by far
the most important healers. The characteristics of these curers, their
number and distribution in Zinacantan, their recruitment to the curing
role, and the general attitudes and beliefs held about them are reviewed.

In Chapter 4, the distinguishing social and economic characteristics
of h'iloletik in particular are presented and analyzed. Here, the curing
role is examined from a purely social and economic standpoint, and in
a comparative way. In other words, we attempt to establish how shamans, as a category of Zinacantecos, operate in their social unit. Chapter
5 offers an extensive comparative analysis of the personalities of a representative group of shamans, using Zinacanteco laymen as a control
group. In analyzing the findings generated by a projective psychological
instrument, we also make use of a variety of social information about
the shamans and their comembers.

Chapter 6 asks how the state of illness is viewed in Zinacantan. The
apparent factors that indicate illness, the way in which illness is handled
in the immediate social group, the various referents of illness, and the
processes that are implicated in given occurrences are analyzed.

Chapter 7 reports the results of two controlled investigations into the
actual knowledge that Zinacantecos have of illness, as viewed entirely
within the native system of meaning and categorization. A group of
shamans and a comparable group of laymen were interviewed about
their understandings of illness, and the data generated from these interviews were analyzed by statistical and information measurement procedures. In Chapter 8 we follow the same comparative approach to
Zinacantecan interpretations of illness, but use Western-defined biological forms and changes (depicted in photographs) as the units of inquiry
and analysis.

Chapter 9 is addressed to the way in which practitioners and their
clients actually participate in the process of medical care; that is, the
rules and processes embodied in the purely medical tasks of diagnosis
and treatment are described and analyzed. The significance of this form
of medical practice is touched upon.

Chapters 10 and 11 give a detailed ethnographic description of the
ceremonies and rituals that h'iloletik perform in Zinacantan, since we
feel that ethnomedicine as such must always consider the behavioral
segments that comprise the fundamental activity patterns involved in a

practitioner's fulfillment of his medical duties. These chapters should be read in light of the alternative approaches adopted elsewhere.

In Chapter 12 we evaluate the role of the h'ilol in Zinacantan. His functions, duties, and obligations in the culture are explicitly stated. We also touch on the theoretical and empirical problems posed by any analysis of a folk system of medical care, hopefully placing the study of such systems in a broader scientific perspective.

The five Appendixes contain information of a more specialized and technical nature, and should be consulted as they apply to particular chapters. We feel they offer the reader a richer appreciation of the perspective and mode of analysis we have chosen. He will find in them finer details regarding illness explanation and differentiation, the mathematical techniques employed in various of our analyses, and the rituals and prayers that punctuate the ceremonies performed by h'iloletik.

Chapter two

The Municipio of Zinacantan

THE MUNICIPIO, or township, of Zinacantan is a community of some 7,600 Mexican Indians located in the State of Chiapas in southwest Mexico. Linguistically and culturally the Zinacantecos share in the Maya cultural traditions, and their language is a dialect of Tzotzil Maya, one of the many Maya languages spoken in the Chiapas highlands (others being Tzeltal and Tojolabal). But although Zinacantecos share many cultural patterns with other Mayas in the highlands of Chiapas and elsewhere, they are distinguished from their immediate neighbors by an exclusive communal religious and political organization and by a distinctive costume.

The highland region of Chiapas is a hinterland almost entirely populated by Indians, and surrounds the valley city of San Cristóbal de las Casas, the economic, commercial, and political center of the region. In the lowlands below the mountain massif in which Zinacantan is located lies the state capital of Tuxtla Gutiérrez, about 50 miles from San Cristóbal via the Pan-American Highway. This city, though larger and more modern than San Cristóbal, is of secondary importance to the Indian population as a governmental and marketing center. Both cities are populated by Ladinos, Spanish-speaking inhabitants who dress in some variant of Western clothing and have a general cultural orientation more "Western" than indigenous. The Ladinos, being politically and economically dominant, tend to maintain superordinate and paternalistic relations with the Indian population (Van den Berghe and Colby, 1961; Colby and Van den Berghe, 1961). However, the distinction is primarily cultural, and Indians can be assimilated by the Ladino world.

The Indian municipios are territorial and political subdivisions of

TABLE 1
Indian Populations of Zinacantan

Hamlet	Population	Hamlet	Population
Hteklum[a]	343	Sekemtik	637
Paste'	1,276	Elamvo'	400
Navenchauk	1,215	'Ats'am	422
Vo'ch'ohvo'	954	Pat'osil	347
Nachih	922	Hok'oenob	299
'Apas	704	Chainatik	121

NOTE: These figures are taken from the official 1960 Zinacantan census; they exclude Ladino residents of Hteklum and the hamlets. Several hamlets recognized as such by Zinacantecos were grouped for purposes of the census.
[a] Permanent population of the ceremonial center; there are many transients.

Chiapas State, and each contains a governmental center and an area of countryside. The administrative centers are typically "vacant" towns, following the prevalent Maya pattern, and most of the people live in scattered rural hamlets. The administrative and/or ceremonial center itself has churches and public buildings, but only a small permanent population. Civil and religious offices rotate, the occupants renting or borrowing a temporary residence in the center during their terms of office. Except during fiestas the center is likely to be quiet and deserted, though there may be a small cluster of officials and litigants in front of the *cabildo* (town hall).

Zinacantan encompasses some 117 square kilometers of mountainous country on both sides of the Pan-American Highway immediately to the west of San Cristóbal de las Casas (see Figure 1). Its ceremonial center, Hteklum, contains three churches, the cabildo and jail, a clinic of the Instituto Nacional Indigenista (INI), and various sacred localities. It includes 15 named hamlets, called *parajes* in Spanish and *paraheletik* in Tzotzil, which are grouped in 12 units for statistical purposes (see Table 1).

Social Organization

The basic unit of residence in Zinacantan is the household, containing one or more families in the same dwelling. The dwellings within a given enclosure constitute a *sitio*, which ideally contains a patrilineally extended family. Clusters of sitios constitute a *sna* (literally "their house(s)") and each such cluster is personally named (e.g. *sna 'akovetik*, "house of the wasps' nests") according to the lineage name of its families. When a

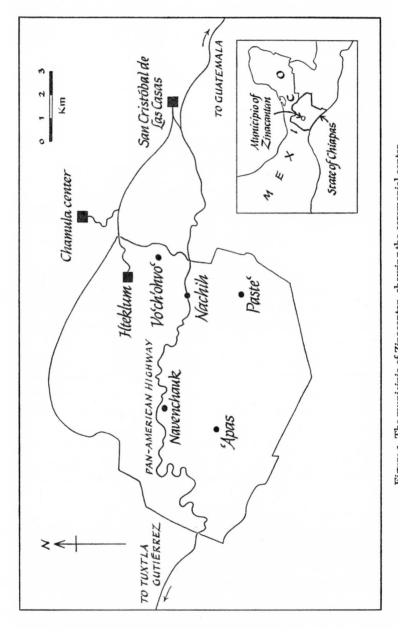

Figure 1. The municipio of Zinacantan, showing the ceremonial center and the five largest hamlets.

sna contains more than one lineage, its name is taken from the dominant lineage. Snas are associated in "waterhole groups" which share a common water supply, and these may change in composition as springs and wells dry up in the dry season and reappear in the rainy season (see Meadow, 1965). Finally, the waterhole groups are subdivisions of the hamlet. Each level of organization—sna, waterhole group, and hamlet— is both delimited and united by ceremonial functions and, in the case of households and sometimes snas, by common economic activities.

Civil and Religious Organization

The municipio of Zinacantan is governed under Mexican law by a complement of civil officials serving three-year terms. They administer the internal affairs of the municipio and form a court that hears minor cases, referring major ones to San Cristóbal. There are also 55 religious officials, each serving a one-year term of office—in Spanish, a *cargo* ("burden"). Each cargo (with the exception of eight positions on the lowest level, whose occupants serve as Indian policemen, or *mayoletik*) involves duties related to the cult of the saints in the three churches in Hteklum and three chapels in outlying hamlets. Each cargo holder undertakes his religious duties at his own expense, usually expending many times his annual income in the process and incurring enormous debts. (See F. Cancian, 1965; Vogt, 1969.)

The cargos are grouped into four levels. A Zinacanteco male progressing through the system will ideally assume a cargo at each ascending level, pausing to recoup his finances between terms of office, until he reaches one of the two top-level cargos. Very few men ever reach the upper levels of the system, and those who do are generally quite old; but many Zinacantecos participate on at least one level. At present the cargos are almost all voluntary, and long-term waiting lists are maintained to give the entire population a fair chance at them. The cargo system is of central importance in Zinacanteco life, and is treated at length in F. Cancian, 1965. Here, we can only summarize the findings that have particular relevance for our study.

1. Cargos are one of the few legitimate outlets for the expenditure of wealth in Zinacantan and are thus a means for ratifying and publicizing one's position in an open-class system based on economic achievement.

2. Because the cargos provide referents, actual or potential, for almost every social position in the system, they are one of the major integrating mechanisms in Zinacanteco society.

3. Optimum or successful cargo performance tends to be related to one's wealth, and also to the wealth and cargo performance of one's father and father-in-law.

4. Population growth is outstripping the slow expansion of the cargo system, and will eventually overwhelm the adjustive mechanisms built into the system.

5. Cargo performance is independent—in formal terms—of any other activity that might be called an occupation, such as holding civil office or being a shamanistic curer.

Religion and Souls

Although the Zinacantecos are nominally Catholic, their religion is in fact a mixture of Catholic and Maya elements, with the latter predominating. Even the many crosses in Zinacantan seem to have little Christian significance, since the cross is also the Mayan symbol of an entrance or doorway into the supernatural world.

The principal deities are the Totilme'iletik (literally father-mothers), ancestral gods who live within the sacred mountains surrounding Hteklum and in mountains near the various hamlets. The Totilme'iletik are seen as physically resembling Zinacanteco senior officials, and they are served by six ghostly mayoletik, the supernatural counterparts of the Indian policemen at the cabildo. Every Zinacanteco has an immanent soul or spirit (*ch'ulel*), residing in his body and containing 13 parts. Animals, plants, and inanimate objects also have souls, and each Zinacanteco shares his soul with an animal spirit companion (*chanul*) who ordinarily lives in the custody of the Totilme'iletik in a corral inside one of the mountains. If a man incurs the displeasure of the Totilme'iletik, he may be punished by the release of his chanul, and will simultaneously suffer any injuries that it encounters.

Also in the hierarchy of supernatural beings are the Pukuhetik, or demons. They are described by some informants as the souls of dead Zinacantecos, the minions of a being called Impierno, who presides over a fiery hell called K'atin Bak (literally, burning bones). The latter concept seems clearly influenced by Christian ideas, and not all Zinacantecos subscribe to it. Whatever their origin, the Pukuhetik are thought of as demonic beings who plague mankind with illness and misfortune.

Immediately beneath the surface of the earth live the Yahval Balamiletik (literally, earth owners), also called Anheletik (angels). These beings resemble Ladinos in appearance and customs. They control lightning and rain, can inflict illness on men, and are immensely wealthy. They use the souls of Zinacantecos, which they either seize or purchase from witches, as servants and beasts of burden. The entrance to their world is through caves and similar places.

Deeper in the earth is another layer inhabited by a race of dwarfs called Koncave'etik. The circuit of the sun and moon passes through this layer after leaving the heavens above the human-occupied surface world. Otherwise naked, the Koncave'etik wear mud hats to protect themselves from the heat of the sun's passing so close above them. These beings seem to have little importance in Zinacanteco cosmology.

Still deeper, according to some informants, is the fiery hell of K'atin Bak, where the souls of sinners are punished. Below this lies the foundation of the world, where four (or possibly eight) beings called Vashakmen (meaning unknown) support the four corners of the world. Earthquakes are caused when the burden becomes too heavy and the Vashakmen shift their load from one shoulder to another.

Above the earth is Vinahel, or heaven. It is occupied by two principal deities: Totik K'ak'al, the sun (also called Kahvaltik ta Vinahel, "our lord in heaven"), and Ch'ul Me'tik (holy mother), the moon. Some informants identify the sun with the Catholic concept of God the Father, and also add to the heavenly pantheon a somewhat vague Christ figure.

The final group of supernatural beings are the Santoetik, or saints. Some 55 saint images, pictures, and sacred objects are kept in the various churches of the municipio. According to Early (1965), these are powerful gods in their own right; their residences are the churches, and they were sent by Totik K'ak'al to help rule the world. Other informants, probably under Catholic influence, see the images merely as symbols of beings whose souls are actually in heaven.

Economic Activities of Zinacanteco Households

The primary economic activity of Zinacantecos is corn farming, mostly on rented land in the lowland, or "hot country," of the nearby Grijalva River valley. Small amounts of corn are grown in the highlands ("cold country"), primarily in small plots adjacent to family houses, and in the temperate country that lies at intermediate elevations. The temperate-country land is mostly in the *ejido*, the communal land holdings distributed to Zinacantan as part of the Mexican government's land reform program (see Edel, 1962). Neither this nor the cold-country household plots provide full subsistence for any but a few households. A family whose only agricultural activities are carried out in the cold country or the ejido usually has some additional source of income.

Land in hot country is typically rented from Ladino landlords, who receive as rent a fixed proportion of the harvest based on the quantity of seed planted. Cultivation is by the *milpa* (field) system of slash-and-burn agriculture; and as a plot of land becomes exhausted after successive cultivations, it may be rented at lower rates until it is finally allowed to lie fallow.

Calculations of planting, harvest, sale, etc., usually follow an old local system of volume measures: one *caldera* equals one metric liter of volume; one *cuarto* equals 5 calderas (5 liters); one *almud* equals 3 cuartos (15 liters); and one *fanega* equals 12 almuds (180 liters). Land is usually measured by Zinacantecos in terms of the volume of seed that can be planted on it. Thus one talks of an "almud" of land rather than a hectare.

Hot-country corn farming is an entrepreneurial enterprise involving the investment of capital, the taking of certain risks, and often the management of complicated organizational problems. Most Zinacanteco corn farmers grow for commercial as well as domestic use. The labor requirements for this scale of production are such that a Zinacanteco farmer, unless he has a large number of sons working with him in the fields, must hire outside labor at certain points in the agricultural cycle. (F. Cancian, 1972, estimates the minimum number of man-days per almud seeded as 30, plus 1.5 days for each fanega harvested. This figure may be much increased by poor land, the vicissitudes of weather, and poor management.)

Differences in the economic success of farming ventures arise from factors of luck and management. Some Zinacanteco farmers are more efficient than others, and the greatest profits come to those who organize their work so as to minimize the labor hired and the number of trips to hot country (each of which may require a day's travel each way). Marketing factors also contribute to the differences in profits among farmers. The price of corn rises and falls in fairly strict conformity to the available supply, and it reaches its peak in August, during the harvest season, when the new corn is not yet in and the supplies of the old are depleted. Obviously, the greatest profits can be made by those who organize their affairs so as to hold back a surplus until this time.

The cultivation of crops other than corn is unimportant in the economy of most Zinacanteco households. Beans are frequently grown in the same fields as corn, but are of less commercial importance. Almost every house has enough fertile land nearby to provide garden crops for domestic use. Flowers and fruit are grown in sitios and in cold-country fields.

For many generations certain Zinacanteco families have had control of the salt trade in highland Chiapas. The salt is purchased at its source in the lowland town of Ixtapa and transported by horse or mule throughout the Indian municipios of the highlands. A smaller number of Zinacantecos engage in merchandising fruits and flowers, either as middlemen or as vendors of their own products. This kind of enterprise has been stimulated in recent years by the building of the Pan-American Highway and the general improvement of transportation in the area.

Wage labor provides a supplemental income for many Zinacantecos, and is the primary source of income for a few. The principal jobs open to Zinacantecos are in road construction, which has provided a fairly steady market for Indian labor in recent years, and in certain construction projects of other sorts. For example, in 1965 the building of a government boarding school in Hteklum provided steady work for many Zinacantecos. A few men go to work as contract laborers on coffee *fincas* in the nearby Soconusco region. This is not a common Zinacanteco practice, however, as it is for the neighboring Chamulas (Pozas, 1959). A few Zinacantecos work as paid laborers for other Zinacantecos. This seems to be more common in some hamlets than in others; in our samples, for example, such cases are reported only in 'Apas.

A few stores in Hteklum and some hamlets are owned by Indians, although most Zinacanteco purchases of manufactured goods take place in San Cristóbal or in the Ladino-owned stores in Hteklum. The native stores rarely consist of more than a small stock of goods kept in the proprietor's house, or occasionally in a separate hut. Other infrequent sources of income include milling (with a gasoline-driven corn mill) and transportation. There are several groups of cooperators who own trucks and rent their services in transporting people and goods; owners of horses and mules often do the same.

The foregoing activities are primarily those of adult males. In a Zinacanteco household all men will ordinarily be engaged in at least one. Most frequently—except in the case of wage labor—all men living in the same household (e.g. a father and his adult sons) cooperate in joint agricultural and commercial enterprises. Certain other activities contribute to the domestic economy, though on a minor scale, and are usually carried out by women. Caring for a small herd of sheep, which are kept for wool rather than meat, is one of these. Another is the raising of garden products, or the keeping of chickens for domestic consumption or sale in the market.

A very few Zinacantecos derive some part of their support from handicrafts. For example, old widowed women, with no other means of support, may weave shirts and other garments to sell to their neighbors.

Chapter three

Zinacanteco Curing Roles

THE H'ILOLETIK are the most numerous and important of the native medical practitioners in Zinacantan. Receiving their powers through divine revelation, and practicing by combined physical and spiritual efforts, they can be called shamans in either a broad or a narrow sense of the term.

Table 2 shows the numbers of male h'iloletik and the total Zinacanteco populations (excluding resident Ladinos) in the six hamlets for which reliable information was available. Table 3 shows the numbers of both male and female h'iloletik in the three hamlets where information on curers of both sexes was available. The populations are based on the official 1960 census (see Chapter 2 for complete figures). For the total population of Zinacantan we can estimate the number of male h'iloletik to be approximately 118, and our figures suggest that the ratio of male to female h'iloletik is about five to two. Thus there are somewhere around 175 practicing h'iloletik in Zinacantan.

The ratio of one h'ilol to 40–45 Zinacantecos, which our figures suggest, is not at all high for the region. Metzger and Williams (1963), for example, report a ratio of curers to general populations of somewhere between 1:10 and 1:25 in the municipio of Tenejapa. In all likelihood our figures from Zinacantan are slightly low. This is the case because in an enumeration of the type we undertook one is likely to miss counting the new, less well-known h'iloletik. Even so, the number of h'iloletik seems to be increasing. For example, one sample to which we had access consisted of 40 male h'iloletik, of whom 13 had made their debuts between 1960 and 1964. Similarly, our figures from the hamlet of 'Apas show an increase of five h'iloletik in about three years.

TABLE 2
Comparative Figures for Male H'iloletik and
Total Population in Six Hamlets

Hamlet	Male h'iloletik	Population
'Apas	14	704
Hteklum	6	343
Navenchauk	13	1,215
Paste'	15	1,276
Pat'osil	8	347
Vo'ch'ohvo'	19	954
TOTAL	75	4,839

TABLE 3
Number of Male and Female H'iloletik in Three Hamlets

Paraje	H'iloletik		Population
	Male	Female	
'Apas	14	7	704
Paste'	15	3	1,276
Vo'ch'ohvo'	19	11	954
TOTAL	48	21	2,934

We should emphasize that it is quite difficult to establish the precise number of h'iloletik in Zinacantan. A new h'ilol usually goes through a period of ambivalent status and furtive activity, during which he engages circumspectly in curing activities but attempts to avoid public recognition of his role, which would entail onerous public duties. It is only when such a person has been discovered and forced to take part in the public ceremonies performed by h'iloletik that one can be sure of his identity as a h'ilol. Our figures, then, in addition to excluding newly recognized h'iloletik probably also exclude a certain number who are in the process of emergence. Finally, the number of female h'iloletik may be underestimated, since women do not participate in the public ceremonies and are therefore unlikely to be known to the general public until many years after their emergence.

As will be observed, the ratio of h'iloletik to laymen is not constant across the municipio. In 'Apas it is approximately 1 to 35. In Vo'ch'ohvo' it is slightly higher (1 to 32), whereas in Paste' it is considerably less (1 to 70). The disproportionate ratio for Paste' seems largely owing to the unusually small number of female h'iloletik reported—only three, as compared to 11 in Vo'ch'ohvo', a hamlet of the same size.

It has become increasingly clear with the acquisition of more information about Zinacantan that there are regular differences of many kinds between the hamlets—in short, that a process of cultural differentiation seems to be at work. Vogt (personal communication) has suggested that these differences go deeper even than the hamlet, distinguishing one sna from the next. In Paste', for which he has detailed information on snas and waterhole groups, he notes a disproportionate clustering of h'iloletik in a few snas, and suggests this may represent a group style of achievement, or possibly a functional specialization. As we shall see, survey data on samples of h'iloletik and laymen show a close association between being a h'ilol and having a parent or sibling who is a h'ilol.

Recruitment

The recruitment of h'iloletik is one of the principal features that lead us to describe the h'ilol as a shamanistic curer. A broad definition of a shaman would include any kind of curer or medical *cum* religious practitioner whose powers come from supernatural sources. A narrower definition would hew more closely to the forms of the original Siberian pattern from which the term shaman is derived (cf. Madsen, 1955). In either case, Zinacanteco h'iloletik are clearly shamanistic practitioners whose characteristics resemble in several important ways the outstanding traits of the classic shamanistic complex.

The Zinacanteco h'ilol attains his position through selection by the ancestral gods, the Totilme'iletik, who command him to become a h'ilol and instruct him in all the information requisite to curing. Informants describe various forms of this supernatural confrontation. In the version first encountered by fieldworkers in Zinacantan (Vogt, 1961), which seems to be the most widespread, the subject experiences a series of three dreams in which he is summoned before the Totilme'iletik in their dwelling inside the mountain peak of Muk'ta Vits. Here he is told that he has been chosen to become a h'ilol and is given patients whom he must cure. If he demurs, in some accounts, he is threatened with illness or death unless he complies. In the course of the three dreams the candidate receives instruction in prayers, diagnostic knowledge, and all aspects of ritual procedure; and he is symbolically given the candles, flowers, and incense burners that he will use in his curing ceremonies.

More intensive interviews with a greater number of informants have revealed some variant beliefs. In one, the selection of a h'ilol occurs before birth; hence certain people are, so to speak, predestined to become curers. This may be revealed early or late in life when the chosen one falls ill. The h'ilol who "pulses" the patient then divines from the blood his destiny as a new h'ilol, and informs him that to be cured he must make his own debut as a curer. The senior h'ilol may take the patient under his tutelage and instruct him in the esoteric knowledge associated with curing, or the patient may come by the necessary knowledge through some further process of revelation.

To some Zinacantecos, seizures or actual epilepsy are signs of the sufferer's predisposition to the role of h'ilol. Confrontation with the Totilme'iletik is said to take place during a convulsion, when the soul leaves the body and travels to Muk'ta Vits to receive instructions. Not all persons with seizures become h'iloletik, however; and, conversely, many h'iloletik give no such history. Thus, a seizure disorder (or any other marked physical disturbance in childhood) can be said to constitute neither a necessary nor a sufficient condition for acquiring the status of h'ilol.

We cannot be certain that these three types of recruitment are either exhaustive or mutually exclusive. It seems most likely that they are considered by Zinacantecos to be alternative, or perhaps complementary, ways of divine election. There may well be others of which we have not heard. In any case, it is interesting to note that these alternatives include several important features of shamanistic recruitment typical of other peoples. Both dreams and epileptic seizures are features of the Eskimo and Siberian patterns. The innate call diagnosed in illness has been described in nearby Chichicastenango (Bunzel, 1952), and is commonly cited in the literature. The only major avenue of known shamanistic recruitment not formally recognized in Zinacantan is inheritance. However, our data show that sometimes the h'ilol status is virtually, if not technically, inherited.

It proved difficult to obtain information on personality characteristics of the would-be h'ilol and his manner of social adjustment during the time before his formal entry into the community as a practitioner. Since the bulk of our data stems from laymen and established h'iloletik, no firsthand depiction of this facet of the h'iloletik's life is possible. What one obtains formally is largely a culturally stereotyped and symbolic representation of how a h'ilol should be selected and confirmed. Our general impression, however, is that sensitive, religious, and more or less introverted individuals are likely to be challenged by the knowledge of their potential association with the role. It is they who are most involved in traditional aspects of life in Zinacantan and least likely to have experienced heavy exposure to Ladino patterns, features that informants consistently associated with the position of h'ilol. Discussions with informants suggest that the period of time during which a h'ilol learns of his destiny is characterized by concern, anxiety, preoccupation, and social withdrawal. In general, it seems that in many instances this period of time is a critical and stormy period in the life of the individual. On the other hand, many h'iloletik spoke of this period of their lives as if their concern had been predominantly a practical one: namely, how to consolidate one's knowledge and expertise regarding medical and spiritual matters. There are a variety of social and political aspects to this question of career selection and professional competence. Unfortunately, because of the secrecy and anxiety surrounding recruitment, it was not possible to evaluate critically the notion that psychological illness promotes and mediates entry into the shamanistic role (Silverman, 1967).

The Debut

Once a Zinacanteco has been apprised of his "divine election" to the role of h'ilol and has learned curing procedures—in a few cases possibly through direct instruction by another h'ilol—he makes his debut. The use of the word debut is not meant to imply a conspicuous ceremony or particular event. In fact, a new h'ilol most commonly practices surreptitiously until he is noticed by the leaders of the community and forced to acknowledge his status. This surreptitious entrance is chosen in large part because of distaste for the public ceremonies held several times a year, in which all male h'iloletik participate. In the local hamlet ceremonies a new h'ilol is usually assigned the most unpleasant tasks. He is also detailed as one of the two or three men sent as representatives of the hamlet to participate in the larger ceremonies in Hteklum, where his duties are even more onerous.

It is therefore to a new h'ilol's advantage to practice furtively at first. Initially, he will cure members of his immediate family, then neighbors, friends, *compadres* (ritual kinsmen), and more distant relatives. When someone sees him engaged in curing activities and reports him to the Bankilal H'iloletik (senior h'iloletik) of the hamlet, they summon him to participate in the public ceremonies, and, if he refuses, complain to the judicial authorities in Hteklum. The authorities will then send mayol-etik (Indian policemen) to arrest the suspected hʻilol and have him brought before the court. He is interrogated, confronted with the testimony of those who have seen him curing, and coerced into admitting that he is a hʻilol. He may even be jailed until he confesses and promises to participate in the public ceremonies. Only after his status is ratified by participation in the ceremonies will a new hʻilol ordinarily display the symbols of his office: the *bish* or bamboo staff, and the *shakitail* (or *batsʻi chamaroil*), a black, red-trimmed blanket worn as a poncho while curing.

In vivid contrast to this pattern of furtive curing and eventual exposure is the rare debut ceremony, Tsvaʻan sba Hʻilol ("to stand up for oneself as a hʻilol"). The prospective hʻilol, having reported his dreams to the Bankilal Hʻiloletik of his hamlet and asked permission to make his debut, finds a senior hʻilol to perform the ceremony with him. Together they make a ritual circuit of the sacred mountains, crosses, and waterholes in Hteklum (and possibly in the curer's own hamlet), where they pray to the Totilmeʻiletik to accept the activities of the prospective hʻilol. The ceremony is apparently intended to avert any divine punishment for practicing without divine sanction, and to ensure the efficacy of the new hʻilol's curing procedures. Actually, the ritual is quite similar to a large-scale curing ceremony (cf. the description of Mukʻta ʻIlel, Chapter 11).

Most hʻiloletik do not undertake a debut ceremony, and many view one as a sign of incompetence, feeling that the new hʻilol who performs it has not undergone an authentic vision and is not *pʻih* (intelligent and spiritually outstanding). Because of his incompetence, he must seek an older hʻilol from whom he can learn the prayers and manipulations that should have been transmitted in his dreams.

Once the debut has been made, the identity of hʻilol is considered permanent, and generally the role cannot be abandoned. A hʻilol is obligated, at the risk of incurring divine punishment, to accept all requests for his services unless they conflict with other necessary activities, such as cargo duties and subsistence pursuits. When hʻiloletik grow old or are otherwise incapacitated, they "retire" gradually as demands for curing duties cease to be made of them. The process is ordinarily informal: the declining powers of the hʻilol make him less desirable as a healer, people stop asking his services, and finally he cures, if at all, only among the members of his immediate household.

We do have a description, however, of a formal retirement ceremony performed by an informant's grandmother. Lacking the strength to make long pilgrimages to the sacred mountains, the old woman made a final circuit of all the ceremonial localities, praying at each for divine permission to give up her duties as a h'ilol. Pleading the feeble condition of her legs, she besought the gods not to punish her for refusing the requests of all but her family. According to our informant, such a ceremony can be used by any h'ilol who finds that ill health or poverty causes him to suffer unduly, but its actual incidence seems to be quite rare.

In general, then, despite the existence of formal ceremonies of debut and retirement, assumption of the role of h'ilol seems to be gradual, informal, and covert. Only the force of public opinion, reinforced by powerful judicial sanctions, can ordinarily bring about a new h'ilol's incorporation in the body of h'iloletik, with their many public responsibilities. Many h'iloletik seem to forestall this event quite some time, and any listing of h'iloletik given by a Zinacanteco informant will typically include the names of several people whose status is doubtful but who have been rumored for several years to be h'iloletik.

The concealment of his curing powers is of great advantage to a new h'ilol, since he can perform private curing ceremonies for whatever rewards or gratifications they may bring him without having to sacrifice time and energy in unrewarding public ceremonies. Moreover, he is not susceptible to being ordered about and disciplined by the Bankilal H'iloletik or the judicial authorities. The period of covert practice allows a new curer time to develop his powers, test his skills, and back out quietly if necessary. It is possible that some h'iloletik enjoy public ceremonies for their own sake. However, seniority is dated from a new curer's first public appearance, and authority among h'iloletik rests on that seniority. This may motivate some new h'iloletik to stage an overt debut.

There are a few cases of h'iloletik who have managed to avoid all participation in public ceremonies. For example, the old h'ilol Shun Vaskis of Navenchauk is a wealthy man with great political influence—enough, it would seem, to insulate him from judicial coercion. In other cases, the persons concerned are owners of "talking saints" (typically, printed pictures of saints who are available for consultation) or other marginal practitioners whose activities smack of witchcraft. But witchcraft as such does not always bar a practitioner from the public ceremonies. One of our informants, observing some poorly clad h'iloletik at a Year Renewal ceremony in Hteklum, asked an official who they were and was told they were h'iloletik but also witches. They were allowed to participate in the public ceremonies so that they could be kept under surveillance; moreover, no one wanted to antagonize them by excluding them from the proceedings.

It should be noted, finally, that the public ceremonies are confined to male h'iloletik. This simplifies the role of h'ilol for a woman, since she does not have to conceal herself and her reputation grows more rapidly than a man's. However, the same factor makes it more difficult to identify the female h'iloletik unequivocally.

Ranking

The seniority of a h'ilol is based on the time elapsed since his first participation in public ceremonies. In common with most other aspects of Zinacanteco culture, the senior position is *bankilal* (older brother) and the junior position *its'inal* (younger brother). Every h'ilol has a rank-position among the h'iloletik of his hamlet, and wherever the h'iloletik gather for ritual purposes the seniority is observed. In ceremonial procession, the most junior member marches first and the most senior last; in ritual toasting, the order is reversed. The actual dimensions of ranking beyond the hamlet are probably unknown to any Zinacanteco. On the municipio level, the fact that no situation arises requiring a ceremonial gathering of all male h'iloletik obviates the establishment of a single, municipio-wide seniority ranking. At the joint ceremonies to which each hamlet sends two or three representatives, there is a sorting and self-arrangement of h'iloletik into the correct order of seniority.

In each hamlet the senior h'iloletik run the collective affairs of the local curers. Our informants give some indications of an ideal situation in which the most senior h'ilol is Bankilal H'ilol and is solely in charge of the rest; but information from many hamlets indicates that in most cases small groups of senior h'iloletik, always including the most senior, are described collectively as Bankilal and exercise authority over the remainder. The boundaries between the two groups seem to follow no set pattern but instead conform to those of cliques and influence groups, changing as older h'iloletik die off.

The responsibilities of the Bankilal H'ilol, with or without a group of senior cronies, are to plan and supervise the hamlet ceremonies, choose representatives to be sent to the public ceremonies in Hteklum, and watch for covert curing activities. In general, the principle of seniority seems to command adherence, but it appears that even here, as in most matters in the highly factional atmosphere of Zinacantan, politics can have a modifying influence.

In the hamlet of Navenchauk, for example, the elderly Petul Tsu (Peter Gourd) claims to have more years of service than any other h'ilol. For many years he acted as Bankilal H'ilol, and his assignments and commands were obeyed by the other h'iloletik. Several years ago, he was deposed from this position by a younger and more junior h'ilol. The mechanism of the coup was informal. Petul arrived at a reunion of the h'iloletik and found the younger man making assignments that were accepted by the others present. Finding no support for his position, and seeing that his own commands were disregarded, Petul was forced to acquiesce and to accept a humiliating position in that year's K'in Krus ceremony.

Petul's own explanation relates this to a deep political cleavage in Navenchauk.* He heads the smaller of two factions in the hamlet, and has a minority of the h'iloletik among his party. Although he was twice Presidente Municipal (the highest civil office of the municipio) in the 1930's and also held the minor position of Pasionero in the cargo system, his successor Manuel Pulivo', has passed the level of Alférez, a much more prestigious cargo. Petul's civil offices are too far in the past to command respect from the younger h'iloletik. This combination of circumstances—being the objectionable leader of a political minority group and not gaining any additional prestige from the cargo system—was apparently enough to outweigh the ideal of absolute seniority in this instance.

It appears that it is always the most senior h'ilol living in the valley of Hteklum who performs certain important duties in directing the annual ceremonies (see Chapter 10). It is he who consults with the Muk'ta Alkalte, the highest cargo official, to set the dates for the ceremonies. It is he who levies a public subscription, via the officials, and calls on

---

* Petul also feels that the problem stems from the introduction of new families to the hamlet through government distribution of Ladino-owned lands. Whatever the validity of this, it seems clear that Navenchauk factionalism is at least partly related to political events in the Ladino world. In the late 1920's Petul acted as a spy for the government forces of Obregón in their attempt to suppress the Pinedist revolt in Chiapas. After the government victory, he was made Presidente Municipal of Zinacantan. A sizeable faction of Zinacantecos apparently supported Pineda.

each hamlet to send representatives. And it is he who directs the ceremonies and takes a leading role, assigning groups of h'iloletik to travel to each of the sacred localities.

This position seems an exception to the "vacant-town ceremonial center" pattern of organization, in which all important ritual offices (excepting the scribes, musicians, and sacristans, who usually live permanently in Hteklum) are filled by rotation, all Zinacantecos being eligible whether or not they reside in the valley of Hteklum. If so, it is an important exception to the principle of seniority that pertains otherwise in the organization of the h'iloletik. It is not clear why this should be so. Unlike the rotating cargo positions, the seniority-based role of Bankilal H'ilol is permanent and might require permanent residence in Hteklum, something ordinarily impossible for a h'ilol from a distant hamlet. However, the actual duties of the Bankilal H'ilol do not seem incompatible with a nonresidency. Nor would the degree of record-keeping needed to determine seniority rankings for the entire body of h'iloletik in Zinacantan be any greater than that currently associated with the maintenance of the cargo system.

Unfortunately, we do not have extensive information about this aspect of Zinacanteco practice. There is no reason why the Bankilal H'ilol who directs the year ceremonies has to be considered superior to all other h'iloletik, and there is no Tzotzil term setting him off from the Bankilal H'iloletik of other hamlets. Perhaps it is merely thought that the shamans of the valley of Hteklum have special responsibilities because their territory includes the principal sacred mountains, waterholes, and churches.

Activities and Defining Characteristics of the H'iloletik

The activities of the h'iloletik include diagnosis through pulsing and divination, the administration of remedies, and the conducting of private curing ceremonies and new house ceremonies. Male h'iloletik, in addition, perform public ceremonies, agricultural rituals, rain-making ceremonies, and certain extraordinary curing ceremonies to avert epidemic disease. These activities will be described in subsequent chapters.

The defining functional characteristics of the h'ilol role can be elicited by using a question of this general form: "What are the things h'iloletik can (or know how to) do that no one else can do?" A series of responses to such a question follow. They are the responses of only one informant, but they adequately represent responses given by many informants under less formal interviewing conditions. Both questions and answers were originally in Tzotzil, but to conserve space only an English translation is given here.

1. Only h'iloletik can pulse the blood; other people cannot pulse.
2. Only h'iloletik know how to speak [pray] at the shrines [the sacred mountains, etc.]; other people do not know how to pray at the shrines.
3. Only h'iloletik know how to leave candles at each mountain. They know how to leave flowers at the crosses of each mountain. They know how to leave the *k'esholil* [a black chicken of the same sex as the patient, which serves as a substitute for the patient's soul]. They know where the patient's substitute is to be left, whether at Sisil Vits or at Kalvario or at Mushul Vits. Others leave it at Muk'ta Vits, and others at Ni Nab Chilo'. The h'ilol says where the substitute is to be left, and how the patient can recover. Those who are not h'iloletik do not know how to do these things.
4. Only h'iloletik know how to see the *sat ishim* [face of the maize—a form of divination with maize grains], how it acts within the water, how to see where the patient's ch'ulel remains and where he was frightened. Those who are not h'iloletik cannot see the sat ishim.
5. The h'iloletik see [in their dreams] where demons are coming from and when illness is coming. They see whether it comes from above or below [i.e. on the upper or lower roads into Zinacantan]. They see whether it comes on foot or on horse, as a forest fire or as a *yahval kuvel* (literally "owner of smallpox," a figure similar in appearance to the Ladino doctor who gives smallpox inoculations and whose presence in a curer's dreams therefore warns of the advent of smallpox). A h'ilol with a ch'ulel that is strong and intelligent can see this. He asks the authorities to order that money be collected in each hamlet and used to buy candles as offerings to ask pardon, so that the disease will come no further and not many persons will die. The h'iloletik can speak thus at the cabildo, and in this manner the order is secured there in the customary fashion. Those who are not h'iloletik cannot see where illness and demons are coming from, and may not talk to the authorities to collect money for a curing ceremony.
6. Only the h'iloletik know how to tell where the ch'ulel of a patient is. The curers know how to pray for the person who has suffered soul-loss, for the one who has fallen ill. They know how to place candles and how to tell from the blood if the patient is going to recover or to die.

The principal criteria distinguishing the h'ilol from the layman, then, are: the ability to pulse and divine; the ability to pray properly; the ability to correctly place candles and flowers in curing ceremonies; the ability to foretell the coming of illness; and the right to initiate public action to combat epidemics.

A similar set of statements regarding differences between h'iloletik was elicited by asking: "What can some h'iloletik do that not all h'iloletik can do?"

1. All h'iloletik know the medicines for reducing fever—*tsotsil habnal* and *chikin cho*—but there are some who do not know how much a patient with a

high fever can take. All h'iloletik know how to give the medicine, but some do not know how much the patient can take. For some, the patient dies immediately. But the other h'iloletik, who know how to give medicine properly, cure their patients. The fever breaks, and the patient's blood cools.

2. Some h'iloletik do not know how to put flowers in the bed of a patient who has sought pardon at all the mountains and all the churches. But others, the good h'iloletik, know how to put flowers in the patient's bed when there is only a little illness and no fever. If there is much illness, if there is fever, no h'ilol puts flowers in the patient's bed or bathes him. But if the illness is minor, the patient can bathe his body in the flowers [i.e. in a broth made from them].

3. Some h'iloletik know how to treat any illness a person suffers, be it sickness or a broken bone. If it is a bone broken by falling in a hole, there are h'iloletik who know how to set it by prayer alone. The bone heals by itself because they set it. It is not necessary to touch it with the hands or to put it in its place. But not all h'iloletik know this; some only know how to pray *k'oplael* [a simple prayer].

4. There are some good h'iloletik [*tukil h'ilol*] and some h'ilol witches [*h'ilol h'ak' chamel*]. The witches know how to cure and how to cause illness. They know how to pray and how to prepare candles, and whether big ones or small ones [a sign of witchcraft] are needed to cure the patient. They know by themselves where to pray—caves that are distinct from the crosses where one can pray. The good h'iloletik do not know how to use the witches' caves.

The range of informants' criteria for distinguishing between h'iloletik is as varied as the h'iloletik themselves. As might be expected, the most pervasive distinction is between good and bad (i.e. witch) h'iloletik. This is followed by distinctions of specialization and distinctions of competence. Specialization distinctions include such major ones as that between h'iloletik who can set bones and those who cannot, and such minor ones as the difference between curers who use three candles per mountain and those who use two (a difference that can loom large in the mind of a thrifty patient). Other informants distinguish between h'iloletik who tell a patient the outcome of their divinations and those who keep them secret. The grounds for judging competence vary widely from informant to informant, although it is generally agreed that some h'iloletik are more competent than others. A distinction is often drawn between h'iloletik who make their debut while young and those who enter the role in their forties or fifties. Some Zinacantecos consider the latter inferior; but many informants consider h'iloletik with long service unreliable, since the consumption of great quantities of alcohol over the years, as part of their curing duties, may have made them forgetful and incompetent.

Many informants express a distinction of particular interest to us:

Some h'iloletik are authentic and competent, having received their powers from the ancestral spirits. Others are spurious and have no abilities; they practice only to get chickens, meals, and liquor by cheating their patients.

Specialized Curing Roles

Bonesetters (*hts'ak bak*). The bonesetter treats fractures and dislocations of bones, as well as various painful conditions that are thought by Zinacantecos to arise from skeletal and/or muscular pathologies. Placing an illness within the purview of a bonesetter involves a complex set of considerations. But ordinarily a fracture, dislocation, sprain, or any well-localized pain in the extremities (even without a history of trauma) will be treated by a bonesetter. One class of "broken bone," however, is the property of the h'ilol. This is *k'asel ta hch'uletik*, a fracture or dislocation encountered by the ch'ulel soul while it wanders in dreams as the victim sleeps. This kind of illness is also believed to result from witchcraft. In either case, because it is an injury to the ch'ulel, it must be dealt with by a h'ilol.

The bonesetters are both male and female. Recruitment to the role is less formally defined than that to the h'ilol role, but it likewise seems to involve supernatural selection and instruction. Some bonesetters, in fact, are also h'iloletik in the fullest sense of the term, and can perform the full range of curing and ritual procedures. These practitioners receive the power to set bones either in the course of their acquisition of curing powers or in a subsequent revelation. There are other bonesetters who rely mostly on spiritual curing methods and are called h'ilol by informants, but who do not perform any of the other activities associated with the role of h'ilol. They, too, may experience a divine call, but of a less elaborate nature. Finally, some bonesetters seem to experience nothing more than a desire to assume the role, with no component of supernatural experience.

The Zinacanteco esteem of bonesetters seems to correspond closely to the degree to which a practitioner can be considered a true h'ilol, in the sense that he uses purely spiritual curing methods. And the most esteemed are those who can perform all the functions of a h'ilol and set bones as well. Also highly regarded are the bonesetters who are sometimes called h'iloletik because they use prayers and other spiritual methods exclusively, even though bonesetting is their only therapeutic ac-

tivity. Both of these classes of practitioners use the same methods in
bonesetting: prayer, the lighting of candles, and the administration of
herbal remedies. As one might expect, the least highly regarded bonesetters are those who use actual physical manipulation of a broken or
dislocated area—in short, a bonesetter who actually sets bones is considered far inferior to one who merely prays over them. Perhaps for this
reason, the actual level of anatomical knowledge among bonesetters
seems to be low. In this respect, Zinacanteco values militate against the
accumulation of empirical knowledge in healing.

The total number of bonesetters in the municipio seems to be quite
low. Their activities are rewarded with gifts of unknown magnitude, but
there are some reports of cash payments running as high as $30.*

Midwives (*htamol*). These are always women, and the information
we have indicates that they are usually old and/or widowed. In the hamlet of 'Apas, for example, there are 11 midwives ranging in age from 58
to 81 years. Of these, one is a spinster, five are widows, and five have
living husbands. Seven midwives in 'Apas are also considered to be
h'iloletik, and one is both a h'ilol and a bonesetter. The distinction between the midwife who is a h'ilol and one who is not rests on whether
or not the practitioner knows how to pray if a baby is not born at the
proper time: if she does, she is considered a h'ilol. When a birth is at-
tended by difficulties, a midwife who is not a h'ilol may send for a h'ilol,
either male or female, to treat the condition.

A pregnant woman usually consults a midwife sometime during the
fifth or sixth month of pregnancy. The midwife then checks the position
of the fetus every two weeks, increasing the frequency of her visits to
once a week as the time of delivery approaches. At the birth she assists
in delivery to the extent of her capacities, calling in a h'ilol if complica-
tions arise. Some midwives are said to have knowledge of medicinal
plants that can be used to assist delivery or to induce labor if the baby
is overdue. After delivery, the midwife cuts off the cord and burns it, and
then bathes the child in an infusion of laurel. She censes the child with
smoke from an incense burner and prays to the Totilme'iletik on his behalf, asking that they take charge of his souls and guard them well. She
also supervises the burial of the afterbirth outside the house, and in the

* Here, as elsewhere in the book, a dollar sign indicates Mexican pesos, not U.S.
dollars. A peso currently exchanges for about 8 cents U.S.

days following delivery accompanies the mother through a series of sweat baths.

The entire sequence of events surrounding a birth is ritualized, and it is accompanied by ritual meals (less formal, apparently, than those for a curing ceremony) that include the traditional rounds of native rum (*posh*). The midwife is first solicited with gifts of rum and food, as a h'ilol would be; and after the birth she is similarly rewarded. Her pay usually consists of one or more chickens, some 30 tortillas, one or more bottles of rum, and occasionally some Ladino bread. Some informants report that a few midwives charge cash fees: $6 if the baby is a girl, $10 for a boy.

Talking saints. The Tzotzil term for the owner of a saint is *yahval riosh* —literally, "owner of the god/saint." There are two terms used to refer to the saint itself: *riosh shk'opoh,* "saint who talks," and *kushul riosh,* "living saint." (Vogt, 1969, gives the term *hk'opohel riosh,* but we have never heard this term used.) The cult of talking saints is an interesting feature of both Indian and Ladino culture in the highlands of Chiapas. Its historical and political background has been described in some detail elsewhere (B. Metzger, 1959; Guiteras-Holmes, 1961; Pozas, 1959), and only a brief outline is necessary here.

A talking saint is typically a small picture of San Miguel, usually taken from one of the cheaply printed religious tracts widely distributed in Mexico. Infrequently a picture of some other saint, or even a small statuette, may be used. The image is kept inside a *cofre,* a small wooden chest of the type used by Zinacantecos to store clothing and valuables. The cofre rests in the house of the owner, on an altar of the kind found in most Zinacanteco homes: a small table or shelf against one wall that is decorated with paper flowers (often with an arch of red flowers similar to the arches of red geraniums that decorate the entrances and altars of churches and chapels in the municipio) and contains printed images of saints, small statuettes, and other ritual objects.

Each talking saint has his own schedule, which is generally known to the public, and at certain designated times he is available for consultation. The client approaches the house, is admitted by the owner, and engages in the normal polite conversation and toasting with rum before he approaches the altar. The degree and kind of this preliminary behavior seem to vary according to how surreptitious the operation is, how busy the saint is, and whether the owner is considered to be a h'ilol. In the last instance, if the saint is considered an adjunct to normal curing techniques, the behavior of client to proprietor follows the highly formal pattern of patient-h'ilol interaction described elsewhere.

On broaching the reason for his visit, the client is usually instructed to deposit money and/or gifts of candles and rum on or near the box. He then addresses the saint, requests advice, and awaits an answer. Informants describe two kinds of communication from the saints: there may be a pattern of knocks, or a voice may actually seem to issue from the box.

Illness is undoubtedly the most common subject on which the saints are consulted, but they also dispense advice on other matters—e.g., marital problems, financial affairs, or the choice of a number to play in the national lottery. All of this information is available only through the proprietor, and possession of a saint can be a highly profitable enterprise. In addition to the fees purportedly collected by the saint before and during the consultation, the proprietor often profits from the sale of herbs and drugs prescribed by the saint. Indeed, certain proprietors are known for their possession of secret nostrums, which they dispense as the saint directs. On a somewhat more sophisticated level, the famous Ladino-owned talking saint at nearby Soyalo draws customers from all over Mexico. Recently, this saint did such a volume of business that four secretaries with typewriters were employed to take down the prescriptions (Holland, 1963); and, according to San Cristóbal merchants, his proprietor was for a time the largest single purchaser of wholesale pharmaceuticals in the entire state of Chiapas.

It is hard to determine how many talking saints there are in Zinacantan itself, since the cult is surrounded with secrecy, at least where ethnographers are concerned. In part, this secrecy arises from the association between talking saints and witchcraft. Zinacantecos differ in their opinions about the legitimacy of the saints and the purity of their owners' motives; but it can safely be said that certain owners are widely suspected of being witches, and that all owners are regarded as possibly, and even probably, capable of witchcraft. For this reason, Zinacantecos are reluctant to talk about the saints or reveal the identity of an owner. Reticence about the talking saints even exceeds that concerning other aspects of witchcraft, probably because there is constant tension between this cult and the public authorities. Talking saints are officially considered shams, and the local police and magistrates have been trying to suppress the cult for years. However, the saints often appear openly as subjects of litigation in the cabildo—usually when a dissatisfied client sues the owner of a saint who has failed to effect a cure.

Modern Zinacantan is rent with dissension and characterized by both a high degree of ideological variation and a growing skepticism about traditional beliefs; hence one cannot always draw the line between legitimate and forbidden practice. At present, the Zinacanteco officials can only take action when the proprietor of a saint is called into court, in which case they demand that he bring the saint to the cabildo and demonstrate its properties. In none of these demonstrations has a saint ever "talked" in the presence of the authorities. The proprietor is often punished and is usually ordered to cease using his saint, and the bystanders are lectured on the manifest untruthfulness of his claims.

From these court cases there has developed the official position that true saints do not take up residence in private houses for the personal benefit of individuals, and that anyone claiming to possess a talking saint is engaged in fraud, witchcraft, or both. Whether this official line is specific to the particular men holding office in the last few years or whether it represents a point of view generally considered appropriate for the authorities and so adopted by each new set of officeholders is an interesting question. For it is clear that many Zinacantecos continue to give credence and patronage to the talking saints, despite a certain amount of skepticism about their efficacy and despite official disapproval. This apparent conflict may be partly explained by some evidence we have gained that Zinacantecos have very different views of the attitudes appropriate to public and private postures. The officials, as representatives of the public good, must oppose the talking saints; but the private Zinacanteco is not thereby restrained from taking advantage of them if he can.

The acquisition of a talking saint is said to involve no contact with the supernatural other than a direct appeal to the saint himself. The prospective owner goes to someone who is already an owner and enlists his help; he then addresses the existing saint, begging that he send one of his companions to live at a new location. This is said to be the way the saints first entered the municipio some thirty years ago, when certain Zinacantecos visited the Ladino-owned saint at Soyalo and successfully petitioned him to send them saints in Zinacantan. Although this story attributes a recent origin to the practice, the talking-saint complex has been evident in the Chiapas highlands for over 250 years, figuring prominently in several Indian rebellions and nativistic movements; so it is likely that the saints have been active in Zinacantan at times in the past (see B. Metzger, 1960).

On receiving the saint's promise to come live in his house, the prospective owner buys a wooden chest and prepares an altar. He then gives a series of three fiestas, complete with musicians, skyrockets, rum, and chicken to eat. The purpose is to impress the new saint with the liberality of his prospective proprietor and to convince him to stay in the new locale. The saint is believed to attend each fiesta and take up temporary residence in the box, where the new owner may talk with him. At the end of the second fiesta the proprietor asks the saint if he is satisfied; if so, a schedule of hours for consultation is established and the date set for a third fiesta, at which time the saint takes up permanent residence in his new home. (In an alternative pattern, reported in Vogt, 1969, some families claim to have found their saints in caves.)

The proprietors of talking saints include both men and women. Some owners are considered to be h'iloletik, and these persons carry the saint with them to patients' houses and use it as an adjunct to more orthodox curing methods. Otherwise, a talking saint remains in the owner's house and is consulted only there. Besides Zinacanteco proprietors, there are several Chamulas (Maya Indians of the neighboring municipio) and possibly one Ladino who operate talking saints within the municipio. There are also numerous saints elsewhere in the region who may be consulted by Zinacantecos; and in some cases, these saints have representatives who travel into Zinacantan and solicit business for them.

Chapter four

Economic and Social Aspects of Curing

IN THIS CHAPTER we analyze the important social and economic characteristics of h'iloletik. This is accomplished by comparing male h'iloletik with a group of male laymen on a variety of relevant indicators that reflect achievement and wealth. The family backgrounds of h'iloletik are also discussed. Some attention is given to the economic benefits and drawbacks associated with occupying the role of h'ilol in Zinacantan. In general, our analyses draw on survey information obtained from approximately 400 households in Hteklum, 'Apas, Pat'osil, Nachih, and Vo'ch'ohvo'. The data from the first three of these are more extensive, and for this reason we have focused on them comparatively. The questionnaire used inquired about the names and ages of all occupants of a house, the background characteristics of the head of household, and the cargo career and economic assets of the head of household.

Economic Indices

Gross household income. This figure was computed by adding all sources of income. The following are the categories of information used and the rationale for each.

1. Amount of corn seeded in cold country. This was converted into income by multiplying the quantity seeded by two constants based on the midpoints of fluctuations in yield and price mentioned by informants. We have used an average yield of 1.5 fanegas for every cuarto seeded and an average price of $110 per fanega harvested; thus one cuarto would yield $165 annual income. The procedure gives results close to those stated by Cancian in his discussion of the economics of Zinacanteco corn farming (F. Cancian, 1972).

2. Amount of corn seeded in hot country. This was given a value of $255 income for every cuarto seeded, based on considerations similar to those for the less fertile cold country. Fifteen pesos per fanega were subtracted in the calculations for transportation and hired labor.

3. Other sources of income. The informants were asked to state all other sources of income for the household head and any other contributing members of the domestic group. These were mostly entrepreneurial profits and wages in cash or kind. Careful questioning in each case elicited the approximate annual value of such income in monetary terms.

4. Fruit trees. In some hamlets fruit trees planted in sitios are an important part of the domestic economy. Generally, however, fruit merely supplements a family's diet, adding little or no cash income. We have considered fewer than ten fruit trees a negligible contribution. Trees in excess of ten are counted at $10 each—an arbitrary estimate, but one based on the rough estimates that informants were able to give.

Household liquid assets. We derived this figure by adding the following two items:

1. The total value of any horses or mules owned by the household head. The consensus of our informants was that the average market value of a horse was $300 and that of a mule $800.

2. The quantity of land owned by the household head. Land owned by a wife through her own inheritance was not counted as a liquid asset of her husband. Land, we have said, is typically measured by the volume of corn that can be planted on it, rather than by area. All responses, therefore, were in cuartos that could be seeded; and we have given one cuarto the value of $500.

Per capita household income. Since not all the persons resident in a house are necessarily part of the same domestic economy or dependent on the gross household income, we use the following general guidelines. Unmarried children are considered to be dependent on the gross income, as are all other unmarried or obviously dependent persons living in the house (e.g. grandparents, in-laws, and stray children). For married children living in the parents' house (almost always a married son living with his father), we tried in each case to determine whether the younger couple maintain a common domestic economy with the rest of the household—that is, the son and father farming together, and the mother and daughter-in-law jointly preparing food from a common supply. In most instances this was the case, and all in the house were counted as depen-

TABLE 4
Economic Comparisons Between H'ilol and Lay Households
(Samples from 'Apas, Hteklum, and Pat'osil)

Category	H'ilol	Lay
Gross household income:		
'Apas	$2,401	$2,653
Hteklum	2,851	3,871
Pat'osil	3,909	3,903
Household assets:		
'Apas	2,392	2,973
Hteklum	2,903	3,189
Pat'osil	3,537	4,004
Per capita income:		
'Apas	800	717
Hteklum	792	944
Pat'osil	798	908

dent on the gross income. When it was possible to separate the income of the parental generation from that of offspring living in the same house, the gross and per capita income figures were calculated only for the senior household male and his immediate dependents.

H'ilol and Lay Households

Table 4 compares the gross household incomes, liquid assets, and per capita incomes of h'ilol and lay households in each of three samples. Although the configurations are by no means the same from hamlet to hamlet, a general pattern is discernible: h'ilol-headed households tend to be less wealthy in both assets and income than those headed by laymen. Before we discuss these figures in detail, it should be noted that the income figures for h'ilol-headed households do not include income derived from curing. A healer is paid by gifts of rum and perishable food; and since these are unmarketable, they cannot be considered in the same manner as the cash and salable commodities on which the household income figures are based, although they obviously affect the economy of the h'ilol's household. Generally speaking, we can regard the present figures as indicative of some economic disadvantage for the h'iloletik.

Household assets. In all three samples the assets of h'ilol households are generally lower than lay households. In 'Apas the lay households average 24.3% higher; in Pat'osil and Hteklum the figures are 13.2% and 9.9%, respectively.

The general tendency for h'ilol households to possess fewer assets than lay households can be ascribed partly to the loss of time involved in curing activities. For example, horses and mules are primarily used either to transport corn from hot country to cold country or to transport the goods of others for a fee. If curing activities reduce the scope of a Zinacanteco's agricultural activities and commercial endeavors, it is likely that he will avoid the expense of maintaining animals; and he may even sell any that he has inherited.

Although we have no direct information about inherited wealth gained by the household heads in our samples, we can draw reasonable inference from two indirect lines of evidence: an individual's birth order and residence after marriage. The ideal pattern is for older sons to leave home on marriage and set up new households on land given them by their fathers, while the youngest son remains at home and inherits the house and sitio after his father's death. When a man unable to afford the customary marriage gifts marries, he lives with his in-laws until he has established some economic autonomy. There appears to be no relationship between a h'ilol's occupation and his place of residence, and there is no discernible tendency for him to occupy any particular chronological position among the male children of his family; these facts suggest that h'iloletik do not start their adult lives at any economic disadvantage in terms of inherited resources. If this is so, then the differences in assets between h'iloletik and laymen must be due either to a curer's dissipation of inherited assets or to his lowered success in acquiring land and animals.

Our figures suggest that the average h'ilol farms on a smaller scale than a layman. H'iloletik own less land and fewer animals, rent less land in hot country, and plant and harvest less corn. The reasons for this smaller scale of agricultural endeavor will be discussed later.

Income. The figures from the 'Apas sample show a somewhat higher gross household income for laymen and a somewhat lower per capita income. In the Pat'osil sample the gross incomes of the two groups are virtually the same, but the per capita income of the laymen is somewhat higher. A more appreciable difference appears in the Hteklum sample, where the layman's gross income is 35.8% higher and the per capita income 19.2% higher. These figures are consistent with our information on liquid assets, although 'Apas presents somewhat of an anomaly. That is, compared to the other two hamlets, h'iloletik in 'Apas show a higher per capita income than laymen. Most simply, this reflects the fact that h'iloletik in 'Apas, although they have a lower average gross income than laymen, also tend to have fewer dependents—a phenomenon for which we have no explanation.

There was no strong association between the size of a household group and whether or not the household head was a h'ilol. But we have found that h'iloletik do tend to live in smaller households (this trend is supported by data collected in the controlled study reported in Chapter 5, which shows that h'iloletik also have fewer children). The average size of h'ilol and lay households, respectively, in our samples was: 3.0 and 3.7 in 'Apas; 3.6 and 4.1 in Hteklum; and 4.9 and 4.3 in Pat'osil.

Since these values do not reveal any striking pattern, it is difficult to relate household size to economic status. The potential role of family size in determining family income can obviously be viewed from two opposing standpoints. Large families tend to lower average income by raising the denominator in the per capita income calculation. But larger families, when they contain teenage or older sons, are an economic advantage insofar as they increase the supply of agricultural labor. We chose to examine the latter consideration by comparing the incomes of h'iloletik and laymen who had sons helping them in the fields. However, our samples do not include consistent data on the ages of sons, but simply state the number and sex of a subject's children. Thus we must use the age of the household head to estimate the role of children in family income. Age 35 was arbitrarily chosen as the point at which it may be assumed that a man's sons begin to be of economic value to him. A comparative tabulation of a sample of cases revealed the same average number of sons per household for both h'iloletik and laymen in this age group. These data, then, offer little support for the hypothesis that ages of children may account for a difference in income.

Able-bodied sons are undoubtedly an asset in farming activity, but it is by no means clear that they are a major factor in determining wealth. Cancian's detailed analysis of the activities of Zinacanteco corn farmers (F. Cancian, 1972) emphasizes that factors of management and inherited assets are much more important than family size in this respect. It seems fair to say that with management skill, good luck, and adequate capital resources (which may be a function of management skill, as through astute borrowing, rather than a matter of inheritance), any Zinacanteco can be a successful agricultural entrepreneur.

Since management skill is crucial to economic success, brothers may be at least as important as sons in explaining income differences. Any pooling of efforts and resources in lowland farming will increase efficiency and lower expenses. Cooperative efforts in Zinacantan often involve friends, neighbors, and/or compadres; but they seem easiest to arrange and most dependable when effected with groups of kinsmen, especially brothers. There is no discernible relationship between being a h'ilol and having any particular number of brothers. One of our tabulations showed a slightly higher percentage of h'iloletik than laymen to be brotherless, but the difference was quite small.

In summary, it appears that h'iloletik have a slight tendency to achieve less economically than laymen. This is particularly evident in the total magnitude of their economic activities (gross household income) and in their accumulation of property (household assets). Apparently, these differences are not explainable in terms of inheritance, differences in family backgrounds, or number of sons and brothers.

Economic Disadvantages and Rewards of the H'ilol

The primary economic handicap associated with the position of h'ilol is that the curing duties of such a role lessen the time available for agricultural and commercial activities. This loss of time is in part unavoidable, since a h'ilol must spend some time conducting public ceremonies, and since many requests for private curing can be difficult to refuse. We can estimate the maximal time devoted to public ceremonies—as experienced by a very junior h'ilol forced to participate in all the public ceremonies or a very senior h'ilol with responsibility for directing them— at perhaps 15 days per year, counting complete days lost to other pursuits but not including hours used for planning and preparations. An ordinary h'ilol, who is neither very junior nor very senior, would spend much less time at public ceremonies.

The time devoted by the average h'ilol to private curing is hard to estimate. But except in special cases where curing is virtually a full-time occupation, the time expended seems to be limited. One sample of Zinacanteco medical histories indicates that a single curing ceremony per person per year would be a very liberal estimate. Dividing an estimated 7,600 curing cases by the 177 h'iloletik thought to practice in the municipio gives a rough estimate of 43 cases annually per h'ilol—less than one ceremony a week. And h'iloletik, when asked how frequently they performed ceremonies, invariably cited an average of 1–2 cases per week.

If we accept Cancian's estimate of 200–250 days per year as the time devoted by a full-time corn farmer to growing and selling his crop (F. Cancian, 1972), then there seems to be little conflict between agricultural responsibilities and the average activities of a h'ilol. Farming, however, is not the only source of income for Zinacantecos, and every day lost in curing is potentially worth further income. At wage labor for other Zinacanteco farmers, for example, one can earn approximately $5 per day, plus meals; work on government construction projects pays $8–12 a day without meals. Besides maintaining a full-time agricultural schedule, then, a h'ilol could earn a substantial additional income during the year if enough work were available. To the extent that curing activities interfere with this type of outside work (as well as with traditional agricultural pursuits), the h'ilol must be seen as economically disadvantaged, since curing earns him only food and liquor.

The economic returns of the curing role come in the form of gifts tendered to the h'ilol in return for his services. These gifts are not conceived of as payment, however, but rather as part of a patient's sacrifices to the gods through the medium of the h'ilol. The quantities given depend on the kind of ceremony, and to some degree on the custom of the h'ilol and his patient. A typical gift sequence associated with a large curing ceremony might be the following:

1. When he pulses the patient, the h'ilol is given a bottle of coffee or rum and a small quantity of *kashlan vah* (Ladino bread); occasionally, he also receives a few tortillas. Some informants mention that 50 centavos in cash may also be given.

2. When the h'ilol returns with his assistant to conduct the ceremony, he is given a bottle of rum, two kashlan vah (worth 20 centavos each), and a bottle or gourd of coffee.

3. After completing the ceremony, the h'ilol departs with a gift of four bottles of rum, four chickens, 80 tortillas, and $2 worth of bread.

4. When the patient's bed is stripped of its flowers after a cure is completed, the h'ilol is given a final bottle of rum.

These gifts are the maximum a h'ilol is likely to derive from any one case he treats. In fact the gifts listed as given after the ceremony is completed are the largest described by any of our informants; most put the gift at this stage of the ceremony at about half the amount we mention. Because the gifts are generally not resalable, it is hard to give them a cash value. The rum is the most easily translatable into cash terms, and possibly can even be resold. If we take Wilson's (1963) estimate of $2 per *límete* (a liquid measure approximately equal to one fifth-gallon), the maximum seven bottles of rum would have a value of $14. The value of the Ladino bread is about $2.50. Eighty tortillas would bring about $3 in the San Cristóbal market. The coffee is of negligible value. The gifts, then, have an aggregate value of about $19.50—approximately what a Zinacanteco could earn in three days of hired farm work. The chickens present more of a problem. At San Cristóbal prices, an average-size live chicken is worth about $20. Chickens, however, are never sold dead, and hence have no resale value. In terms of the h'ilol's domestic economy, the chickens will provide about two meals for his family.

Generally speaking, if we consider all the gifts a h'ilol receives as the equivalent of two family meals, their cash value (i.e. the expenditure they replace) is reduced to somewhere between $10 and $15. However, chicken is a luxury food ordinarily eaten only on festive and ceremonial occasions. The Zinacanteco consumption of rum is such that we can credit the seven bottles against a normal household's expenditures, but chickens are an item that would not otherwise be consumed.

The h'ilol's gifts, then, contrast strongly with the pay earned through other economic endeavors. They cannot be saved, invested, or stored against future needs. The h'ilol who loses two days' work while performing a large ceremony in return for comestibles that would cost up to $90 in the market but replace only some $15 of domestic expenditure is actually somewhat worse off than the layman who earns $15–$25 in cash in the same amount of time. Moreover, the layman can invest his extra money in agricultural enterprises, in gaining prestige through the cargo system, or in any of a variety of potentially rewarding activities. The h'ilol, by contrast, must still accumulate enough cash to finance his agricultural and commercial enterprises, buy goods that cannot be produced at home, and underwrite his own participation, if any, in the cargo system.

The real contribution of curing to the average annual incomes of h'iloletik is hard to estimate, since we lack information on the exact frequency and type of curing ceremonies that are performed. Earlier, we mentioned 43 curing cases a year as an average, but only a few of these will be major ceremonies for which large gifts are given. We can roughly estimate the incidence of major ceremonies from our own observations. During no 12-hour ceremonial circuit in Hteklum did we ever observe more than two other curing parties. If we make a liberal estimate of five parties a day (to take account of major ceremonies in the outlying hamlets), or 1,825 such ceremonies a year, the average number per h'ilol is slightly in excess of 10. Letting each major ceremony replace two meals, each remaining ceremony replace one, and giving a family meal the cash value of a little over $7, the average value of a h'ilol's gifts comes to about $400.

The $400 estimate is more than enough to eliminate any differences between h'iloletik and laymen in our 'Apas sample, but it does not cover the entire gap in the Hteklum sample. The average income of h'iloletik from Pat'osil, however, would actually be raised above that of laymen by the addition of this amount. Generally speaking, then, our evidence suggests that the incomes of h'iloletik are relatively comparable to those of the rest of the population. But from a remunerative standpoint their time and income is not spent optimally. The same days devoted to wage labor or commercial activity would bring in a somewhat larger income, and in cash. The h'ilol, although roughly equal to others in terms of providing meals for his family, has fewer liquid assets. This may be reflected in his failure to accumulate assets as fast as others do, and in his inability to engage in large-scale agricultural enterprises.

Economically Specialized H'iloletik

A very few h'iloletik are essentially full-time practitioners. A number of these with whom we are familiar are extremely poor, having virtually no other sources of income and no assets; and they are widely known either as acknowledged witches or as suspected witches who can cure "bad" illnesses. Their special powers and their willingness to treat cases other h'iloletik will not handle make them highly sought after—to the point that some are even consulted by Indians from other municipios or Ladinos. Zinacantecos themselves recognize the association between poverty and witchcraft. Thus it is said that h'iloletik who wear dirty, shabby clothing (a sign taken to reflect poverty) are witches; their poor appearance and their poverty are a punishment from God and a sign of their evil intentions. (To some extent, a shabby and dirty appearance may be used by the witch to dramatize his association with powerful, though evil, forces.)

Curing, for the ordinary h'ilol, is at best a small aid to the domestic economy; but it is, we think, the major support of this small group of practitioners. If one is unwilling to expend any effort on the ordinary

TABLE 5

The Influence of H'iloletik Among Parents and Siblings

(Samples from 'Apas, Hteklum, and Vo'ch'ohvo')

H'ilol among parents or siblings	'Apas		Vo'ch'ohvo' and Hteklum	
	Laymen	H'iloletik	Laymen	H'iloletik
H'ilol in family	46	19	17	9
No h'ilol in family	161	31	110	17
TOTAL	207	50	127	26

NOTE: For 'Apas, $X^2 = 4.5$, $p < .05$; for Vo'ch'ohvo' and Hteklum, $X^2 = 5.5$, $p < .02$.

agricultural or commercial endeavors of Zinacantecos, the occupation of a witch h'ilol can provide an alternative means of subsistence. It is characteristic of these people that they live from hand to mouth, usually having no houses of their own and no land under cultivation. Their full-time curing activities, however, keep them amply supplied with food and liquor, and often with cash. Their reputations as witches cause them to be feared but at the same time make people reluctant to refuse them loans of cash, a bed for the night, and so on. In return, they sacrifice reputation and personal security. They are marginal men in Zinacanteco culture, often hounded into temporary exile by their enemies or the public authorities and always running the risk of imprisonment or even assassination. Only some half-dozen cases are known to us, too few for any statistical analysis. On an impressionistic basis these witch h'iloletik seem to have similar personal characteristics. Although we have too little data from which to draw general inferences about them, their existence does yield some support for the often-quoted notion of shamanism as a refuge for the economically and socially unsuccessful. It is to be emphasized, however, that they represent but a small subset of the h'iloletik in Zinacantan.

The H'ilol's Family

The figures in Table 5 show a positive association between the role of h'ilol and having a h'ilol among one's parents or siblings. The statistical relationship is significant at the .05 level in the case of 'Apas, and at the .02 level in Vo'ch'ohvo' and Hteklum.

This finding confirmed our impression that h'iloletik tend to cluster in families. It is not at all uncommon to find groups of brothers, parents and children, or husbands and wives sharing the h'ilol role. The phenomenon is by no means pervasive in Zinacantan, however: for instance, only 38%

of the h'iloletik in the sample have parents or siblings who are also h'iloletik. Thus, the shamanistic role can in no way be said to be inherited, and this is reflected by the fact that there is no formal concept of such inheritance in Zinacantan.

At least two interrelated factors must be considered in explaining the tendency for some h'iloletik to be clustered in families. First, proximity to a h'ilol may stimulate a person to choose the role himself. He may perceive the occupational specialization as part of a general role model; or there may be active demonstration in his own experience of the rewarding aspects of the role, leading to a predilection in its favor. Second, the psychodynamic influences on occupational selection must be considered. Certain types of psychological conflicts or personality traits that lead to selection are no doubt created in the household environment. Unfortunately, we were not able to employ this framework of analysis. (The difficulty of gaining access to those who are in the process of consolidating their identity as h'iloletik should be emphasized; see Chapters 3 and 5. Besides the strictly sociolegal considerations in this respect, one must also consider the dangerous association that Zinacantecos see in contacts with the supernatural.)

Another possibility suggested by Vogt, on the basis of his detailed data from the hamlet of Paste' (Vogt, personal communication), is that various families, snas, and even waterhole groups might maintain certain kinds of ritual and occupational specializations. He identifies a clustering of certain cargo and other ritual positions in Paste' groups, and there is increasing evidence for cultural differentiation and specialization between hamlets. Just as our present data show a clustering of some h'iloletik in family groups, the same samples reveal a strong association between being a *comerciante* (a middleman in fruits, flowers, or salt) and having a father or brother in the same specialized occupation. In the case of salt merchants, informants state explicitly that the occupation is passed down from generation to generation in certain families.

All these factors tend to show that a Zinacanteco has a better than chance likelihood of resembling his father and brothers in occupational specialization, wealth, and cargo career. In the case of cargo careers, this is bound up with the maintenance over generations of economic and social rankings, which are largely reflected and determined by cargo participation (F. Cancian, 1965). Our impression is that becoming a h'ilol is unrelated to the economic ranking of one's father. As will be demonstrated, however, the status of h'ilol seems to facilitate a level of cargo performance higher than one's economic status alone would warrant. It is possible, then, that the continuation of the role in families is bound up with a larger perpetuation of a social standing that cannot be achieved otherwise.

A third factor that may be operative in the tendency of individuals to follow the occupational choices of their parents and siblings is the availability of information. The h'ilol role demands control of a fair quantity of esoteric knowledge, including ritual manipulations and prayers in which the h'ilol is supposed to be word-perfect. In theory this information is exclusive to the h'iloletik and is imparted to them directly by the gods. In fact, it is of course learned in purely natural ways, and many laymen are familiar with the proper way to light candles, pray, and so on. It is because of this very fact—that his clients are likely to have a fairly strict standard of shamanistic performance (allowing always for certain areas of permissible variation)—that a h'ilol must learn the prayers and manipulations used by other h'iloletik rather than merely making up his own. The prayers and basic ritual operations, in other words, are largely outside the areas of permissible deviation. Unique revelations to h'iloletik seem to lie primarily in the area of diagnostic knowledge.

Curing knowledge, except for the possibly rare (and, according to some informants, reprehensible) cases where a new h'ilol is tutored by an older one, seems to be acquired simply through exposure to curing ceremonies. The greatest opportunity for this exposure comes to those who have a h'ilol living in the same household. Many curing rituals, especially pulsing and K'oplael (a simple ritual of saying prayers), can take place in the h'ilol's own house. In addition, it is not uncommon for a h'ilol to take children, siblings, or spouse along on his curing missions— often for the purpose of seeing that he gets home safely after a ceremony in which ritual drinking has been heavy. Having a h'ilol as parent or sibling, then, is an advantage in terms of opportunity to acquire the experience necessary to become a h'ilol oneself. If we assumed that the entire population of Zinacantan was equally situated in terms of motivations to enter the h'ilol role, then having a parent or sibling who is a h'ilol would provide a subgroup of people with easier access to the necessary training.

No other aspect of family structure that can be adduced from information in our samples shows any differences between h'iloletik and laymen.

TABLE 6
Cargo Performance
(Hteklum and Pat'osil Samples Only)

Category	No cargos	1 or 2 cargos	3 or 4 cargos
All men in sample:			
Laymen	182 (74%)	54 (21.9%)	10 (4.1%)
H'iloletik	28 (59.6%)	15 (32%)	4 (8.5%)
Men over 35:			
Laymen	64 (53.8%)	47 (39.5%)	8 (6.7%)
H'iloletik	17 (47.2%)	15 (41.7%)	4 (11.1%)

NOTE: For the entire sample, $X^2 = 34.33$, $p < .01$. No significant chi-square relationship for men over 35.

There is no relation between being a h'ilol and having any particular number of sons, any particular number of brothers, or any given position in the birth order of male children. The last is true even if single children are lumped with youngest sons on the assumption that either position will increase one's inheritance.

These findings regarding family composition are important in two respects. First, as discussed earlier, they contribute to our conclusion that the economic situation of h'iloletik cannot be attributed to family structure. If h'iloletik tend to be smaller agricultural entrepreneurs, it is not because they lack sons or brothers, nor is it because they are disadvantaged in terms of inheritance (as far as we can tell indirectly from our economic data). Second, the lack of association between family structure and being a h'ilol is important because it can be used to draw psychological inferences. We can say, in general, that if any psychological differences exist between h'iloletik and laymen, they are not traceable to differences in birth order, number of brothers, and the like. They could, however, involve such things as nurturance-succorance needs, independence-dependence, or sex identity, which may or may not be related to family structure, composition, or position.

Unfortunately, we lack data on the most illuminating aspects of the Zinacanteco family situation for the purpose of making psychological inferences, since we have no comparative information at all on the nature of interpersonal relations in the households of h'iloletik and laymen. Our fieldwork did not elicit data on female siblings, for example, or assess the presence or absence of the father from the household during crucial early periods of the h'ilol's life. It can be said that since there is no difference in male birth order between h'iloletik and laymen, one factor that may be associated with the absence of a father in early child-hood is not present (i.e., the lower down a child is in birth order, the greater the likelihood of his father dying while he is still in infancy).

Cargo Performance

Table 6 shows the distribution of cargo performances for all men in the Pat'osil and Hteklum samples. It is clear that h'iloletik outperform laymen in the system, and the difference is significant at the .01 level. Some 40% of h'iloletik participate at some level, as opposed to 26% of lay-men. These data include males of all ages. The level of performance therefore looks lower than it really is, since participation in the cargo system generally begins after 40. In a sample of men over 35 almost half the laymen have held at least one cargo; but h'iloletik remain slightly in the lead. What this reflects, in part, is the fact that a h'ilol apparently makes an earlier start in the cargo system.

These data have interesting implications. First, they tend to contradict the hypothesis that the h'ilol role is an alternate avenue to prestige for Zinacantecos who cannot manage successful cargo careers. It appears that h'iloletik are more likely than the average Zinacanteco to enter at least the first level of the system (and at an earlier age) and are no less likely to reach the upper levels. Second, it must be remembered that the participation of a h'ilol in the cargo system is carried out in the face of an economic disadvantage that makes any cargo a much heavier burden. The whole matter of financing cargos needs further elucidation. It is clear that the system is maintained by intricate patterns of borrowing, and in some cases it is questionable whether all debts are repaid. Infor-mation is needed on the degree to which loans made by young Zinacan-tecos at a high earning level are the foundation for their borrowing after age 40, at which time they are entering on cargo positions but are earn-ing less.

We can only speculate. But it is possible that the h'ilol role itself plays an important part in the establishment of the network of debt relations on which financing a cargo depends. The h'ilol, through his practice, has a greater opportunity than most Zinacantecos to achieve early in life a large number of personal relationships that carry some sort of obligation with them; and it is possible that he can claim from his patients loans and assistance that the ordinary Zinacanteco can obtain only by spend-ing a much longer period loaning money and assistance to older men.

Similarly, it is possible that the prestige and supernatural powers of the h'ilol insulate him somewhat from strong pressure to repay his loans, so that he can spread his debt relations farther in time and over a wider social network than the ordinary layman.

In this light the h'ilol's role seems to be not only a possible alternative avenue to prestige but also an alternative avenue to the cargo system itself. For those who are economically disadvantaged but nonetheless desire the prestige of cargo participation, the h'ilol role may be quite useful. In this sense, the prestige that attaches to the h'ilol role per se may be expressed through the cargo system. Cargo performance and prestige generally relate closely to a Zinacanteco's economic ranking (Cancian, 1965); but this is not true of h'iloletik, who peform more cargo duties than laymen with comparable incomes. If the respect (and fear) they inspire by being h'iloletik is an operative factor in making this over-performance possible, we may make the prestige-ratifying function of the cargo system more general. To wit: the cargo system expresses prestige rankings that can be attained either through economic performance and/or through being a h'ilol.

Chapter five

The Psychological Characteristics of H'iloletik

IN THE PREVIOUS chapter we reviewed some of the economic and social background of the h'iloletik; in this chapter we will deal with their psychological characteristics. As we pointed out in Chapter 1, there is a growing literature on the psychological aspects of shamans, centering around their adjustment and adaptation within their respective sociocultural units. We address ourselves to this topic chiefly by comparing groups of male h'iloletik and male laymen in terms of their responses to a projective personality test. To interpret the psychological results it was necessary to collect specific information on social background; and by establishing how comparable the two groups were in social terms, we obtained a framework for the analysis of psychological characteristics. In the final section of the chapter we will review more recent contributions involving the cognitive features of h'iloletik.

Our study sample contained 43 Zinacanteco males chosen by two informants who were associated with the Harvard Chiapas Project. The informants were simply asked to enlist the cooperation of the Zinacantecos who made up the sample, and no other criteria were used in delineating potentially eligible subjects. Of the 43 subjects, 20 were known to be h'iloletik practicing in the municipio, and the remaining 23 were engaged in differing types of work, mainly agricultural.

The Tests

Each subject was administered a questionnaire dealing with background information. The questionnaire items included the following: (1) Age. When informants were unable to give their precise age and it was not possible to "locate" their birth dates by reference to known past events, their ages were estimated by the investigators. (2) Economic level. As in the survey described in Chapter 4, each subject's relative personal wealth was estimated from his total income, and also by taking into consideration the number of his children and other dependents. (3) Social status. The data for this category consisted of economic level measures combined with the subject's past history and anticipated future performance in the cargo system. (4) Educational level. Years enrolled in the Mexican educational system and number of grades completed were used as the measures. (5) Acculturation or identification with Mexican cultural values. Besides education and degree of fluency with the Spanish language, the following factors were used to estimate an individual's level of acculturation: frequency and type of social transactions with Ladinos, number of household items or possessions of a non-indigenous type, and frequency of visits to nearby Ladino urban centers. (6) Principal occupation (healer, agriculturalist, etc.). (7) Marital history and stability. To assess this variable, the number of previous marriages was the major consideration, although the number of years married was also used. (8) Family size (number of living children).

Each subject was also administered the full complement of cards that make up Form A of the Holtzman Inkblot Technique (HIT).* In almost all instances, the subjects had enough command of the Spanish language that it was possible for either of the two investigators to administer the test and feel that the subjects were involved in a meaningful task. With the few subjects who had a poor command of Spanish we used the native dialect. For all subjects, however, the initial instructions were given in both Spanish and Tzotzil, in most cases by one of our principal informants. The reason for this was to insure that the subjects clearly understood the instructions. Occasionally, the subjects volunteered responses that they were unable to translate into Spanish, and in these cases we relied on a principal informant for Spanish translations.

Using the HIT, we evaluated 22 standard variables and 2 additional variables applied to this survey as follows:

1. *Reaction time (RT)*. The time in seconds from the presentation of the inkblot to the beginning of the primary response.

---

* One subject, a h'ilol, refused further testing after responding to the first 15 cards. He gave poor physical health as the reason for this refusal. His responses were scored and showed no striking differences from those of others, but he is not included in the overall sample.

2. *Rejection* (*R*). Failure of the subject to give a scorable response. Range: 0–45.

3. *Location* (*L*). A 3-point scale used to measure the tendency to fragment the inkblot into smaller areas. The greater the area used, the lower the score. Range: 0–90.

4. *Space* (*S*). This variable is scored when there is a true figure-ground reversal (e.g., when the white part of the card is used as the figure in the percept with the inkblot serving as background to delineate the form of the white area). The higher the score, the higher the tendency to reverse figure and ground. Range: 0–45.

5. *Form definiteness* (*FD*). A 5-point scale measuring the definiteness of the form of the concept reported, regardless of the appropriateness of this form to the structure of the inkblot. The greater the score, the more definite the concept. Range: 0–180.

6. *Form appropriateness* (*FA*). A 3-point scale indicating the fit of the form of the percept to the form of the inkblot area used. The higher the score, the better the fit. Range: 0–90.

7. *Color* (*C*). A 4-point scale measuring the primacy of both chromatic and achromatic color in determining a response. The higher the score, the more color is used as a primary determinant. Range: 0–135.

8. *Shading* (*Sh*). A 3-point scale measuring the primacy of shading as a response determinant. The higher the score, the more shading is used as a primary determinant. Range: 0–90.

9. *Movement* (*M*). A 5-point scale indicating the movement energy level the subject voluntarily ascribes to his percept regardless of its content. The higher the score, the greater the movement energy level. Range: 0–180.

10. *Verbalization* (*V*). A 5-point scale measuring 9 qualitatively different types of autistic and pathological thinking. The higher the score, the more deviant the thinking. Range: 0–180 plus.

11. *Integration* (*I*). A 2-point scale indicating the presence or absence of the organization of adequately perceived inkblot elements into a unified response. Range: 0–45.

12. *Human* (*H*). A 3-point scale measuring the amount of human content seen. Each inkblot is scored 0 for no human content, 1 for parts of a human, and 2 for whole humans. Range: 0–90.

13. *Animal* (*A*). A 3-point scale measuring the amount of animal content seen. Each inkblot is scored 0 for no animal content, 1 for parts of animals, and 2 for whole animals. Range: 0–90.

14. *Anatomy* (*At*). A 3-point scale measuring the amount of anatomy content seen. Each inkblot is scored 0 for no anatomy content, 1 for bone structures, and 2 for visceral and crude anatomy responses. Range: 0–90.

15. *Sex* (*Sx*). A score (0–2) of degree of sexual content verbally reported in each perceptual response. The higher the score the more overt and blatant the reference to sexuality. Range: 0–90.

16. *Abstract* (*Ab*). The score (0–2) reflects the degree of abstraction expressed in the response, ranging from no abstract concept to a wholly abstract response. The higher the score, the greater the abstraction. Range: 0–90.

17. *Anxiety* (*Ax*). A 3-point scale measuring the amount of anxious content seen. The greater the score, the more anxious the content of the response. Range: 0–90.

18. *Hostility* (*Hs*). A 4-point scale measuring the amount of hostile content seen. The greater the score, the more hostile the content of the response. Range: 0–135.

19. *Barrier* (*Br*). A 2-point scale measuring the presence or absence of body image boundary definiteness in a response. Range: 0–45.

20. *Penetration* (*Pn*). A 2-point scale measuring the presence or absence of body image boundary diffusion or disruption in a response. Range: 0–45.

21. *Balance* (*B*). This variable is scored either present (1) or absent (0) and indicates the concern of the subject for the symmetry-asymmetry dimension of the blot. Range: 0–45.

22. *Popular* (*P*). This is scored when the subject's response to a certain area of the blot coincides with a response that is frequently given to that same area of the blot. A score of 1 is given for each popular response. Twenty-five cards are scorable on Popular. Range: 0–25.

23. *Pure anxiety* (Ax_p). Nonstandard. Anxiety score with references to religious and diabolical themes left out of total.

24. *Genetic level score* (*GL*). Nonstandard. Total score obtained by configurally scoring responses for *L, FD, FA, V,* and *I* variables.

All protocols were scored without knowledge of the identity of the subject (i.e. h'ilol or layman). For most responses, a translation between the native and scientific (scoring) categories was accomplished without much difficulty. In some instances, notably with regard to the Anxiety variable, it was difficult to determine whether a particular response, viewed from the perspective of Zinacantan, reflected anxiety as it is ordinarily understood when this variable is scored. For this reason, the variable was first scored using the content of the response exclusively— i.e., disregarding the possibility that some responses might not reflect anxiety in this setting. Then responses touching on supernatural themes (which are automatically scored for Anxiety in the standard HIT evaluation) were excluded creating a separate variable that is here termed Pure Anxiety (Ax_p). Finally, for each subject a genetic level score was computed in the manner outlined by Becker (Becker, 1959; Steffy and Becker, 1961). Briefly, this is a rating based on configurally scoring each inkblot for the variables Location, Form Definiteness, Form Appropriateness, Verbalization, and Integration. This score yields a measure of perceptual organization or maturity for each subject in terms of his responses to the HIT.

Results

Social background. The h'ilol subject group was slightly younger than the lay group, but these differences were not significant in a statistical sense. When the two subgroups were compared in terms of family background, the size of the family of procreation (number of siblings), the number of female siblings, and the subject's rank or position in the sibling hierarchy did not differ across the subgroups. Approximately half the members of each group indicated that their fathers had been present in the house during their formative years. Although differences in educational attainment did not reach a significant level, the h'iloletik tended to have less education than the laymen. A proportionately greater number of h'iloletik had no prior schooling whatsoever, and both the average highest grade completed and the average total years in the educational system were higher in the lay group.

With regard to marital stability, no striking differences were noted. Most subjects were middle-aged men with only one marriage. Four subjects were unmarried. The two of these who were not h'iloletik were quite young (ages 21 and 18); however, the two unmarried h'iloletik were 26 and 28 years of age. It is possible that a subset of healers enter marital relationships later, perhaps forming heterosexual relationships with difficulty or in a different way. That there is something different about the marital relationships of Zinacanteco shamans is suggested by the fact that the mean number of children per married subject differed significantly in the two subgroups, with h'iloletik having a significantly smaller number of children. All four married subjects who were childless were in the h'ilol subgroup, and only three h'iloletik (as compared to eight laymen) had more than three children.

The two groups were also evaluated in terms of their performance in the cargo system. The age of entry into the system, the relative status of the position(s) held, and the status of future positions applied for were considered in this evaluation. About half of each subgroup had not participated by the time of our survey. Considering each subgroup as a whole, there were no differences in the proportion of levels passed or aspired to. Next, the performance or lack of performance of each subject was examined with reference to his current age. In the group aged 30 or less, a slightly greater number of h'iloletik had participated. In the group over 30, however, the laymen were overrepresented in the cargo-participation cell. In general, the cargo performance of the two subgroups failed to reveal statistically significant differences, although from this sample of subjects it appears that healers may enter the cargo system at an earlier age than nonhealers. Very few of the subjects fall in the high-performance class; but of the few that did, most were h'iloletik. We also obtained a history of the cargo positions held by the subjects' fathers. This information was analyzed on the basis of the prestige ratings of the various positions. The patterns of the ratings did not show any differences suggesting that the fathers of subjects in either subgroup were characterized by higher cargo prestige ratings.

The average current socioeconomic level of the two subgroups (as judged by total assets, total income, and the income/dependent ratio) did not differ in a statistically significant sense, nor were clear trends suggested by careful inspection of the various economic measures evaluated.

Participation in Ladino culture. Here, we will focus on each of the separate facets of participation that were studied, as well as on the composite ratings formulated.

Each Indian municipio in Chiapas has its own governmental system and set of committees through which the political and civil affairs of the municipio are administered. Although the various governmental tasks in Zinacantan are to a large extent performed by Zinacantecos, the supervision of these tasks is in charge of Ladinos representing the Mexican national government. Political involvement thus to some extent means involvement in the Mexican national system. The extent of current and past participation in various political activities (civil offices, school committees, etc.) did not differ appreciably between h'iloletik and laymen. Using the number and relative significance of the various offices held, as well as the nature of the duties performed by the subjects, we formed a rating reflecting our subjects' degree of political leadership in the community (or the political responsibility given them by the community). In general, the two groups did not differ significantly, although there was a slight trend suggesting that laymen were politically more active.

Subjects were also compared in terms of the pattern and frequency of their transactions with Ladinos in social activities and in activities like marketing, employment, and middleman commercial transactions. No significant differences emerged from this analysis. Fluency with the Spanish language and the extent of exclusively native modes of dress (as opposed to the use of various items of Ladino clothing) were also similar in both subgroups, as was the overall ownership of Ladino artifacts. An analysis of the frequency distributions of particular Ladino items (e.g., radio, tile roof, or shotgun) owned by members of each group failed to reveal statistically significant differences.

Lastly, we tabulated the number and frequency of visits to San Cris-

TABLE 7
Comparison of Groups on HIT Projective Test Data

Variable	Group means	
	H'ilol (N = 20)	Layman (N = 23)
1. Reaction time	29.50	34.57
2. Rejection	0.25	0.74
3. Location	37.80	30.26
4. Space	0.90	0.17
5. Form definiteness	69.15	62.04
6. Form appropriateness	32.15	35.43
7. Color	9.90	10.70
8. Shading^a	0.70	2.00
9. Movement	20.70	12.52
10. Verbalization^a	12.35	5.30
11. Integration	3.00	2.52
12. Human	21.60	13.30
13. Animal	26.75	23.04
14. Anatomy	3.45	3.09
15. Sex	0.20	0.04
16. Abstract	0.00	0.00
17. Anxiety^a	16.15	7.04
18. Hostility	12.55	4.91
19. Barrier	5.30	7.83
20. Penetration	4.80	3.57
21. Balance	0.10	0.22
22. Popular	5.55	4.87
23. Pure anxiety	8.95	4.70
24. Genetic level score	111.31	118.45

NOTE: The groups were compared by use of the Mann-Whitney U test.
^{a} Probability level <.05.

tóbal, the principal city in the area and, for many Zinacantecos, the economic center of the region. These visits inevitably entail meetings and social transactions with Ladino merchants and a general exposure to the urban Mexican social system, and they thus express one form of interest or participation in Ladino affairs. In this analysis, answers were coded in terms of visits per year and the median test was applied. The lay group reported a larger number of visits per year, which proved to be statistically significant. The frequency of trips to Tuxtla Gutiérrez (the Chiapas state capital, in the lowlands about 6o miles from Zinacantan) was also analyzed; but results did not reveal statistical differences or suggestive trends. Most subjects actually visited Tuxtla rather infrequently.

Psychological test data. Because of the small size of our sample, a nonparametric statistical test, the Mann-Whitney test (Siegel, 1956), was used to compare the groups on the various HIT variables. In Table 7 are listed the mean scores of each subgroup on the set of variables analyzed, together with the results of applying the statistical test. The Mann-Whitney test yielded statistically significant values (<.05) on the variables Anxiety, Verbalization, and Shading. The h'ilol group had a substantially higher mean score on the variables Hostility, Human, and Movement, though the *U* value obtained from the use of the Mann-Whitney test did not reach the level required for significance.

An *F* test was applied to compare the groups' variances on each HIT variable (McNemar, 1955). On 11 of the 22 standard HIT variables, the subgroups differed significantly in dispersion about their group mean; and in 9 of these 11 instances, the h'iloletik showed the significantly greater dispersion.*

Discussion

Our analysis of the information on social background showed that the h'ilol and lay subgroups were relatively similar in age, family, economic level, and general prestige in the community; nor did the extent of acculturation to Ladino dress, language, or material possessions differ significantly between the subgroups. However, when exposure to or participation in Ladino society was evaluated by educational experience in the Mexican school system, political leadership, and frequency of visits to San Cristóbal, the laymen proved to be somewhat more "acculturated." There is, of course, no firm reason to believe that measures reflecting participation or involvement in a "contact culture" necessarily imply commitment to or identification with the underlying values of that culture. As classic anthropological literature asserts and recent investigative work confirms, the meaning and assessment of acculturation is a complex matter (Doob, 1960; Chance, 1965; Graves, 1967; Broom et al., 1967).

Perhaps a tentative statement based on our results should simply (1) emphasize the apparent lack of correlation between the various features

---

* The variables with significant differences in dispersion were: probability <.05 for Human and Anatomy; probability <.02 for Rejection, Space, Movement, Verbalization, Integration, Sex, Anxiety, Hostility, and Penetration. The h'iloletik had the higher dispersion for all variables except Rejection and Anatomy. Our two added variables also produced significant differences, with a probability of <.05 for Pure Anxiety and one of <.02 in Genetic Level Scores; on both of these the dispersion of h'iloletik was higher.

thought to reflect acculturation and (2) note that the groups were similar in terms of the active use that was made of aspects of Ladino culture (radios, Ladino clothing, tile roofing, language, etc.), although (3) the lay group showed a somewhat greater participation and exposure to social aspects of Ladino culture.

The importance of the h'iloletik in Zinacantan—specifically, their ability to communicate with the ancestral gods—makes them key persons in the traditional cultural system. Consequently, one might anticipate that h'iloletik would manifest a greater identification with Zinacanteco values and, by extension, a lesser tendency to accept Ladino patterns. This formulation may explain why h'iloletik as individuals showed somewhat less social involvement and participation in Ladino culture.

Before we analyze the projective responses, a brief mention should be made of our information on the characteristics of the marital relationship. As will be remembered, marital stability (estimated by counting previous marriages and considering the age of the subjects) was similar in the two groups. Married h'ilol subjects, however, had a statistically smaller mean number of children than did married laymen. We had no background data or impressions that allowed us to anticipate this finding. In general, not enough is known about the many factors affecting family structure and family size in Zinacantan (Collier, 1966; Cancian, 1966). Certainly it should be stated that a large number of sons can be considered an advantage for those Zinacantecos who are primarily farmers, insofar as land and farming activities can be distributed to allow higher productivity. Unfortunately, we did not collect data on the sex or current age of the children in our sample, hence the economic effect of having fewer children cannot be evaluated. It may be that h'iloletik, who are slightly less dependent on agricultural activities for income when compared to laymen, may be less motivated to produce large families. But this type of reasoning alone obviously cannot explain the significantly smaller number of children in h'ilol families. Factors having greater psychodynamic relevance in general, and sexual identity considerations in particular, are probably involved. One is reminded of other investigations that have suggested possible sexual identity conflicts in shamans. Further and more precise investigations of this question are needed.

In general, the absence of striking differences between the two groups in terms of social characteristics is consistent with the material we reviewed in the previous chapter. In the present sample, the economic level and cargo performance of the h'ilol group were more like those of other male Zinacantecos than was the case in our earlier analyses, which showed that h'iloletik were relatively more successful cargo performers despite their somewhat lower incomes. This inconsistency, however, could easily be the result of random fluctuations. We feel that our subgroups are representative of male h'iloletik and laymen in Zinacantan. In addition, we believe that our analyses confirm the general similarity in social characteristics that exists between h'iloletik and other Zinacanteco males. Our analysis of the psychological test data, then, will proceed on the assumption that the groups are both representative and suitably matched.

Statistically, our sample groups differed only on the variables Anxiety, Verbalization, and Shading. Moreover, these differences were only at the .05 level of significance. When a series of statistical tests are performed, as in this study, several significant statistics can be expected to occur on the basis of chance alone (Sakoda et al., 1954). Consequently, if one adopts rigorous statistical criteria, it must be concluded that there is no strong evidence differentiating h'iloletik from laymen in terms of psychological parameters. This conclusion is consistent with those derived from our background data. However, there are still a number of points that can be discussed regarding the psychological material.

The subgroups, it will be remembered, did not differ significantly on the variables of Form Definiteness, Form Appropriateness, Location, and Integration. The genetic level scores, obtained by configurally scoring these variables together with Verbalization, also did not differ significantly. This can be taken to mean that the groups are similar in terms of the degree of differentiation and hierarchic integration manifested in their responses to the inkblot stimuli. The genetic level score is a way of rating perceptual responses in terms of structural features that conform to the theoretical ideas of Werner (1948): response differentiation is judged by criteria related to the levels of functioning of children at different stages of mental organization. When applied to schizophrenic protocols, the score is used as a measure of personality organization (Fabrega and Swartz, 1967). In this study, it is used as a measure of perceptual maturity. Following this line of reasoning, it can be said that male h'iloletik and laymen apparently function at a similar level of perceptual-cognitive maturity.

Color, Shading, and Form Definiteness represent the major determinants of responses involving direct stimulus correlates in the inkblots. Of these three variables, the groups differed significantly only on Shading. It should be noted that a Sh score was assigned only infrequently in either group ($\overline{X}$ = 0.7 and 2.0), so it cannot be said that shading was a frequent determinant of the responses. Our results do show, however, that shading or texture characteristics were less frequently observed in h'ilol responses. Although movement may be classified as being in part a determinant of responses, it obviously has only faint psychophysical correlates in the stimulus. The relatively higher mean score of h'iloletik on the Movement variable should be viewed as resulting almost entirely from the nature of their fantasy activity. It can be said that h'iloletik apparently tend to display greater movement and activity in their projective responses.

The h'iloletik had substantially higher scores on the Human variable. This suggests that people and situations involving interpersonal relations occupy a more prominent part in the fantasy life of these shamanistic healers—that is, h'iloletik are more person-oriented. The groups did not differ significantly in scores on the other "content" variables: Animal, Anatomy, Sex, and Abstract. It may appear somewhat surprising that the At score was so similar in the two groups, since the healing activities of shamans expose them to an apparent concern and preoccupation with bodily ailments and functioning, as well as with lesions and growths of various types. It should be remembered, however, that in the Zinacanteco medical system (as in the medical systems of related Chiapas indigenous social units) disease etiology, mechanism, and explanation do not involve notions of physiology or anatomy, regardless of whether these two domains are viewed scientifically or in a folk-taxonomical manner (i.e. ethno-anatomy. Fabrega et al., 1970; Holland, 1963).

It is important that h'iloletik obtained higher scores on Anxiety, Hostility, and pathognomic Verbalization. These factors together suggest that certain personality characteristics may be more frequent in this group. To the extent that inkblot responses manifest anxiety and hostility, for example, they imply that these dimensions or traits are characteristic of the perceptual and ideational lives of the subjects. The pathognomic component of Verbalization includes elements such as fabulized combination, autistic logic, contamination, and deterioration color. Generally speaking, when these features are "reflected" in a response, the stimulus has perhaps evoked percepts that the subject is unable to organize and synthesize while maintaining the requirements of form, balance, articulation, and logical consistency. This is another way of saying that the subject, in attempting to make sense of the blot, has shown a poorly integrated mode of perceiving, thinking, and feeling. Viewed abstractly, then, our results suggest that h'iloletik more frequently manifest this mode of functioning. In sum, h'iloletik, when compared to laymen, show greater evidence of anxiety, hostility, and deviant verbalization (or what has been termed pathological thinking). Because these results relate closely to clinical issues that have been traditionally associated with shamanism, it seems useful to discuss them further.

With regard to the Verbalization variable, when features touching on pathological modes of thinking are very prominent in a set of projective responses produced by a subject, it is legitimate to speak of psychological dysfunction or disorganization. The validity of this assertion would be strengthened if the subject's performance on the whole test demonstrated a similar level or type of functioning, in which case a diagnosis of psychosis or schizophrenia could be entertained. Several factors about the psychological functioning of Zinacanteco h'iloletik, as revealed by the HIT, argue against these possibilities. First, in any one subject the number of responses scored for V was generally quite small. Second, a large proportion of the 20 h'iloletik offered responses that received no scores on the pathognomic element of Verbalization. Finally, and most important, the intensity or degree of "pathological thinking" (i.e. the actual V score) per response was quite low.

For example, the h'iloletik produced 153 responses that received a V score, as compared to 69 for the laymen. And of these, 85 h'ilol responses and 21 lay responses received a V score of only one. In general, there is no reason to regard these responses as "pathological," although almost all of them reflected fabulation—according to HIT standards, a tendency in the subject to "unduly elaborate on the feeling element of a response." There were no significant group differences in the number of responses scored two for V. The h'iloletik did produce almost all the responses that received a score of three on V; but there were only 12 of these in all, out of the approximate total of 900 h'ilol responses. No responses received a V score of four.

On the whole, then, there is little in these protocols that could be called evidence of "pathological thinking" as reflected by the Verbalization variable. There does appear to be a clear difference in fabulized responses and a trend toward the undue elaboration or expression of feeling, with the h'iloletik investing their responses with more affect; but only infrequently do they show evidence of what one would clinically term disordered thinking.

Responses that received Anxiety scores were commonly encountered in both subgroups. It should be noted, however, that all responses touching on supernatural themes automatically receive an *Ax* score on the HIT.* Though the nature and content of some responses we obtained clearly indicated anxiety, many simply reflected what might otherwise be termed "supernaturalistic labeling"—reflecting, perhaps, a religious disposition or orientation. Religious and supernatural themes are pervasive features of Zinacanteco experience, and are especially central to the work of a h'ilol. It is questionable, then, whether evidence showing that these themes affect the thinking and perceiving of h'iloletik should be viewed as an indication of anxiety in the dynamic or personality sense. And when responses showing supernatural themes were excluded, the groups did not appreciably differ on the *Ax* score. It seems preferable to say that although content anxiety is a more prominent feature of the perceptual responses of Zinacanteco shamans, it is difficult to be precise about the extent to which shamans differ from laymen on this variable, and about the significance to be given to any putative difference in view of the HIT scoring criteria.

Hostility is a variable that appears to distinguish the two groups. Not only did the statistical test suggest this, but inspection of the frequency distributions showed that very few laymen received a high total *Hs* score as compared to h'iloletik. Of the 78 responses that received a *Hs* score of two, 63 were made by h'iloletik. A great many of the responses manifesting hostility involved interpersonal situations; and in general, it can be said that the fantasy projections of Zinacanteco shamans frequently include people in hostile interactions. In the performance of his medical role, which involves the diagnosis and treatment of illness caused by malevolence, the h'ilol is often confronted with hostile situations. Further work is needed to explore the meaning of this finding. It is possible that a prominence of hostile feelings characterizes the would-be shaman

---

* It was possible to differentiate the supernatural responses into two types: those referring to religious objects (e.g., cross or church), situations (e.g., church scenes or processions), or personages (heavenly beings or angels), etc.; and those referring to diabolical themes (those involving devils and witches). Both types were more common in the h'ilol group.

even before his social identity is crystallized, and that a need to channel these feelings adaptively may play a role in the shamanistic recruitment process. The mean *Hs* score of younger h'iloletik, however, did not appreciably differ from that of older ones, or from that of younger laymen; hence one should be cautious in adopting this line of reasoning.

Social background factors must be taken into account when interpreting the HIT results. Since h'iloletik had lower measures on the indices of acculturation that involved interpersonal contact with Ladinos, it is possible that they perceive and respond to this contact with greater distrust, suspicion, and fear, owing to their lesser familiarity. Perhaps a h'ilol's greater identification with native and traditional values is primary, entailing a "negative" definition of the Ladino (dangerous, distrustful, etc.). At any rate, any tendency to show this kind of psychological response to the Ladino would probably be carried over into the experimental situation itself, since it is likely that Zinacanteco subjects perceived the investigators in large part as Ladinos. Projective responses suggesting greater emotional arousal and psychological interference in the h'iloletik group (i.e., Anxiety, Hostility, Movement, and Verbalization) may have resulted from this factor. In other words, the testing relationship (which involved sitting close to a "Ladino" for two or three hours in the Ladino's home) may have been more threatening to h'iloletik; and the possibility that this threat may have affected a h'ilol's performance on the test should be considered. Thus we must not be too quick to conclude that the test results necessarily point to significant and enduring personality traits.

The discussion thus far has implicitly relied on clinical psychodynamic principles in interpreting the differences between the test groups. These differences, however, can also be explained in an altogether different framework, a framework that takes into account the behavioral requirements of the shamanistic role. It could be said, for example, that because a h'ilol is repeatedly involved in interpersonal relations with his "patients," he tends to perceive human figures on the HIT cards, and also, perhaps, to elaborate on feelings. Similarly, the contingencies of his work may force him to look for hostile interactions when explaining culturally defined illnesses and other social events, since hostile interactions are typical Zinacanteco explanations for these phenomena. Because a h'ilol must treat illness and resolve human conflicts involving people in circumstances of considerable stress and anxiety, he may be more inclined to attribute this behavior dimension to the inkblot. By this last interpretation, the h'iloletik's higher scores on many of the variables would be viewed largely as time-bound consequences of the performance of their role, and not as personality differences in the classic sense.

Deciding which of the two alternative frameworks is the more suitable for explaining observed differences is obviously a complex matter. It involves issues such as the theory of projective techniques, dynamic explanations of personality, and the relation of these to the influences of language and experience in cognition and perception. The second analytical framework we offer suggests that older h'iloletik, when compared to younger ones, might receive higher scores on the various dimensions likely to be affected by role performance, since they have spent a greater amount of time performing their various duties. To test this possibility, however, the scores of the lay group also had to be analyzed in the same way in order to exclude the possibility that age alone, independent of role status, might be associated with higher scores on the various dimensions. We performed a two-way analysis of variance (shaman-nonshaman vs. old-young); and, although there were some main effects due to age, there were no interaction effects that proved to be statistically significant. Thus it appears that age is not associated with role status in any specialized way.

This does not mean that an analytical framework derived from consideration of a h'ilol's work experience is untenable. It is possible that the amount of time needed to become "sensitized" to the various behavior dimensions is actually quite small, and that thereafter the psychological effects of work experience are not related to time. In this context, it should be remembered that h'iloletik typically "practice" surreptitiously for an indeterminate period of time before publicly acknowledging their social position. The younger h'iloletik in the sample, in other words, may already have been affected by such work experience, since they had all practiced their profession for at least 3–4 years. If this is the case, dividing the h'ilol group on the basis of age would not be a conclusive test of the possibility that their work experience could explain observed differences on the psychological variables. To directly test the possibility that experience in the role accounts for elevated scores in those variables of potential psychodynamic significance, the actual number of years in practice would have to be used as the independent variable. Unfortunately, we did not include this question in our protocol.

Further studies, focusing on recently recruited h'iloletik and potential h'iloletik, could resolve many of the questions we have raised in this study—provided a means can be devised to identify potential h'iloletik, or samples could be large enough to guarantee that they would include a sufficient number of subjects on the point of becoming h'iloletik.

Finally, we must comment on the group differences that were observed where the *F* test was used. It will be recalled that on 9 of 11 variables the h'ilol group showed greater dispersion or heterogeneity than the lay group; that is, the h'iloletik demonstrated a greater scatter or dissimilarity in overall performance level. H'iloletik are a well-defined social segment of Zinacantan society: people entrusted with highly specific responsibilities and believed to possess equally specific abilities and powers. As a group, however, h'iloletik are more variable in their psychological characteristics than members of a male Zinacanteco "control group." If significant personality attributes are actually being tapped by the HIT, this group variability would urge a certain amount of caution in accepting the assertions of informants (or investigators) that members of a specific subgroup within a culture are "alike." The greater dispersion in psychological functioning of the h'ilol group strengthens the argument that members of a native culture respond to important and respected "others" using social-structural rather than psychological criteria. In other words, it appears that in Zinacantan attitudes and dispositions toward h'iloletik may be mainly determined by implications of the h'ilol role or social position itself rather than by the personality attributes of the individual h'iloletik.

The Cognitive Features of H'iloletik

We have stressed in earlier chapters the unified way in which Zinacantecos construe all illness—i.e., that illness links with, has implications for, and at times symbolizes the diverse preoccupations of the Zinacanteco. In later chapters we will draw explicit attention to the close relationship that illness has with social relations, emphasizing that illness can express the moral concerns of the Zinacanteco and pose deep problems for him. In many ways, illness represents that which is least under his personal control. These issues all point to the emotional implications of illness and curing. A visit by a patient to the h'ilol can thus be interpreted in a purely psychological framework. At the very least, the visit can be seen as an attempt to gain security: by seeking the help of the h'ilol the Zinacanteco expresses his emotional need for a mediator who will secure for him some form of supernatural confirmation and social validation. At the same time, the visit can be interpreted cognitively as a search for some form of order, structure, and control. Illness, because it is threatening and has uncertain implications, involves a loss of structure, order, and control.

Issues related to the question of structure that is imposed on experience led Richard Shweder (1968) to evaluate the cognitive aspects of the h'ilol's performance under conditions of stimulus ambiguity. Drawing on the ideas of Lévi-Strauss (1963a, 1963b, 1966), Geertz (1966), Bruner (1968), and Bruner and Potter (1964), he assumed that a key psychological function of the shaman was to provide and communicate order to those seeking his services. Novel or extraordinary situations prove threatening either because they deviate from structured and organized cognitive models that have created expectations, or because their significance is difficult to interpret. "In the face of those contingencies of the environment which threaten the group intellect [culture] and the individual who makes his life meaningful in terms of that group intellect," the shaman is the person who "provides a response, interprets the uninterpreted, and reorders the occurrence in terms of accepted patterns of meaning" (Shweder, 1968: 1).

Shweder analyzed the responses of a group of h'iloletik and laymen to six series of photographs, each a number of prints that developed from blurring and ambiguity to full focus on an object familiar to Zinacantecos (a horse, a market scene, etc.). By first using independent judges, he was able to determine the earliest photo in each series that was sufficiently recognizable to allow "objective" confirmation. He then compared the way h'iloletik and laymen coped with the task of identifying the content of each series. During four of the series (the so-called no-choice series) the subjects were allowed to volunteer any response; in the other two series they were provided with choices and alternatives. For all series, they were told that if they were uncertain about the nature of the photo they were to respond "I don't know."

In general, h'iloletik were found to offer the "I don't know" response significantly less often, although this tendency was less striking in those conditions when alternatives and choices were provided. They also classified or categorized photos significantly earlier in the no-choice series; and they generated and produced significantly more unique categorizations, often going outside the experimenter's given choices.

Shweder's impression is that these cognitive features of the shaman's performance represent true personality traits. That is, because the shamans were not recruited to perform rituals, the test situation did not constitute a role situation but instead allowed existing personality characters to become manifest. Of course, the shamans may have felt that their position and role in the culture nevertheless required them to appear knowledgeable, and that this expectation was implicit in the testing situation. Their performance, in short, can be seen in the light of constraints and expectations tied to their role in Zinacantan. Still, Shweder concludes that shamans appear to manifest a greater need for order and structure—or conversely, to avoid experiencing bafflement and uncertainty—and he attributes this to personality and not to social-role factors. In other words, when shamans are confronted with stimuli that are ambiguous, problematic, and not readily identified, they consistently tend to seek closure and impose control. Shweder relates these personality characteristics, as well as the shamans' greater generativeness and productivity, in terms of the shaman's time-honored function as a mediator between the natural and supernatural realms. One function of the h'ilol in Zinacantan, he asserts, is to impose organization and regularity on experiences and circumstances that are ambiguous and chaotic. This often requires a form of inner-directedness and improvisation, as well as the ability to creatively reorder that which is enigmatic and puzzling.

The results obtained by Shweder are interesting and offer some support for the hypothesis described above. It should be reemphasized, however, that Shweder's approach, like our own, does not allow one to determine whether the observed personality differences express innate personal characteristics (what one would term dispositional traits) or whether they result from experience in performing the shamanistic role. His study, nevertheless, is valuable and contributes greatly to an understanding of shamans generally and h'iloletik specifically.

Summary of Psychological Differences

We have thus far presented essentially contrasting interpretations of the psychological characteristics of h'iloletik. In other words, we have viewed the projective data as reflecting either personality traits or sociocultural factors. Using the perspective and orientation presented in Chapter 1, we felt compelled to draw attention to the sociocultural factors that influence a subject's psychological adjustment. A h'ilol, after all, is a special type of shamanistic medical practitioner, and we feel that it is important to consider his unique role duties in explaining how he interpreted the inkblot stimuli. Obviously, however, any person's style and adjustment to life must be seen as involving a compromise between both personal and social factors. From this psychosocial perspective, it is the synthetic and creative strivings of the individual that are brought into focus.

The empirical information we have received in this chapter and in the preceding one sketches the h'ilol as certainly no more pathological or disturbed than his lay counterpart. There is virtually no telling evidence that h'iloletik are psychiatrically ill or disabled; nor are they poorly adapted in their social settings. On the contrary, we would submit that h'iloletik, from a psychosocial standpoint, appear to be essentially freer and more creative. Persons, feelings, movement, and novelty characterize their fantasied projections. They accomplish as much socioeconomically as their lay counterparts, and with less effort. Their position in Zinacantan requires them to "see" beyond that which is naturalistically given and to reinterpret everyday worldly circumstances in terms of other-worldly values. This essentially social task is made easier by the h'ilol's ability to relax ordinary (so-called secondary-process) constraints on thinking and feeling, to delve creatively into the everyday affairs of men, and to compose novel interpretations of these in line with both humanistic and magical considerations. This, we have seen, h'iloletik also seem to accomplish in the testing situation. To the extent that this mode of perceiving and construing "reality" promotes the expression of personally suppressed feelings or facilitates such expression in others, we would say that h'iloletik, psychosocially, are predisposed toward cathartic abreaction. As we shall see, the Zinacanteco view of illness and medical treatment makes this mode of adaptation and orientation both appropriate and useful.

Chapter six

The Meaning of Illness in Zinacantan

IN ZINACANTECO THOUGHT, illness is seen as reflecting and expressing the status of a man's relations with himself, his social group, and his deities. For example, hostility and envy, two feelings that can pervade and structure interpersonal relations, are believed to be the motivations that lead others to promote illness and injury, either directly (by alleged poisoning or compacting with the devil) or indirectly (through the services of a sorcerer or witch). Similarly, transgressions of the spiritual and/or social code are believed to be punished by divinely sent illness. The individual himself, his worldly contemporaries, and the gods are locked in a triple web of relationships; and a frequent expression of disarticulation in this web is illness, or *chamel*. It is in this sense that one can speak of illness in Zinacantan as having a moral basis: the individual's essentially sacred and spiritual view of himself and others requires that he behave appropriately and in conformance with socially validated rules; but chamel both reflects and symbolizes a disarticulation of his triple balance.

In a strictly physiological as well as moral sense, Zinacantecos, like other Maya Indians in Chiapas, generally distinguish two principal states of ill health: a person can have either a "strong" or a "weak" illness (Fabrega, Metzger, and Williams, 1970). These two states appear to be differentiated primarily by the degree to which they exhibit symptoms and constrain the sufferer's pursuit of his life activities. Some distinguish a third type of illness, the "simple." Because it is brief and in no way incapacitating, however, simple illness is of little more than momentary concern to some and may not properly be regarded as a chamel by others. The label of illness is applied when a Zinacanteco perceives himself, or is perceived by those responsible for him (e.g., by his parents), to be in pain, unable to work, and showing impairment of bodily function, lassitude, loss of appetite, etc. Such a situation presents the individual with a number of possible choices. These, in turn, relate to the kind of knowledge about his illness that he can be expected to have.

Illness, generally speaking, is of great personal concern to a Zinacanteco. Our observations and general discussion suggest that when a person develops illness, he (and to a considerable extent his family) experiences great concern and uncertainty—in some instances feelings that resemble guilt or self-derogation. This constellation of unpleasant feelings may be relieved if the h'ilol, when summoned, diagnoses that the illness is benign (i.e. not due to witchcraft) and performs the appropriate ceremony. If the diagnosis is that the illness is not benign, anxiety and concern may be alleviated by the curing ceremony, but the feelings of guilt may not be alleviated and may even be reinforced. This is likely to be the case if the h'ilol diagnoses witchcraft as the cause of the illness, and more so if he implicates a family member as the witch. Even if an outsider is indicated as the witch, the successful completion of a curing ceremony may not relieve the patient and his family of the fear that the outsider will again use witchcraft against the family.

The conditions of impaired well-being usually regarded as illness, then, seem to be associated with anxiety, self-doubt, and uncertainty stemming from an inability to explain the condition. These psychological accompaniments of the illness state are apparently caused by the social and/or moral implications that illness has for a Zinacanteco, and not by the fact that his highly unified and interdependent social unit is seriously handicapped by an illness. Disabilities resulting from trauma or accidents (e.g., fractures or wounds) are not accompanied by the same feelings of apprehension and self-doubt, and often are not regarded as illness at all; yet they may be equally disruptive and economically damaging to the person and his family. Zinacantecos appear to draw a logical distinction between real illness and disabilities with easily explained "natural" causes. To the extent that illness, besides signifying moral factors, also involves a psychologically altered state, we can speak of Zinacantecos as espousing an integrated or unified view of illness. Chamel, in short, is a perceived failure or deviation in an individual's psychosocial adaptation that is partially manifested by bodily infirmities.

As we pointed out earlier, there are several types of practitioners in Zinacantan. Here, we focus primarily on health and illness concerns that involve conditions labeled as chamel by our informants and are treated by the most important type of medical practitioner, the h'ilol. Chamel is regarded as endemic in the world of man, having existed since the beginning of time; and the existence of disease is linked directly to the Zinacanteco belief that man is imperfect, corruptible, and prone to misbehave and do harm to others. More specifically, the symptoms of chamel can be said to fall into three classes.

1. Some symptoms are clearly recognizable as belonging to a single, named condition. The presence of the symptoms alone is enough to indicate the nature of the illness to any layman, without the necessity of a curer's diagnosis. One such symptom is *hak'ob 'ik'*, a minor skin ailment that is extremely itchy but is easily cured by various ointments.

2. Some symptoms are clearly recognizable as indices of a given illness, but in this case an illness whose exact nature, it is generally agreed by Zinacantecos, can only be unequivocally established by a h'ilol. For example, a fever and skin eruption are characteristic of the illness *sarampio*; but only a h'ilol can properly say that they constitute sarampio.

3. Some symptoms are too ambiguous to attribute to any named condition without a curer's diagnosis. Loss of appetite, chills, lassitude, or weakness, for example, can be characteristic of so many different illnesses that they ordinarily present no clue to their underlying cause.

These three categories operationally reduce to two: illness that must be cured by a h'ilol and illness that one can cure oneself. In general, illnesses too minor to require a h'ilol's attention are those whose identity is immediately recognizable from the symptoms. Illnesses that must be treated by a h'ilol are those whose symptoms cannot readily be associated by the layman with cause, name, and cure. It is within this second type of illness that Zinacantecos attach the qualities of strong (serious) and weak (minor or not serious, with recovery predictable). A Zinacanteco patient, however, does not start with a named identified illness about whose properties he inquires. Rather, he finds himself afflicted with one or more symptoms and must make a decision about them. In only a very few cases can one predict that a given symptom will be taken by almost any Zinacanteco to indicate a given condition whose treatment is appropriately handled by the patient himself. In theory, almost any symptom can be due to witchcraft or divine punishment, or to some underlying cause whose nature can only be divined by the h'ilol and whose cure depends on that knowledge.

The man who is chamel, then, must first decide whether he can treat his own illness or whether he must have its underlying cause divined by a h'ilol. Most of these decisions seem to be primarily idiosyncratic. Every Zinacanteco has a slightly different set of ideas defining the boundaries between the various classes of symptoms. One man with periodic fevers may diagnose his own illness and treat it with patent medicines; another will go to a h'ilol, who may tell him he is suffering from *shi'el* and prescribe a *lok'esel ta balamil* ceremony. The difference may be due to personality factors or to ideology. Some Zinacantecos are visibly more skeptical than others about the efficacy of traditional curing, and some are more suspicious of witchcraft and therefore seek a h'ilol's diagnosis of symptoms that another Zinacanteco might consider straightforward and minor. Knowledge of proper treatment is another factor. Some remedies are generally known to most or all Zinacantecos; others are known only to h'iloletik and to a few laymen who have observed the h'ilol's prescription for a particular condition.

As another alternative, there is the Ladino pharmacy. San Cristóbal abounds in drugstores, although few, to our knowledge, are under the supervision of a trained pharmacist. Most are well supplied with pharmaceuticals ranging from steroid preparations and antibiotics to a plethora of patent medicines. Most preparations in these stores appear to be sold without prescription, although our information on this account is fragmentary. To be accurate, then, we should include the drugstore clerk as one of the medical practitioners a Zinacanteco may consult in case of illness, especially if the ministrations of a h'ilol do not seem imperative to him. Some h'iloletik, indeed, have begun to add drugstore remedies to their repertoires, and their patients may be sent into San Cristóbal with a general or specific prescription for some purchasable remedy to supplement the curer's prayers and herbal potions.

Our continuing work in the Chiapas region has identified a good many lay healers who practice in San Cristóbal—not only Ladino curers, but Indian practitioners as well. Some moved to the city for "positive" reasons; that is, they saw economic and occupational advantages (either as a practitioner or otherwise) that could be enjoyed there. Others made the move to escape from persecution by dissatisfied customers and civil officials, and simply set up shop in San Cristóbal. The more disreputable of them (i.e. suspected witches) practice in the peripheral and ecologically marginal areas of the city. Much of their clientele consists of Mayas from the surrounding municipios, including Zinacantan.

During a visit to the city, then, a Zinacanteco may seek a diagnosis and cure from a lay healer; and he may stay overnight in the healer's house (for a "hospital" charge) in order to obtain repeated care. Even while pursuing the advice of a San Cristóbal pharmacist and using "prescribed" medicines, the sick person will be receiving shamanistic treatment from a "displaced" h'ilol, and perhaps from a renowned Ladino folk practitioner as well.

When a sick man believes his illness does not demand the treatment of a h'ilol or some other lay practitioner, he may also consult a Ladino physician, although this is a relatively infrequent occurrence. In Hteklum, the government maintains a small medical post with a resident Zinacanteco male nurse, who is supplied with a hypodermic needle and large quantities of penicillin as well as similar medicaments. Injections, no matter what their content, are generally considered by both Indians and Ladinos to be an effective therapeutic procedure; and the service of the INI nurse and his needle is often sought by a Zinacanteco patient as an additional measure to supplement some other curative procedure.

To recapitulate, when the diagnosis of a curer seems necessary, the preferred consultant is a native Zinacanteco h'ilol. Zinacantecos do, however, make use of many other curers—including Chamula shamans, both Indian and Ladino owners of talking saints, Ladino herbalists and spiritualists, and so on. But these are ordinarily patronized only after some attempt has been made to have the illness treated (or at least diagnosed) by native personnel. A more formal and analytic statement of the process and dynamics that surround the delivery of medical care in Zinacantan will be discussed in Chapter 9.

General Features of Zinacanteco Medical Knowledge

One finds no indications anywhere in Zinacanteco curing that h'iloletik or their patients think or act about illnesses on the basis of concepts that involve the body as a system composed of functionally interrelated parts and processes—with the possible exception of body temperature, to be discussed below. The greater part of shamanistic curing is entirely spiritual, and illness, though given the significance and interpretation mentioned earlier, is believed to arise from various supernatural events acting on one or both of the victim's two souls. The translation of supernatural causes into physical symptoms is taken for granted, without reference to intervening explanations that involve anatomical or physiological considerations.

There is an area of Zinacanteco curing where remedies are directed primarily at the relief of symptoms rather than at the propitiation of supernatural forces, and where concepts of cause of illness involve what we would call "natural" phenomena—e.g., overeating, contagion, and exposure to weather. Even here, however, the concepts we could term physiological are unimportant. Despite the existence of an extensive herbal pharmacoepia, the effects that Zinacantecos describe for various herbal remedies are directly linked to symptoms and do not touch on mechanisms that are "physiological." One hears statements like *"posh nibak* cures swelling," but almost never a statement like "herb X stimulates circulation of the blood." The knowledge of direct relationships between the administration of a remedy and the relief of a symptom, furthermore, is said to have its origin in supernatural revelation rather than empirical observation. Even a simple herbal treatment, then, is related back to the underlying spiritual nature of the medical system.

A limited exception to this general rule is the symptom of body temperature, especially "blood temperature" (Madsen, 1955). In common with most Middle American cultures, Zinacanteco medical belief stresses the opposition between "hot" and "cold" conditions of the blood, which are intimately related to the hot and cold properties of a variety of natural phenomena in the universe. Foods are variously hot, cold, or neutral, as are herbs and other remedies. The same is true of climatic conditions and physical experiences (e.g., a cold bath), and these often are linked to illness for this reason. Zinacantecos associate the underlying condition of the blood with body temperature, but it is the blood that is the important factor. Hot blood, for example, is said to cause high fevers, whereas chills are caused by cold blood.

The condition of the blood can be both a cause and an effect of illness. Conditions such as exposure to hot sun or cold winds are considered to affect the temperature of the blood and thereby to cause illness; or the cause of the illness may be supernatural, and the blood temperature merely a symptom or an intervening factor. In either case, however, certain remedies and ceremonial procedures are specific for the condition of the blood. Ingesting "hot" plants, for example, is prescribed as a treatment for cold blood, and vice versa.

These aspects of blood and body temperature are virtually the only place in Zinacanteco medicine where notions of cause and effect involving bodily events and processes are linked in a clear and specific manner to illness and to the actions of remedies. Elsewhere, they are to some extent implied, as in the belief that certain illnesses are contagious, or that others arise from the ingestion of "bad" substances. Informants do not speculate, however, on the actual connections involved. Contagion is reported, but there is no theory to account for it. Bad food somehow spoils inside the body and affects the "stomach" and surrounding areas, but the mechanism of these effects does not seem to be considered important. The appearance of anatomical terms in a Zinacanteco discussion of illness usually marks nothing more than location. *K'ush o'on*, for example, is a pain in the "heart" or chest; the location implies nothing about the physiological background of the condition.

Generally speaking, then, systematic ideas about the structure and function of the body are not important in Zinacanteco medical knowledge. What are important are concepts of causality, and other attributes whose nature, in an ultimate sense only comprehensible by a h'ilol, determines the form to be taken by the curative procedures. These concepts, which we will term dimensions of illness, are outlined in detail in Appendix 1. They are the basic conceptual materials with which both h'iloletik and patients operate in the system. A second major area of medical knowledge is that necessary for the performance of curing ceremonies. This is described in Chapters 10 and 11. In this chapter we are mainly concerned with the general features of medical knowledge, and with how this knowledge is used by Zinacantecos.

One of the salient features of medical or health-related behavior in Zinacantan is that despite the existence of a somewhat elaborate and systematic body of knowledge regarding illnesses, Zinacantecos generally show little confidence in applying this knowledge when they or their family members become ill. The h'ilol is usually consulted for evaluation and treatment, regardless of how similar a particular episode of illness might be to previous ones. One way of explaining this is by stressing what we touched on earlier, namely, the essentially affective component of illness. Illness has both life-threatening and, perhaps more importantly, moral implications; it implies, in other words, that the key relational transactions (i.e. to the gods and to his fellowmen) binding a person to a relatively predictable future are in disarray. Illness in this sense is a fearful and unpredictable event in an otherwise highly ordered life. Medical knowledge may be patterned and shared, but it does not offer much comfort to those caught in and threatened by illness. A spiritual consultation is required, and the hʻilol is needed to perform this. This reliance on the hʻilol can be explained by what appear to be two implicit principles of Zinacanteco medical ideology, which may be formally stated as follows:

First, with the exception of certain minor illness, the legitimate application of all diagnostic knowledge is in the hands of the hʻilol. The patient cannot properly say, even from previous experience with the symptoms, what his illness is and what therapy is needed. The true nature of an illness lies in an underlying cause, usually spiritual, that expresses itself in the blood. The blood "speaks" to the hʻilol, who knows how to pulse, and reveals the nature of the illness and the cure that is demanded. The layman cannot be certain of these; hence the services of a hʻilol are imperative in any major illness.

Second, diagnostic and therapeutic knowledge is revealed directly to each new hʻilol through contact with the Totilmeʻiletik. Although the general body of curing practices ordained by the Totilmeʻiletik is known to all hʻiloletik, new and unique aspects of knowledge may be granted to any given hʻilol; these individual revelations account for variations in practice between hʻiloletik.

Sociological Aspects of Illness

Like other nonliterate groups, the Zinacantecos do not have what we could term a medical care system that is a clearly delimitable and independently functioning unit within their culture. In other words, the beliefs, practices, personnel, and facilities available for dealing with occurrences of illness are not easily separated from those that serve other institutional functions in the society. Hʻiloletik, as we shall see, serve a variety of functions that we could term religious, social, and ethico-moral. Despite a rather broad definition of what constitutes illness, hʻiloletik are asked for advice on many problems that neither outside observers nor the Zinacantecos themselves would necessarily associate with illness. Conversely, problems that an observer would ascribe quite unambiguously to disease are not the exclusive concern of medical practitioners in Zinacantan, but are given political and social importance by civil authorities and village elders respectively.

Zinacantecos tend to adopt what might be described as a sociological interpretation of illness. This does not mean that illness is not a personalized event of significance to the individual, or that phenomenologic experiences do not punctuate and in fact guide and mediate the behavior of persons who are ill; as has been pointed out, this experiential dimension of illness is quite evident among Zinacantecos. What must be emphasized here is the extent to which an occurrence of illness provides the context for acting out a drama with important social implications and functions for the group.

In Zinacantan, illness is frequently regarded as a sign that the sufferer has sinned or otherwise misbehaved and has been duly punished by the gods. It may also indicate that a known or suspected enemy has actually plotted with demons and witches to inflict harm on the person who is ill. In the first case, the illness itself is interpreted by others (including the village elders) as evidence that the sick person has misbehaved. As a result, either because of external prodding or because of a purely inward motivation, he and his family will ordinarily make the necessary social, moral, and religious amends. In the second case, the occurrence of illness may serve one or both of two functions. It may allow one to justifiably direct his hostility in the form of witchcraft, violence, or personal insults, at the human agent believed to be responsible for the illness. Or, in some instances, it may actually constitute the necessary evidence that an act of malevolence has been perpetrated, in which case the victim merely has to report his illness to the civil authorities. If the social friction involving the "assailant" is clear and easily documented, or if an independent evaluation by a chosen h'ilol confirms the nature of the underlying illness, the suspected person will be reprimanded, physically punished, or placed in jail.

We see, then, that an instance of illness (defined generally as an episode of pain, weakness, impaired bodily function, and/or social inhibition and withdrawal) is the beginning of a process that involves both individuals and various operations of the social system. We could depict the illness graphically as a pattern that extends across space and time; an individual's impaired functioning constitutes one element of the pattern, but the significance of this element is clearly small if it is not examined in the context of the other elements and social processes that give the pattern design and meaning. To support this view of illness among the Zinacantecos, we collected observations and interview data about the causes and consequences of illness, participated with families in activities aimed at curing illness, and tried to determine how individual Zinacantecos viewed their bodies and their own personal identities. The last of these points requires further elaboration.

The Zinacantecos do not view their bodies as units composed of elements that can be differentiated in mechanism and function but harmoniously interact. The body, for Zinacantecos, may be depicted as a "black box"—undifferentiated, unarticulated, and unrefined. It contains a very general potential to be affected by evil (or good) and crudely signals when this evil (or abnormality) is assuming concrete form. People may swell, have pain, and experience many degrees of change in bodily functions; these "evils," however, do not represent the disordered workings of a machine that is capable of variable levels of functioning and interdependence. Inside and outside sources of bodily changes are not differentiated or are not clearly separated. Instead, visible changes in bodily appearance and function assume relevance when they are associated with the experience of chamel.

With regard to what an outside observer might term bodily functioning, then, illness is judged to be present when disordered function produces or is associated with an altered experiential state—that is, a state involving changes in awareness, consciousness, and strength that signify social happenings. When significant diminutions in these levels of feeling and felt competence occur (with or without more specific bodily symptoms), illness is diagnosed. This diagnosis or judgment begins the systematic unfolding of a socially significant episode. It is because a Zinacanteco sees illness as a direct or indirect extension of the workings of the social system and in time acts on the illness itself as if it were a social fact that one can term his view of illness "sociological." The body is not seen as a functional entity having any exclusive importance to the self, to one's personal identity; nor is it subject to much influence, modification, and control by the person himself.

To some extent, Zinacantecos also lack the concept of a self that is internally housed, autonomous, and separate from the selves of other "objects" (i.e. persons, things, deities, or animals). A man is seen as tied to his family, his land, and his activities; to a large extent he is as he behaves and acts. The ideas of self, personality, or mind as entities somehow separate from the concrete person and able to order, monitor, and control human actions are not as important. Each person's animal spirit (*cha-nul*) is capable of wandering, but it appears to be seen as a passive agent. It can be the object of injury and harm (which is reflected in the owner's body), but it is not a controlling agent under the owner's influence. Feelings, too, are not thought of as housed within the individual person; nor are they separate entities that affect choice, influence bodily concerns and human motivations, and exist as circumscribed reactions to interpersonal or impersonal occurrences. Instead, the prevailing view appears to be that pain, sadness, anger, happiness, envy, and the like are concomitants of life and are rooted in social occurrences; people experience these reactions in certain types of situations, and the situations in turn channel one's actions in particular directions. We might describe the Zinacanteco's view of self and person, like his view of the body, as equally "spread out" onto his family and group.

Clearly, illness and medical care in Zinacantan are bound up in the processes of social control; for what we have seen are beliefs and consequent actions about illness that establish persons and bodies as working participants of the social system. A real illness (whether of dysentery or pneumonia, for example) is an affliction that may affect one's body; but it is also a reflection of how the social system functions. Specifically, since an occurrence of illness often constitutes evidence on the basis of which sick persons, village elders, or civil authorities punish others, it allows for the implementation of social sanctions and rules. Illness, in short, often expresses personal wishes and actions, and serves to control the behaviors and actions of others within the bounds deemed appropriate by the culture. In a metaphorical sense, illness and bodily states may be seen as part of the social machinery that implements norms, just as the fear of punishment and other legal sanctions (symbolized in part by illness) serve to promote harmony and resolve conflicts. We could view the treatment of an illness as an occasion for removing pain and restoring of function to a person. However, given the Zinacanteco view of illness as well as the actual mediatory activities of the h'ilol during curing ceremonies, we are equally justified in terming this treatment an occasion for the execution of social, legal, and moral precepts. This aspect of the h'ilol's activities will be dealt with in Chapter 12.

Biomedical and Zinacanteco Views of Illness

Several different but related emphases in the scientific community deal conceptually with health and disease, and all are strongly influenced by the behavioral sciences. Engel stresses the need for a unified view of disease, and has lucidly described the arbitrariness and pernicious consequences of traditional definitions (Engel, 1960). In his view, health and disease, rather than representing discrete states or conditions, should be described as phases of the continuously changing, multilevel set of processes (e.g., cellular, chemical, and behavioral) that at any one moment constitute human striving. Feinstein, by contrast, prefers to conceptualize disease in purely morphological, physiological, and chemical terms (Feinstein, 1967). What the physician directly observes in his dialogue with the patient he terms the illness, which consists of subjective sensations (symptoms) and certain findings (signs). The illness results from the interaction of the disease with its host; and the physician should emphasize the mechanism by which the disease develops, and by which it "produces" or is associated with the illness. One implication of this conceptualization is that a physician treating a patient is engaged in two related transactions, one with the disease (controlling or eliminating it) and the other with the illness (alleviating its distress). Mechanic (1962) has introduced the concept of illness behavior to help explain the diverse ways in which people behave when they perceive sickness in themselves. He sees this behavior as influenced not only by the meanings and response tendencies that the sufferer has learned to associate with intraorganismic sensations, but also by the sociocul- turally determined interpretations that are placed on concepts such as health, disease, and medical care.

Substantively, these three viewpoints have a great deal in common. All are alike in that the cause of the disease or illness is seen as multi- factorial, with both genetic and environmental factors playing important roles. The empirically derived and experimentally tested knowledge acquired by the various scientific disciplines is used to generate mecha- nisms that explain the correlates of impaired well-being, and these mech- anisms are structured in terms of necessary and sufficient conditions.

The practice of the Zinacanteco curer also requires that he define and explain illness, but he does so in supernatural and moral terms. Illness, as the h'ilol sees it, is directly caused by an imbalance or lack of harmony in his patient's psychosocial and moral state; thus the patient's relation- ship to the ancestral gods and to his fellowmen is the critical consider- ation. In subsequent chapters we will see that medical treatment in Zinacantan in fact involves the restoring of balance to this relationship. The h'ilol explains the development of a patient's symptoms in terms of factors like wrongdoing, punishment, or envy.

Notions of cause, disease, and illness, which are logically separated in the scientific system, are fused and condensed in Zinacantan. A patient's symptoms and signs are both disease and illness, and they are both seen as the objectification of spiritual or malevolent agencies. This is a sufficient explanation for the h'ilol. If probed, he says the disease-illness traveled and entered in the way that smoke or wind spreads and diffuses in and around an object. He would agree with the notion that the body's functioning has been disturbed, but he does not explain this disturbance in biomedical terms; instead, he uses concepts analogous to force, damage, injury, and evil.

Zinacantecos seem to conceptualize health and illness as time-bound, sharply demarcated, and mutually exclusive conditions: one is either sick or not sick. This conception is isomorphic with the one that appears to be held about treatment. Zinacantecos seem always to be in search of the right curer or the right herb for an illness, assuming that illness simply enters into or descends on a person and must be removed. The notion of a chronic illness that can improve or is subject to remissions and exacerbations does not appear to exist. During a remission one is well and not sick, and subsequent symptoms are viewed as manifestations of a new illness, or of the same illness improperly cured. A good cure, in other words, is one that eliminates symptoms permanently and makes one well; a reappearance or recrudescence of symptoms that might be taken to reflect the same illness implies an ineffective treatment and consequently a weak h'ilol.

Chapter seven

The Structure of Medical Knowledge in Zinacantan

IN OUR INTRODUCTION we mentioned the need for precise information on how the members of nonliterate social units interpret and organize medical problems. To reiterate briefly, most work that focuses on medical beliefs is descriptive, general, and cast in the framework of descriptive ethnography or structural-functional analysis. The content of the beliefs is examined in relation to other cultural activities and institutions; and case studies or participant observation techniques are by and large the predominant method of approach. We know little of how the subjects themselves evaluate bodily symptoms, or how medical beliefs are distributed across subjects. In particular, whether practitioners in different cultures, when compared to laymen, have a different, more specialized, or more highly structured basis for their approach to medical problems is largely unknown.

Researchers have dealt with medical problems as if they invariably represent natural and ecological "givens"—facts and imperatives that the subjects must cope with in some way, however exotic the approach adopted. Few have tried to depict the medical domain in a differentiated manner that at the same time preserves the specificity of native conceptual categories. In this chapter we will address ourselves to this need for close and culturally relevant analyses of medical problems by first examining the semantic content of the medical terms used in Zinacantan.

Interpretations Placed on Symptoms (Study A)

Two bilingual Zinacantecos served as the principal informants in this study. They in turn enlisted 30 male h'iloletik and 30 laymen as subjects. Several representative hamlets were chosen, and within each hamlet an attempt was made to select all the males who were practicing h'iloletik. Laymen were recruited in the same places, except that proportionately fewer of the eligible males were selected from each hamlet. Only adult laymen who resided in separate households were chosen, in order to avoid sampling persons with very similar medical experiences.

Each subject was asked verbally, in Tzotzil, a series of questions dealing with medical issues. The questions included 18 Tzotzil terms, each defining an illness condition in Zinacantan; these were selected from the list of 76 illness terms described in Appendix B. Following the formulation of Rubel (1964) these 18 terms can be regarded as designating specific folk illnesses, and they include as part of their meaning references to causation, severity, treatment requirements, etc. Our questions also included 24 items referring to behavioral events and to disturbances in bodily processes and functions. These items were chosen after pretest interviews with informants had indicated that they represented meaningful units of Zinacanteco discourse regarding behavior and bodily concerns; from the perspective adopted here, they can be regarded as potential symptoms and signs. For each of the 18 illness terms, each subject was asked separately whether each of the 24 potential illness manifestations was seen in or constituted an element of that illness.*

The information used in this study can be represented in matrix form (see Table 8). We have roughly translated the various bodily and behavioral symptoms; and the letters heading the columns refer to Tzotzil illness terms with no precise equivalent.† We selected terms that were diversified, referring to many different bodily abnormalities as well as to notions of morality and social processes. These terms, we believe, offer a reasonable cross section of Zinacanteco folk illnesses. The first part of our study compares the responses of the h'iloletik with those of the laymen by applying the chi-square test to find differences in the proportion

---

* Two additional variables were used, one asking whether the illness had a predilection for men, the other asking the same for women. These two items were so rarely said to be characteristic of any of the 18 illnesses that we dropped them from the ensuing analyses. The importance of these findings, however, should be acknowledged: for all intents and purposes, no folk illness in Zinacantan is said to be associated with a particular sex.

† The illness terms are detailed in Appendix B. Our letter references designate the following terms: A, *k'elel*; B, *ta skuenta*; C, *sarampio*; D, *tashk'a srinyon*; E, *sim nak'al*; F, *tup'em sat*; G, *komel ta balamil*; H, *taki chamel*; I, *chuvah*; J, *sak obal*; K, *sik k'ok'*; L, *pumel*; M, *mahbenal*; N, *me vinik*; O, *ip hsekubtik*; P, *k'ush holol*; Q, *makel*; R, *hik'ik'ul obal*.

TABLE 8

Matrix Showing Association of Symptoms with Folk Illness Terms

Bodily disturbances (symptoms)	A	B	C	D	E	F	G	H	I	J	K	L	M	N	O	P	Q	R
1. Sleepiness							‡											
2. Excessive urination		‡	‡															
3. Poor hearing									‡									
4. Stomach (abdominal) distension																		
5. Lack of appetite		*									*		*		*		‡	*
6. Chills		*	*	*	*			*			*		*		*	*	*	*
7. Pain while defecating	*	*	*	*	*			*										
8. Headache	*	*	*	*	*			*	*	*	*	*	*	*	*	*	*	*
9. Leg pain		*	*	*				*			*		*					
10. Throat pain	*		*	*	*	*		*	*	*	*	*	*	*	*	*	*	*
11. Crying, sadness	*	*	*	*	*	*		*	*	*	*	*	*	*	*	*	*	*
12. Weakness	*	*	*	*	*			*	*	*	*	*	*	*	*	*	*	*
13. Blood in stool					*													
14. Blood in urine				‡														
15. Pruritus (with/without skin eruption)									*									
16. Chest pain	*	*		*	*			*		*	*	*		*	*	*		*
17. Quarrelsomeness, excessive hostility									*									
18. Poor vision						*												
19. Vomiting	*	*	*	*				*		*	*	*	*	*	*		*	*
20. Coughing	*	*	*	*				*		*	*	*	*	*	*	*	*	*
21. Fever	*						*								‡			
22. Pain while urinating					*			*				*			*			
23. Stomach (abdominal) pain	*	*		*				*			*			*	*		*	
24. Arm pain	*	*		*														

NOTE: In cells marked * 80% or more of the respondents linked disturbance with illness term. In those marked ‡ we give the illness term to which respondents most frequently linked disturbance where no strong consensus was noted (i.e., no term was linked to disturbance by at least 80% of respondents).

of each group that associated a particular sign or symptom with a particular illness. In the second part of the study the responses of both groups are combined, and we analyze the manner in which the subjects generally associate illnesses and their manifestations. In particular, whenever 80% or more of the 60 subjects link a particular disturbance with a folk illness, we assume that the linkage is a typical or meaningful one in Zinacantan. The reader should keep this in mind whenever we refer to the particular components of Zinacanteco illnesses during our discussion.

Results

H'ilol/lay differences. The proportion of those in each group associating each of the various symptoms and signs with the various illnesses was compared by the chi-square test (18 × 24, or 432 comparisons). In only one instance was the value obtained statistically significant—a result that could certainly develop from chance fluctuations. We concluded that there was no evidence differentiating the groups' associations of discrete symptoms with discrete illnesses.

We next attempted to determine whether the subjects of either group had a greater tendency to agree about the various symptom-illness linkages. First, focusing on each individual symptom, we noted whether one group more frequently had a larger proportion of its members linking that disturbance with any of the illnesses. We repeated this procedure using the illness terms as units of analysis; that is, we determined whether one of the groups consistently tended to have a larger proportion of its members linking various disturbances with each illness term separately. No consistent patterns emerge from either analysis. We conclude, then, that there are no consistent differences in the way h'iloletik and laymen associate symptoms with folk illnesses.

The general Zinacanteco view of illness. The responses of both groups were combined for this part of the study. Each entry in Table 8 is either blank or contains one of two symbols: one symbol denotes the level we have defined as a "typical" linkage of symptom with illness term (i.e., an 80% or greater consensus among respondents), and the other denotes the term to which a given disturbance was most frequently associated when no typical linkage occurred.

By concentrating on the horizontal rows of the matrix, we can evaluate how broadly a potential illness manifestation is construed. For example, symptoms 8, 11, 12, 19, and 20 are all typically linked with most of the 18 folk illness terms. These manifestations, then, can be regarded as relatively undifferentiated units of illness. If we assume that our selected terms are actually representative of illness conditions in Zinacantan, this cluster of symptoms can be said to bear a strong association to the general Zinacanteco conception or model of illness. The actual content of two symptoms, weakness and headache, in fact refers to what scientific medicine would regard as a general and/or systemic manifestation of disease; two others, vomiting and coughing, are specific and highly visible manifestations of gastrointestinal and respiratory disease, respectively. The very broad associations of symptom 11, sadness and crying, reflect the well-known fact that in Zinacantan there is a strong affective or emotional dimension to any condition of impaired health.

Symptoms 5, 6, 9, 10, 21, 23, and 24 are also quite general, though not so much as the five already mentioned. Given the relatively high association of these symptoms with Zinacanteco illness, they also appear to be constituent parts of the general model of illness. Four symptoms refer to pain localized in different parts of the body. It would appear that pain, even though it certainly may be explicitly referred to a segment of the body, signifies a relatively general and undifferentiated construct. Many "illnesses" can include pain, but there does not appear to be a unique medical significance to explicitly localized pain. (Two exceptions should be noted. First, "pain while defecating" is linked exclusively with illness *E, sim nak'al.* The description of this illness (see Appendix B) suggests that it may sometimes refer to biological changes a physician could term dysentery. Second, the symptom "pain while urinating" was not characteristic of any one illness, although it was principally linked to illness *O, ip hsekubtik.*)

We conclude, then, that various bodily pains unassociated with any discrete physiological functions are common ingredients of many folk illnesses. This may reflect the common clinical observation that generalized aches and pains are components of many diseases (usually infectious). Abdominal pains and cramps seem to be commonly linked with illness conditions in Zinacantan; but highly localized pains tied to excretory functions are rarely associated with the folk illnesses. We cannot, of course, exclude the possibility that illnesses not included in our questionnaire might relate to these "physiological" pains. But if our findings are valid, we can say that Zinacantecos do not identify pains and discomforts tied to particular physiological functions as key elements of illness. Our data suggest that highly specific pains such as these are not commonly among the complaints of the patient who seeks a h'ilol, and it is possible that the actual prevalence of the complaints in Zinacantan is low. At any rate, excretory pains do not appear to "demand" special illness terms. We are here implying that one must view the illness terms as labels used by Zinacantecos to identify important and recurring elements in their lives; and it may be that some physiologically based symptoms are not important enough for such formal marking.

Symptoms 6 and 21 (chills and fever), in the Western biomedical framework, are regarded as typical accompaniments of infectious and/or inflammatory processes; and their application by our subjects suggests that infectious processes may frequently accompany the conditions labeled by many Zinacanteco illness terms. Symptom 5, loss of appetite, is also a frequent correlate of infectious processes, and in addition can be regarded as a general and relatively nonspecific symptom of illness.

For the remaining symptoms, the subjects only infrequently demonstrated a consensus on possible associations with illnesses. That is, these particular symptoms and signs are not regarded as general accompaniments of illness in Zinacantan. Some signs (7, 13, 15, 17, and 18) have very distinct associations with particular illnesses. Others (4, 14, and 22) have no generally acknowledged link with any illness, and it may be that they are infrequently encountered or reported in Zinacantan (abdominal distention is especially perplexing in this regard). We cannot exclude the possibility that some symptoms are simply not recognized as accompaniments of illness as such; or that they are, though verbalizable and hence to some extent meaningful, rarely encountered as culturally organized units (sensations, events, or perceptions).

Symptoms 11 and 17, the two symptoms of a symbolic nature (i.e. involving social behavior), bore very different relationships to the illness terms. One, sadness, was associated with virtually all illnesses, which reflects the essentially psychosocial view of illness prevalent in Zinacantan. Illness is a threatening, frightening, and emotionally troublesome state that indicates a serious social disarticulation of the sufferer, and it seems to produce worry and despondency. The other "social" symptom, aggressiveness, was associated only with term *I, chuvah.* This illness actually signified changes that a Western physician could describe as an intellectually disorganizing acute psychosis (see Fabrega, Metzger, and Williams, 1970). We note, then, that in Zinacantan changes in the intensity of a person's aggressiveness or a propensity toward irritability and quarrelsomeness are not features of the general model of illness, but instead are singled out for special attention (i.e. are diagnosed as chuvah). Despondency, sadness, and crying, however, are typical accompaniments of the model "illness role."

The information so far presented can be summarized by using the illness columns as units of comparison. From this perspective, it is obvious that subjects tend to link a relatively large and fixed proportion of the symptoms with most of the illnesses. Sixteen of the illness terms are linked with 7 to 13 symptoms each. Terms F and I ("spot in the eye from staring at the moon" and "madness") are the exceptions.

The symptom "poor hearing" was most prominently linked with chuvah, or madness—no doubt reflecting the fact that a man suffering from chuvah is not amenable to ordinary forms of social control and does not hear or "respond" to others. However, even though chuvah is most strongly marked in the minds of Zinacantecos by striking behavioral changes of a social sort (and we have recorded several case histories pointing this out), headaches and weakness are also said to be key components of the illness; and we observed several other "physiological" symptoms strongly associated with chuvah, notably coughing, lack of appetite, and chest pain. This clustering of physiological or bodily complaints in what an observer might regard as an essentially "psychiatric" disorder may reflect the holistic way in which illness is viewed (and perhaps expressed) in settings like Zinacantan.

The Western dualistic system of medical perception seems to tell us that psychiatric or behavioral disorders, in general, should not be associated with bodily symptoms (pain is a clear exception to this generalization; see Merskey and Spear, 1967). But in Zinacantan, where this dualism is not observed, there is no such dichotomization of symptoms. Our data from Zinacantan (especially those bearing on chuvah) suggest that what we term a psychiatric disease in some fundamental sense may actually represent a failure in a person's *total adaptation* (defined as his response to a situation of stress, which he shows in an *integrated* manner). In this sense, our data support the convictions of medical theoreticians who hold an essentially psychosomatic orientation, that is, a unified view of disease. (Engel, 1960; Lipowski, 1969.)

All terms except the pairs C-M and L-N are associated with a distinct number and/or clustering of symptoms. Because of this, one could say that in Zinacantan a very large proportion of folk illnesses have a unique or distinct "manifestational" profile—although the bulk of these manifestations, to be sure, are shared by many illnesses. Conversely, one could claim that the pair of illnesses *C-M* share the same manifestational profile even though the illnesses in Zinacantan mean quite different sorts of things (see Study *B*, following, and Appendix B). This pattern is also observed in the illness pair *L-N*; that is, the terms have identical manifestations but quite distinct meanings in the culture.

The illness *sim nak'al* illustrates a point not unrelated to that described for chuvah, although we suspect that it reflects somewhat on our assumptions and perhaps on a limitation of our methods. Sim nak'al is uniquely associated with two symptoms that are not strongly linked with any of the other illnesses: pain during defecation and blood in stool. Despite its lack of association with vomiting, this illness term apparently labels changes one could describe as gastrointestinal. However, the subjects also associated "coughing" with this illness, a symptom that biomedically signifies respiratory difficulties. In theory, this could mean that illness in Zinacantan does respresent a physiologically more interconnected state. Our Western scheme tells us that the "combination" of system-disturbances is unusual, reflecting "hysterical" problems or a generally deteriorated physiological state. In the present case, the pattern may simply mean that a very general view of illness prevails in Zinacantan, and that the meanings of more specific folk illnesses are grafted on to the general picture. On the other hand, it could be that folk taxonomies (in this case the medical one) are not composed of airtight categories, that their terms have overlapping meanings or extensions, and that they are used differently by different members of the culture (see Frake, 1961).

That the pattern may result from our arbitrary use of 80% concurrence to designate "critical" symptoms is no doubt true, but problems can be expected to arise with any percentage one would choose in defining critical components of a taxon. The important point, it seems to us, is that studies of this nature bring out interesting and important questions that will require a sharper method of analysis in future ethnomedical studies. We must find ways to distinguish between logical categories, empirical categories, and "true" components of events that occur in nature, and must know how all of these matters are interrelated in given situations.

Summarizing, then, if we assume that our terms are representative of all illness terms in Zinacantan, a folk model of illness symptoms emerges: generalized pain; evidence of debility, toxicity, and infection; depressed emotional tone; and certain highly salient or visible manifestations of system dysfunction. This model or empirically derived profile of manifestations would appear to correspond to the Zinacanteco perception of chamel.

Further Implications of Study A

It must be emphasized that we did not directly question subjects about the *actual* physical or bodily correlates (i.e., symptoms and signs) of specific folk illnesses. To investigate this question, one must, for each illness, limit the sample to persons who have actually been diagnosed as having that illness; and each sampling should be undertaken with explicit instructions that the subject use the particular illness episode as his unit of observation or reference. The procedure used in the current study inquires instead about the subject's *general* knowledge of symptoms and illnesses. The responses we obtained, therefore, were probably a composite result of direct experiences with some illnesses, indirect experiences through exposure to friends and relatives who had been ill, and general Zinacanteco knowledge about illness that subjects had learned during the process of enculturation. Rather than determining the actual bodily correlates of folk illnesses, strictly speaking our study should be viewed as investigating the modeled or proposed relationship that Zinacantecos establish between specific bodily disturbances and natively construed states of illness. The information reviewed, however, does raise questions about illness occurrences, since we must assume that the "knowledge" a subject has or acquires reflects real-life experience with happenings in nature.

The close resemblance between the responses of h'iloletik and laymen in our sample is, in our estimation, an important finding, and one supporting our impression that knowledge about the features of illness (i.e. illness manifestations) in Zinacantan is widely shared among the male members of the culture. There seems to be no conceptual discontinuity across the groups, and the group-proportion differences that do occur are explainable as chance fluctuations. We would suggest, then, that h'iloletik in Zinacantan do not deal with medical phenomena by using specialized knowledge about illnesses and their manifestations.

When the responses of the two groups were combined it was noted that Zinacantecos generally linked a relatively large and fixed number of symptoms with almost all the diverse illnesses we used as examples. These symptoms, then, appear to make up the Zinacanteco model of illness, at least with regard to sensory-motor and behavioral concerns. It should be emphasized that the critical features of the complete illness model may well refer to moral or social identities, as others have suggested and as we ourselves mentioned in Chapter 6. However, these identities seem nevertheless to be associated or correlated with a fairly general but distinct model of bodily and behavioral elements.

Our results could be interpreted from an ethnocentric standpoint: namely, from one that emphasizes the semantic profile of folk illness terms viewed against the "universality" of the Western biomedical scheme. From this standpoint, one would conclude from our results that folk illnesses in Zinacantan, although they are labeled by separate terms and also appear to have diverse semantic dimensions (e.g., notions of cause and severity), share much meaning in that a large proportion of them are viewed as exhibiting the same distinct cluster of bodily manifestations. Most of these manifestations, it is true, are general and nonspecific when analyzed from a scientific perspective. But since two manifestations broadly linked to illness terms by the subjects (i.e., vomiting and coughing) reflect disturbances or malfunctioning in very different and separate bodily systems, one might assume that Zinacanteco illness terms and labels are relatively loosely tied to specific bodily events. (What was mentioned earlier should not be forgotten, however; and that is that this general or holistic model of illness has altogether different implications involving contemporary orientations in biomedicine.) At the same time it should be remembered that a few malfunctions have a very definite association with specific illnesses. As we have already seen, only two pairs of terms (*C-M* and *L-N*) have identical symptom profiles; thus one could argue that there is some specificity of meaning at the level of bodily symptoms. Further considerations of importance bearing on this point were discussed earlier.

So far, we have implied at least three aspects to the notion of specificity in a folk illness. First, an illness in Zinacantan can in fact be specific with regard to sensory-motor or bodily events; that is, a specific subset of symptoms and signs of their behavioral correlates may justify the application of the illness term. Second, a folk illness can be specific at an explanatory or interpretive level. A sociocultural group's key components of illness may not relate at all to physiological symptoms, but may instead rely on folk notions of cause, morality, imputed severity, and therapeutic demands. In earlier chapters, we have included these factors as illness dimensions. The consistent application of a set of values for illness dimensions, regardless of what the patient experiences or manifests, may be what is specific about a particular folk illness. Finally, a folk illness may be specific in both of the first two senses. That is, its specific meaning may result both from its invariant association with certain bodily disturbances and from the culture's interpretive or explanatory mechanisms.

In general, a conservative interpretation of the results of Study A suggests that when one emphasizes bodily and behavioral symptoms and uses a high level of consensus to determine cognitive associations, folk illness terms seem relatively nonspecific. However, a closer inspection of our raw data showed that a few subjects tended to interpret the illness terms in various ways; that is, a small proportion of Zinacantecos associated the terms with symptom profiles that were not recognized by their fellows. We contend that the concept of a folk illness is useful whenever its meaning in a cultural group is specific in any way—that is, when it denotes something that members of the culture will agree on. Tentatively, our study supports the notion that members of a cultural group will reliably label events of ill health at the symptomatic level, provided one's viewpoint is a configurational one (i.e., provided that it emphasizes the pattern of symptoms associated with illness terms). It must be clearly understood that to a subset of subjects illness terms will have contrasting and shifting referents.

Our study, then, suggests that at least some native illness terms current in a culture are specific with respect to symptoms. But we would admit that the various symptoms relevant to a folk illness are not mutually exclusive (i.e., those applying the term probably do not evaluate each symptom separately); and also that the symptoms are probably not evaluated solely in terms of their presence or absence but rather in terms of their intensity. In short, the symptoms of an illness must be intricately and exhaustively mapped out, not only in relation to the symptoms themselves but also in relation to other domains and premises, in order to specify their relevance in any particular illness.

Our efforts, then, must be taken as no more than an exploratory attempt to evaluate the effect of culture on illness manifestations. Clearly, we are also limited by our reliance on salient, visible, and to some extent posited categories of symptoms. We began with a large group of known symptoms and searched for a subset of these our subjects could regard as important and that we could translate into equivalent units of meaning (i.e., that we could refer to clearly specified bodily and behavioral disturbances). We cannot exclude the possibility that we may have overlooked key Tzotzil terms referring to culturally specific behavioral events and patterns of bodily perceptions; and these omissions may well be the very things that determine the application of folk illness terms.

The Organization of Medical Knowledge (Study B)

In our second study, we tried to evaluate the pattern inherent in Zinacanteco beliefs about illness. Necessarily, we did this by comparing the beliefs with categories (i.e. specific physiological systems) articulated on the basis of the Western biomedical system.

The goal of a purely intracultural analysis of medical knowledge is to portray the relationship between the various elements and conceptual dimensions of a given folk system, and, by extension, to describe how members of the culture in question think and act regarding medical concerns (Metzger and Williams, 1966; Goodenough, 1957; Pike, 1954). A different understanding of the native medical system obtains when the conceptual dimensions of the system are analyzed and compared with information that is contextually similar but is organized on a different basis. In the present study, Western biomedically organized knowledge is also used as the "external" information. More specifically, we apply biomedical knowledge about the particular symptoms, signs, and syndromes that are labeled and recognized in Zinacantan in order to highlight the important features of the native conceptions.

The reason for using Western scientific medical knowledge in this analysis is twofold. First, it reflects a conceptual system differing in content but having the same general purposes and functions as the folk system. Second, Western medicine, because it has succeeded in controlling some diseases, can contribute specialized meaning to any particular segment of folk knowledge with which it can be conceptually linked. Analyzing a native body of knowledge by means of this independent informational grid should help to clarify the functions and dynamics of the folk system in its own culture.

Our underlying assumption is that all taxonomic systems can be said to "exist" for specific purposes and functions. A domain in question may *appear* to be classified and defined mainly in terms of salient physical criteria (i.e., color, shape, consistency). Careful studies of native taxonomic systems, however, have indicated that culturally determined rules or conventions are the real basis for delimiting conceptual categories (Lounsbury, 1956; Conklin, 1954, 1955). Intensive and extensive knowledge of the sociocultural unit involved should thus disclose the underlying reasons for category boundaries. Some social domains clearly reflect the cultural determinants of classification and conceptual organization; and medical knowledge is one of these, even though it appears to be structured according to causal, functional, or utilitarian considerations (Fabrega, Metzger, and Williams, 1970; Frake, 1961; Feinstein, 1967). What makes the classification of medical knowledge particularly complex is that the content of this knowledge refers to behavior, which is fluid and often involves verbalizations about subtle personal sensations, as well as to natively structured moral and existential premises. The units of the medical knowledge system are often vague, sometimes complex, and rarely mutually exclusive; and they can usually be grouped in overlapping hierarchical sets.

In Study *B*, as in the previous study, bilingual Zinacantecos were our principal informants. They enlisted the cooperation of 33 male h'iloletik and 36 laymen as subjects. As before, several representative hamlets were used, and analogous sampling procedures were followed.

Each subject was asked 10 questions about each of the 76 illness terms that are described in Appendix B. These questions and the response options presented the subjects (both dealing with the relevant Zinacanteco dimensions of illness reviewed in Appendix A) were as follows:

A. Is ———— an instance of *chamel?*
    0. No
    1. Yes

B. Which of the following most closely corresponds to the cause or explanation of the illness?
    1–5. [Five references to the involvement of deities—e.g., illness sent by ancestral gods]
    6–14. [Nine references to the involvement of witchcraft and demons]
    15–22. [Eight references to naturalistic events—e.g., illness caused by bad food, chill, or drinking]

C. Is the illness a major or a minor one?
    1. Major
    2. Minor
    3. In between

D. Is there a remedy for this illness?
    1. Yes
    2. No
    3. A curing ceremony is the only remedy

E. How is the illness cured?
    1. A h'ilol must be asked
    2. The illness will cure itself
    3. A Ladino doctor must be asked
    4. A h'ilol must be asked, depending on the course of the illness
    5. Both a h'ilol and a doctor are necessary
    6. No cure

F. Is the sufferer's blood hot or cold in this illness?
    1. Hot
    2. Cold
    3–5. [Intermediate states]

G. Does the h'ilol use candles to cure this illness?
    0. H'ilol not involved
    1. Yes
    2. No

H. How many sacred mountains must be visited during the cure?
    0. None, or no ceremony needed
    1–9. Number of mountains

I. Do only adults or only children get this illness?
    1. Adults only
    2. Children only
    3. Both

J. Do only males or only females get this illness?
    1. Males only
    2. Females only
    3. Both

As in Study *A*, the subjects' responses can be depicted in rectangular matrices showing the responses of (1) h'iloletik, (2) laymen, and (3) the two groups combined; each matrix has 76 rows representing the illness terms and 10 columns representing the medically relevant questions that were asked. An abbreviated sample of the third matrix appears in Table 9.

Two types of measures were used to summarize the responses of the members of each group to the various questions. First, the modal re-

TABLE 9
Example of Analytic Matrix Employed

	Medically relevant questions									
Illness terms	A	B	C	D	E	F	G	H	I	J
	MODAL RESPONSES									
1. Simal 'obal (grippe-like syndrome)	1	1	2	1	2	1	2	0	3	3
2. Sik k'ok' (fever and chills)	1	1	1	1	1	1	1	4	3	3
3. Espanto (soul loss from fright)	1	6	1	3	1	2	1	0	3	3
· · ·										
	DISPERSION									
66. Vahbal (itchy rash)	0.92	2.69	0.45	0.41	1.13	1.76	1.30	0.51	0.78	0.11
67. Ti'ol (weakness, lassitude)	0.27	2.30	0.87	1.19	0.65	1.78	0.72	2.15	0.60	0.20
68. Ch'ich' k'abnel (blood in urine)	0.00	2.83	0.84	0.38	1.39	1.13	1.19	1.42	0.80	0.29
· · ·										
76. 'Uma' (muteness)	0.98	1.38	0.99	0.70	1.38	1.94	1.35	0.93	1.01	0.00

NOTE: This table shows the basic structure of the matrices for the different analyses involved in Study B. Two matrices were examined for each of three groups: h'iloletik, laymen, and the two combined. The first matrix of each pair contained the group's modal response to a particular question, and the second used the group's dispersion across response options (information variable *H*, as in terms 66, 67, 68, and 76).

sponse of each group was used as a measure of central tendency: that is, each group was collapsed and its modal response was taken as the response of a typical group member. Thus the element h_{ij} of matrix *H* represents how the h'iloletik responded (i.e. their modal response) to the *j*th question when it was asked of the *i*th illness term. Second, a nonmetric measure of dispersion or variability was used. This information variable, *H*, indicates the amount of uncertainty or information, expressed in bits, that inheres in a set of responses (Attneave, 1959; Garner, 1962); it is calculated by the formula

$$H = - \sum_{i=1}^{n} p_i \log p_i$$

A group's distribution of responses to each question that was asked about each illness term was expressed in percentages, and these percentages were used as the set of probability values for computing the H measure. For each question that was asked about each illness term an H measure was computed. This yielded, for example, a matrix N where an element l_{ij} represented the laymen's uncertainty or dispersion associated with the jth question when it was asked of the ith illness term. An elevated value of H indicates that the responses to a particular question contained a great deal of information, which is another way of saying that the members of the group responded heterogeneously to that particular question. A low H reflects low uncertainty, which indicates that the group had high agreement on or sharing of that particular item of information.

Analysis of illness terms across ten questions. The first analysis involves comparing the modes of the two groups—that is, the typical h'ilol and layman—across the 10 questions on each of the 76 illness terms. Diagrammatically, this is done by examining the horizontal rows of each group's respective matrix. The modal responses of the two groups to all 10 questions were the same on 29 of the 76 illness terms. For 22 additional terms, the modal responses differed on only one question. Thus the two groups showed substantial agreement on two-thirds of the illness terms when this agreement was assessed by modal response. For the remaining 25 terms, the groups differed on two questions 21 times and on three questions three times; on only one illness term did the groups differ on four questions.

We next compared the relative value of the H variable of the two groups across the 10 questions for each illness term; that is, we determined on how many illness terms the responses of the h'iloletik, compared to those of the laymen, consistently showed more or less dispersion or scatter across the questions. On no one illness term did the H measure of the groups tend to differ consistently; and on only six terms was there any semblance of a pattern in terms of this type of analysis. Since we were running 76 comparisons, we know that this many occurrences can be expected simply on the basis of chance. In other words, we were not able to uncover any striking differences in group dispersion across illness dimensions. H'iloletik and laymen, it appears, do not tend to differ from each other with regard to variability when we focus on all the items of information that bear on any one illness term.

Analysis of questions across 76 illness terms. Here we compared the same responses of the groups, but this time across the 76 illness terms on each of the 10 questions separately. First, we examined the modes of the 2 groups vertically down each of the 10 columns. The aim of this analysis was to determine on which question the groups showed the greatest disagreement or agreement across the 76 terms. Both groups answered question A in the same way for 74 of the 76 terms, indicating virtually complete agreement that these terms represented states of illness. The agreement on D and I was also marked, 72 out of 76; and on question J there were no differences at all. A moderate degree of intergroup disagreement was found for questions C (12% disagreement), F (14%), E (16%), G (9%), and H (11%). The greatest disagreement was associated with question B, which dealt with diagnosis or cause: the groups had a different modal response on roughly one-fourth of the illness terms.

The group of h'iloletik was then compared with the lay group in terms of the degree of dispersion associated with a particular question across the 76 terms. We asked whether, on a particular question, the H values of the two groups differed randomly across the 76 illness terms, or whether one group was consistently associated with lower (or higher) H measures on this question.

Question A was associated with low values of H: on more than one-half of the terms (41), all members of each group responded that the condition in question indicated an illness state. On 35 terms the H values of the groups differed, and on 23 of these the h'iloletik were associated with the lower value. Although we did not obtain a significant value when we applied the chi-square test, we can conclude that on this question there was a moderately strong tendency for the h'iloletik to show higher intragroup agreement than did the laymen. On the two questions asking about medical personnel (E) and existence of a remedy (D) the h'iloletik also showed a strong association with lower H values across all the illness terms. They agreed more often on who (i.e. a h'ilol) should be sought for treatment ($X^2 = 3.9$, $p < .05$), and on whether a remedy (i.e. yes) existed for the illness ($X^2 = 9.86$, $p < .005$). On questions B and H, the h'iloletik tended to be associated consistently with higher H values, indicating that they tended to disagree among themselves more than did the laymen about the cause of an illness and the necessity of visiting any sacred mountains during the curing process ($X^2 = 4.76$, $p < .05$ for question B; $X^2 = 34.22$, $p < .001$ for question H). On the five remaining questions, each group's H value seemed to fluctuate randomly; and on none of these questions was either group consistently associated with higher or lower H measures across the 76 illness terms.

We chose to examine more closely the notion of causation as conceptualized by these Zinacanteco males. Three broad categories of causes (deities, witchcraft, and naturalistic) were formed. When we applied the chi-square test to determine if the distribution of group modes in these three categories differed, we obtained a value that was not significant. We concluded that if one focuses on the modal response and classifies the various causes of illness broadly, no significant group differences emerge. We next looked at the *proportion* of the members of each group who chose one of the three response categories on each of the 76 terms. Here the groups did differ: on a significantly larger number of terms, the h'iloletik tended to have a larger proportion of its members choosing the response category of Deities ($X^2 = 10.78$, $p < .005$) and a smaller proportion choosing the Naturalistic category ($X^2 = 11.29$, $p < .001$). There were no significant differences in the proportion of each group choosing the witchcraft option.

Subject consistency. In order to conduct this analysis, each subject's 76 responses to each of the 10 questions were collapsed. A subject's responses to a given question were then expressed as a frequency distribution indicating the proportion of his responses in each of the various response options to this question. Using these distributions, we computed an H measure on each question for each subject and then ordered these, combining the subjects of both groups. This yielded 10 ordered listings of H measures: subjects at the bottom of the distribution had small H values, reflecting greater consistency (or less response variability) across the 76 terms; those at the top showed the highest variability in choosing responses to the terms.

To this array of ordered H measures, we applied the median test to determine whether the groups differed in the consistency of each member's responses to the 10 questions. In only one case did the test yield a value that was significant (question E, where a greater proportion of the h'iloletik had lower H measures: $X^2 = 5.27$, $p < .025$). Again, this finding could be the result of chance fluctuations, since a long series of tests was involved. On inspecting the raw data, however, we noted a tendency for h'iloletik to be overrepresented below the median *H* value and underrepresented above; this occurred on 9 of the 10 questions. Our tentative conclusion on the basis of these observations is that there is no strong evidence differentiating individual h'iloletik from individual laymen in terms of the consistency or diversity of their responses to each question across the 76 illness terms. However, we feel that the definite tendency of h'iloletik, as individuals, to be more consistent in their responses should be more closely examined in subsequent studies of this nature.

Western medical-scientific correlates of Zinacanteco beliefs. To the extent that we move away from the inherent structure and organization that obtains in native knowledge and attempt to link it with a language that is governed by scientific medical criteria, our analysis becomes more difficult. We approached the problem by first determining the bodily or physical referents of native terms, then classifying these referents on the basis of Western scientific criteria, and finally attempting to link this classification scheme with the Zinacanteco one. Whatever linkage is possible, of course, is likely to take place at relatively general levels or on a restrictive basis, since both the intensive and extensive organizational characteristics of the two systems differ.

This point requires elaboration. Earlier studies in highland Chiapas have shown that subjects' descriptions of the symptoms associated with various illness terms include references to visible, salient, and very generalized characteristics (Holland, 1963). Thus a symptom of gastrointestinal disturbance, such as diarrhea, or vomiting, may be reported as the principal bodily referent of a particular illness terms. The same is true of specific respiratory symptoms (e.g., color of sputum produced by a cough, difficulty in breathing) or general systemic symptoms (e.g., wasting away, lassitude). The cognitive implications of the illness episode (e.g., its severity or the nature of its presumed cause), however, are what appear to be regarded as critical aspects of the "illness," and it is these dimensions that Zinacantecos may use to grade and perhaps classify illnesses.

In other words, it seems that to a Zinacanteco an illness, regardless of its specific bodily correlates, "is" or "means" what it connotes, mostly in terms of its severity and its socio-moral implications. To the scientifically trained physician, by contrast, an illness usually implies a set of molecular, biochemical, and physiological processes or events. He groups illnesses in terms of cause, organ system affected, and/or pathological process. In view of these considerations, it will be appreciated that an attempt to link the native system of medical knowledge with the scientific system entails associating highly discrepant meaning systems.

In order to make our analysis meaningful, we concentrated on the dimensions of cause, severity, and condition of the blood, and on the therapeutic issue of visits to the sacred mountains (questions *B*, *C*, *F*, and *H*). Together, these accounted for most of the variance present in the responses. Both groups were first combined, and the response mode for each question-term coordinate was determined, yielding a 76 × 4 matrix. This, in effect, was a matrix of information representing the "typical" Zinacanteco male's response to these four questions when they were asked about each of the 76 illness terms. Using descriptions of each illness term provided by five informants outside the test group, we performed a content analysis utilizing the key "biological" referents of the terms (i.e. those denoting specific bodily disturbances). From these referents we were able to place certain of the terms into one of the following subgroups: gastrointestinal, generalized skin eruptions, discrete lesions (e.g., localized swellings and tumors), permanently altered bodily states (e.g., blindness or deafness), and respiratory infection. These results are shown in Table 10.

In only a few instances was it possible to link the native and the scientific frames of reference in a manner that suggested consistency. The terms in the category of generalized skin eruptions are by and large believed to be associated with hot blood. Discrete lesions are believed to be caused by witches, and they tend to be regarded as serious. Permanently altered bodily states are believed to be caused mainly by the deities and tend to have no associated remedy. And respiratory infections are seen as caused by the deities and are associated with hot blood. By and large, these observations are not striking and could be due to chance factors. In addition, several of the Western medical categories show no meaningful correspondence with the various dimensions.

The patterning of medical knowledge in Zinacantan. In this section we will describe our attempts to delineate the relationship between the dimensions that Zinacantecos use to qualify or interpret illness, and also

TABLE 10
Sample Analysis Linking Zinacanteco and Scientific Illness Categories

		Questions			
Scientific category	Illness terms	B Cause	C Severity	D Remedy exists	F Condition of blood
Gastrointestinal:					
Diarrhea	5	deity	major	yes	hot
	12	deity	major	yes	cold
	32	deity	major	yes	hot
Constipation	16	witch	major	yes	hot
	29	witch	major	yes	cold
Stomach worms	39	natural	minor	yes	cold
	42	witch	major	yes	cold
Generalized skin	8	deity	major	yes	hot
eruptions	9	deity	major	yes	hot
	10	deity	minor	yes	hot
	24	natural	minor	yes	cold
	50	natural	minor	yes	hot
	65	witch	major	yes	hot
	66	natural	minor	yes	hot
Discrete lesions	19	witch	major	yes	cold
	20	witch	major	yes	hot
	21	witch	major	yes	hot
	49	witch	minor	yes	hot
	60	witch	major	yes	hot
	62	witch	major	yes	hot
	69	witch	major	yes	cold
Permanently altered	45	deity	major	yes	hot
bodily states	46	deity	minor	no	cold
	48	deity	major	no	hot
	63	deity	major	no	medium
	72	deity	minor	no	medium
	73	witch	minor	no	cold
	76	deity	minor	no	medium
Respiratory	1	deity	minor	yes	hot
	6	deity	major	yes	hot
	7	deity	major	yes	hot
	18	witch	major	yes	hot
	28	deity	minor	yes	hot
	43	deity	major	yes	hot

the relationship between the 76 illness terms. The original set of responses associated with each question was recoded in such a manner that an ordinal system of measurement was established. For example, the 22 response options that were originally provided for question *B* (the cause of an illness) were collapsed into three main categories: natural, witchcraft, and deities. This ordering reflects our assumption that there is a meaningful continuum in the dimension of cause, extending from the earthly-naturalistic through the interpersonal-malevolent to the deity-supernatural. Similarly, the three responses to question *C* (severity) were ordered into minor and major. An analogous ordering rationale was followed for the responses associated with each question. The two groups of Zinacanteco subjects were then combined, and, using the new ordering system, we obtained the new modal response associated with each illness term for each question. The result of this condensing and ordering procedure was to reduce the amount of dispersion or variance associated with the responses, thus rendering the modal response a more representative measure of central tendency. The new modes for questions *A* and *J* were the same for each of the 76 terms, and we used only the remaining eight questions in the analysis.

Using the above matrix of information, a correlation coefficient was computed for every pairing of questions, reflecting the nature of the association between the respective questions (Table 11). For example, the correlation coefficient of 0.68 between question *E* and question *G* indicates a high positive association between these dimensions—i.e., when the subjects felt that a h'ilol was needed to treat an illness condition, they very often tended to feel that candles were also necessary.

An inspection of Table 11 shows that whenever subjects explain the cause of an illness in categories removed from the naturalistic and straying toward the supernatural or deity category, they also tend to

TABLE 11

Correlation Between Questions Across Illness Terms

Question	Question							
	B	C	D	E	F	G	H	I
B	1.00							
C	0.34[a]	1.00						
D	−0.37[a]	−0.10	1.00					
E	0.36[a]	0.57[a]	0.00	1.00				
F	−0.22	−0.14	−0.21	−0.11	1.00			
G	0.43[a]	0.66[a]	−0.15	0.68[a]	−0.11	1.00		
H	0.28[b]	0.29[a]	−0.43[a]	0.27[a]	−0.10	0.27[b]	1.00	
I	0.00	0.02	0.00	0.04	0.07	0.03	0.10	1.00

NOTE: The modal responses of both groups combined were used for these correlations. The modes on questions *A* and *J* were identical across the 76 illness terms; consequently, these questions were not used in the analysis.

[a] Correlation coefficient significant at $p < .05$.

[b] Correlation coefficient significant at $p < .01$.

classify the term as serious ("major") and to acknowledge that h'iloletik (as opposed to other practitioners) are needed for treatment. Associated with this type of causal explanation is the conviction that candles are likely to be required in the curing ceremony itself. Conversely, when subjects settle on a naturalistic explanation as the basis of a particular illness, they also tend to assert that it has no remedy. It can be seen that Zinacantecos tend to believe that h'iloletik are the persons qualified to treat serious illnesses.

Using the same matrix of information, we next computed a correlation coefficient for each pair of illness terms. This, in effect, allowed us to determine how the illness terms were interrelated; and we were able to group the terms that showed a high relationship to each other, that is, those on which the group's modal response pattern across the various questions tended to be very similar. A correlation of 1.00 between a particular pair of illness terms indicates that by the response mode, Zinacantecos construe those terms equivalently. Conversely, a low correlation indicates that the illness terms are construed in a discrepant fashion. Since we listed the illness terms in such a way that those with high correlations were placed contiguously, it was possible to note the groups of terms that shared the same semantic dimension.

This analysis yielded several "clumps" or groups of illness terms that had a unity correlation. With regard to the particular Zinacanteco illness dimensions that were used in this study, then, these terms seem to have equivalent meaning. We have already pointed out some of the correspondences between the Zinacanteco and the scientific medical perspective, and indicated the generally narrow and truncated nature of these correspondences. The bodily referents of the illness terms comprising each of the high-correlation clumps highlighted the essentially divergent perspectives involved. For example, one group includes terms that refer to (1) severe gastrointestinal upset, (2) serious respiratory infection, (3) chest pain, (4) deafness, (5) earache, and (6) toothache. If we view these ailments from the Western scientific perspective, they have little in common, except the fact that they can be incapacitating. Another group contained (1) constipation, (2) chronic coughing, (3) inflammation of the hand, (4) madness, (5) growth or tumor, (6) boil, and (7) blood in urine. Again, from the standpoint of the bodily system or process that is disturbed, it is difficult to single out a commonality of meaning.

Implications of Study B

First, we should emphasize that particular identities or values associated with the various illness dimensions were not invariably associated with separate illness terms by the subjects. Neither group of subjects agreed completely about the folk medical knowledge evaluated in this study. (The reader can determine the extent of group consensus by examining Appendixes A and B.) The linking of certain dimensions, such as cause and condition of the blood, was heterogeneous; but the subjects linked other dimensions, such as who was vulnerable to an illness or who should be consulted for treatment, almost always in the same manner to the various terms. In other words, knowledge about illness, at the level tapped by our study, is distributed unevenly in Zinacantan. This suggests that one should be critical toward reports about the specificity of socioculturally peculiar syndromes (Rubel, 1964). Illness beliefs and natively construed health-crisis episodes no doubt exist, and at a general level of measurement (e.g., the mode) unique and consistent patterns can be demonstrated on certain dimensions. It appears, however, that subjects apply these beliefs rather loosely to certain dimensions, and that even on dimensions where a strong consensus exists, some of the members of a cultural group will always manifest different responses. The results of study *A*, which involved the direct use of symptoms, essentially confirm this picture.

In general, the results of comparing the responses of h'iloletik and laymen support our impression that much of the knowledge involving illness in Zinacantan is generally shared by the male members of the culture. There were some intergroup differences, principally on the dimension of cause. On the rest of the dimensions, however, both groups showed considerable agreement on measures of central tendency and relative dispersion, and the differences observed were primarily of degree and not of type.

When we examined the sample group's response variability across the illness terms, h'iloletik produced smaller H measures on certain questions and larger H measures on others; but on most questions there was no consistent pattern across the terms. This characteristic of h'iloletik as a group should not be confused with the slight but definite tendency of individual h'iloletik to be associated with greater response consistency or clustering—i.e., to have, individually, lower H measures. Clearly, each individual h'ilol could have an *H* measure of zero if in answering a question he chose the same response across the 76 terms. But if each h'ilol gave a different response to each term, the group would have greater variability than a lay group who did the converse—that is, who individually chose differing response options across terms but as a group always chose the same response to the same term.

In view of our findings, it would appear that at the group level h'ilol response variability differs according to the nature of the question, whereas at the individual level h'iloletik tend to have a more consistent or uniform response pattern regardless of the question. In other words, individual h'iloletik, compared to laymen, tend to be more conservative and to restrain their answers, perhaps because their knowledge of medicine is more crystallized and patterned. However, at the group level h'ilol response variability on a subset of the questions differs from that of laymen, although the difference is not uniform and appears to be affected by the content of the questions.

The implication of these results would seem to be that with regard to the dimensions tested h'iloletik as a group do not validate their social position generally, nor their medical functions specifically, by commanding and sharing a specialized body of knowledge about illness. Their validity as healers appears to be a consequence of their *consistently* applying private knowledge on an individualistic basis. Much medical knowledge, however, is shared with other male Zinacantecos. The sanctions that h'iloletik exercise would thus seem to inhere in their ascribed powers and in capacities that at the sociocultural level can be seen as the result of factors like spiritual revelation, presumed natural endowment, and the processes of recruitment and socialization directly associated with training. Given the exigencies of medical care delivery in Zinacantan, we cannot exclude the additional possibility that h'iloletik owe their success as practitioners to the properties (pharmacologic or otherwise) of their remedies, but this seems highly unlikely (see Chapter 12). The potential influence of personality factors on a h'ilol's role performance and on curing functions was discussed in Chapter 5 and will be reviewed from another perspective in Chapter 9.

We assume that our illness terms portray in an extensive manner the semantic field or domain of medical phenomena in Zinacantan. As has been touched on earlier, Zinacantecos, in receiving medical care, have many options besides the traditional one involving a h'ilol (see Chapter 9). Given the representative medical vocabulary of a culture and the knowledge that physicians can be and are consulted, a formal linkage between the native and the scientific medical systems might be anticipated. Such a linkage was, in fact, observed in Zinacantan but its scope was narrow. Specifically, there was no illness term on which the group of respondents showed a high consensus (i.e., greater than 80%) when judging that the services of a Ladino physician were required, although five terms produced this care option as the modal response. Interestingly, laymen tended to choose this option more frequently, suggesting that they are more receptive to non-Zinacanteco medical ideas. It should be emphasized, however, that the "physicians only" option was chosen relatively infrequently.

Since the set of illness terms used in this study is fairly comprehensive, we can conclude that "nontraditional" identities are, to a limited extent, a formal part of medical knowledge in Zinacantan. But the fact that there was no prominent negative association between the personnel category (the zero unit in this binary variable includes physicians) and other conceptual categories of the Zinacanteco system suggests that nontraditional identities are not consistently integrated into this system. In the light of these results and previous observations dealing with the manner in which Zinacantecos obtain medical care, the following formulation can be offered. Ladino physicians are consulted when the native belief system ceases to be sufficient, and the system includes units and identities that allow for transitions of this type. Linkages between the conceptual systems, however, are minimally developed in a formal sense, and the process by which the transition takes place is difficult to specify. Stated differently, when the Zinacanteco medical system fails, alternate conceptual systems (embodied in explanations as well as coping options and strategies) are used. The "failure" may be one of omission (a new health crisis that somehow cannot be articulated within the native system of knowledge because of its discrepant elements) or commission (something previously conceptualized and explained in an articulated fashion begins to be judged as different, discrepant, and hence outside the native system).

The rationale of the procedure followed in our Study *B* is summed up in Figure 2, which depicts four different but related analytical levels of the domain of medical concerns. *A* represents the behavioral level (including both social and physiological) and merges with the whole spec-

LEVEL D: DIMENSIONAL PATTERNING OF ILLNESSES	Illness Type A: Witchcraft cause Minor illness Blood is hot Etc.	Illness Type B: Naturalistic cause Major illness Candles used for cure Etc.	Illness Type X: Deity cause Minor illness 4 mountains used for cure Etc.

LEVEL C:
DIMENSIONAL
CLASSIFICATION
OF ILLNESSES

Illness dimension	T_1	T_2	T_3	T_4	T_5	T_6 ... T_n
D_1	1,1	1,2	1,3	1,4	1,5	1,6 ... 1,n
D_2	2,1	2,2	2,3	2,4	2,5	2,6 ... 2,n
.	.	.	.	.	.	. .
.	.	.	.	.	.	. .
D_m	m,1	m,2	m,3	m,4	m,5	m,6 ... m,n

Illness Terms

LEVEL B:
ILLNESS TERMS
OR DESCRIPTIONS

LEVEL A:
BEHAVIORAL
TERMS

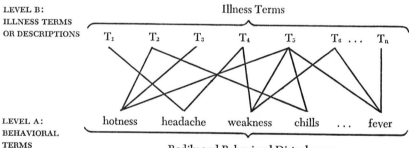

Illness Terms

T_1 T_2 T_3 T_4 T_5 T_6 ... T_n

hotness   headache   weakness   chills   ...   fever

Bodily and Behavioral Disturbances

Figure 2. Four analytical levels involved in investigating the domain of medical concerns. On level A are the various bodily disturbances or symptoms that may indicate illness. The terms on level B are those assigned by informants to clusters of one or more behavioral symptoms. On level C these terms are analyzed in relation to the major illness dimensions recognized by Zinacantecos (see Appendix A, pp. 229–37); each term will usually have a specific value or position on each of the relevant dimensions. Finally, on level D, the illness terms may be sorted into types on the basis of similar patternings of the dimensional values.

trum of human functioning. By far the largest proportion of human be- havior is functionally productive, organized, and patterned in routine ways, in no way requiring interpretations beyond that which is usual and expected given the norms and regulations of the group. Some of this behavior, however (often linked ultimately to biologically altered states), disturbs the processual equilibrium of a person and his group at the same time that it threatens his existence; and perhaps because of this it is judged as "illness." What the critical determinants of this judg- ment are, we do not know precisely, although we have already referred to specific factors that appear important (Chapter 6; see also Chapters 9 and 12). We suspect that the behavior in question includes statements referring to altered feelings, sensations, and bodily processes, and at the same time overtly or symbolically communicating functional im- pairment. The person's perceived relations with his fellows and with the gods are critically important, as are any concurrent events (e.g., dreams) that can be taken to reflect supernatural happenings. How discretely and explicitly a person perceives the functioning of his body, and how the various elements of this perception relate to the definition of illness, are empirical problems that have not been closely examined. The exact role of situational or contextual variables should also be explicated.

Level *B* in our diagram depicts the medical vocabulary used by mem- bers of the sociocultural unit to describe and refer to that which they define as illness. This level, in essence, can be regarded as a descriptive one, made up of language terms than enable labeling and discourse.

Levels *C* and *D*, finally, we arbitrarily call the interpretive or theoreti- cal aspects. They contain the relevant dimensions of illness; the rules for classifying, organizing, and interpreting the previous descriptive level, and various action directives (whom to consult, proper treatment, etc.). Our efforts in this study have been aimed primarily at the relation- ship between level *B* and levels *C* and *D*—that is, at depicting the or- ganization and specificity of medical knowledge at the descriptive and interpretive level. Our attempt to study the folk-scientific linkage, dia- grammatically, can be seen as an effort to associate level *A* with levels *C* and *D*, using medical scientific language to crudely relabel concepts that Zinacantecos furnished us at level *A*. We saw that destructive and circumscribed lesions are regarded as the result of malevolent forces (witchcraft), whereas respiratory infections are said to be caused by punishment from the gods. Some suggestive correspondences were also noted regarding the presumed condition of the blood. However, when we grouped or correlated illness terms using the whole spectrum of native knowledge (i.e. using all the dimensions) and then inspected the bodily referents (level *A*) of the various terms, we noted little correspondence. (Relations between levels *A* and *B* were analyzed in Study *A*, and have already been described.)

Chapter eight

The Perception of Altered Bodily States

THUS FAR in our evaluation of how Zinacantecos view medical problems we have focused primarily on the content and patterning of beliefs. By and large, our strategy has been to uncover Zinacanteco medical categories by using as analytic units the linguistic forms that are important to the subjects themselves. Descriptions of the symptoms recognized and labeled in Zinacantan have been related to illness terms that form a part of the native taxonomy of illness, and the native interpretations placed on these illnesses have been analyzed. Finally, the relations between the various dimensions of illness and between the illness terms themselves have been examined.

In this chapter we will describe two studies that employ an altogether different approach, although they are aimed at elucidating the same basic problem, namely, how Zinacantecos interpret medical illness. This time we inquired about native judgments by using photographs of persons who were ill and photographs of different types of skin lesions. To the extent that we introduced the units of analysis (the "diseases" depicted in the photographs), we can be said to have anchored our evaluations of native perceptions to externally derived biomedical forms of reference. For this reason, a different class of theoretical questions becomes relevant and should be briefly discussed before we describe the results of the studies.

Medical Ecology and the Biology of Disease

We mentioned earlier that the question of how the individual members of a nonliterate culture classify and respond to medical phenomena has long challenged behavioral scientists, as well as biologists and physicians. By far the largest proportion of earlier work in this area has focused generally on conceptions about the causes of illness, although the characteristics of curing practices have also received much attention. In general, illness has been described as having moral implications; and the material we have presented confirms that this is also the case in Zinacantan. Another concern of earlier ethnomedical work has been the sociopsychological changes produced by curing ceremonies that in turn seem to affect health status. But investigators have already reported whether bodily manifestations or changes have an influence on the native diagnoses and classification of illness. Indeed, in ethnomedical studies illness has usually been handled as a cultural category and for this reason has been termed "folk illness."

When studies have focused on what we could justifiably call the biological correlates of disease, it is usually the case that rather general components have been used as referents (e.g., pain, fever, weakness, or sleeplessness) (Frake, 1961; Rubel, 1964). Several methodological factors account for this. The first is the obvious lack of medical training among social scientists. This, of course, could easily be remedied: there is no reason why social scientists could not train themselves in specialized apects of medicine in order to carry out their studies. We believe that a more serious constraint on the social scientist who wishes to study medical problems is the nature of the domain he is exploring. Other domains, such as firewood, the color spectrum, or botany, may allow the investigator to present concrete specimens to the subjects in an orderly manner (Berlin, Breedlove, and Raven, 1968; Conklin, 1955; Metzger and Williams, 1966); but the investigator wishing to study how illness is classified is forced to adopt one of two limited strategies. He may analyze his subjects' responses to a natural occurrence of disease, which is problematic, since illnesses are infrequent, judged to represent crises, and regarded as highly private affairs; or he may rely on interviews conducted after the fact.

The consequence of these inhibiting factors is that it is difficult to obtain precise and reliable data about the components of illness episodes, and in particular about the specific indicators that underlie native forms of illness diagnosis and classification. In short, an investigator wishing to study how native subjects classify medical phenomena is usually constrained by the general difficulty of observing specific and concrete instances of illness occurrences. This constraint must be taken as an inherent limitation of prior ethnomedical studies.

An equally serious limitation, which we have already emphasized, is that medical data elicited and organized as part of an ethnographic inquiry are rarely analyzed in terms of external systems that bear directly on the domain under investigation. Our attempts to achieve such a comparison so far in this study may have clarified at least a few of the theoretical questions important to ethnomedicine. In each instance we have applied the alternative classificatory framework, Western medical knowledge, to information generated from interview data. But the items classified have stemmed from the subjects' cultural views or recollections of past illness episodes, not from what we could term observable manifestations of disease.

It is true, as social scientists who study medical problems assert, that much of what transpires during episodes of illness and medical care is organized in frames of reference we would term social, psychological, or cultural. However, we gain little by going on from this to assume that biological and physiological factors are completely irrelevant to native medical orientations and practices, or that social and cultural events are seldom related to concrete biological happenings. One unfortunate consequence of analyzing folk medical beliefs or perceptions without the precise and rigorous use of reference points that are external to the native system and grounded in theoretical frameworks dealing with the biological correlates of disease is that many questions of concern to medical ecologists and population biologists cannot be meaningfully answered (Alland, 1970; Dunn, 1968; Neel, 1970).

One such question that has been repeatedly raised is how diseases operate or may have operated as selective agents in the evolution of human society—and more importantly, how cultural factors have influenced the objective population-environment exchange involved in illness and healing. There are at least two general strategies that may be applied to such questions. First, general cultural practices and institutions that may bear on the development, propagation, or treatment of specific endemic diseases can be analyzed in relation to population trends and distributions in particular geographic settings (Cockburn, 1971; Livingston, 1958; Wiesenfeld, 1967). In analyses of this type, the interaction between a cultural group and a particular disease or group of diseases is generally approached at a rather high level of abstraction; consequently, one cannot determine whether members of the culture recognize either the value of a particular medical practice or the specific features of the disease that they may be controlling.

The second approach, with a view toward generalizing to earlier historical periods, attempts to analyze how representatives of particular "nonliterate" cultures actually respond to medical phenomena: that is, how they define and treat illness, how they organize their social lives when they judge an illness to be in their midst, and above all how various actions taken in response to native categories of meaning may affect the social group biologically (Hughes, 1963; Vayda and Rappaport, 1968). The requirements of this analytic strategy are quite different from those of the first one, since the focus is now on specific groups, and the investigator must usually be present within the culture in order to make direct observations. He hopes to demonstrate that cultural responses to disease have significant consequence to the group's survival, and thus it is imperative that he be able to systematically compare his observations regarding native classification schemes with knowledge of the actual biology of disease. To study the influences that cultural practices have on the effects of disease, he must carefully delimit native illness categories, using the biologically significant components of disease as referents (Gajdusek, 1964; Alland, 1970; Fabrega, 1972).

The goal of the studies reported in this chapter was to arrive at an understanding of how members of a preliterate group classify medical data when the manifestations of disease that we choose to view as "more biological" are made evident. Consequently, we excluded from the studies a number of highly important social and psychological factors that affect illness-related transactions in nonliterate settings, so that we could determine the extent to which native views were influenced by factors we could tentatively label as more physical and biological. As stimulus material we used photographs of the faces of persons who showed evidence of disease and also photographs of dermatological conditions, relying on these to depict the phenomenal domain of "disease." Clearly, our intent was not to answer broad questions that touch on evolutionary or population concerns; to do this, we would have to conduct more intensive investigations of diseases that are likely to have striking and profound sociobiological consequences. Instead, we simply tried to clarify the nature of the judgments that Zinacantecos make about disease when the visible biological components of disease are evident, and to analyze these judgments in terms of the Western scheme of medical classification.

Judgments of Illness Severity (Study C)

For this study, male h'iloletik and laymen were asked to judge and rate photographs of persons who showed various physical characteristics of disease. One specific aim of the study was to assess the extent to which these physical signs could influence native medical judgments of a disease's severity. Our hypothesis was that h'iloletik, because of their greater experience in treating illness, might be more sensitive to parameters that reflect severity. We first compared the judgments of h'iloletik with those of laymen since our hypothesis led us to expect group differences in these judgments. We then compared the judgments of both groups with those of academic physicians of various medical specialities who were given a similar task. Here, we anticipated that the judgments of h'iloletik would be closer to those of the physicians. Our avoidance of many important features related to medical evaluation and care was obviously a powerful constraint on the study, but one that would hopefully allow us to test the specific hypothesis that was posed. A second and more general aim of the study was to explore the relationship that exists between native judgments of illness severity and illness cause.

Our sample included 35 practicing male h'iloletik and 31 male laymen. The manner of selecting subjects for the study was similar to that described in Chapter 7. Background material, which included age and socioeconomic status (F. Cancian, 1963), was collected from each subject, and analysis showed no significant differences between the two groups in these respects.

The test, which was administered individually in either Spanish (to bilingual subjects) or Tzotzil, consisted of seven color photographs: three of faces of males, three of faces of females, and one of a pair of hands.* The faces showed local lesions and/or manifestations of systemic disease; the hands showed evident arthritic changes. The photographs were displayed together on a table top, and each subject was asked to rank them according to how seriously ill he thought the person depicted was. Following this, he was urged to discuss the nature of the

---

* All photos were of dark-skinned *mestizos*. Pictures of Zinacantecos should have been used, but circumstances make this impossible.

underlying condition, in particular its presumed cause. Illness severity, the "size" of an illness, is a construct Zinacantecos use when addressing themselves to the consequences and implications that illnesses have for the life of an individual. "Danger to life" is one suitable paraphrase of the meaning Zinacantecos ascribe to severity.

Descriptive aspects. From the combined responses of the two test groups, we computed a mean severity rank for each photograph. Photograph *C*, which depicted a terminally ill woman with scleroderma, received the highest rank, and photograph *D*, a woman with the classic facies of hypothyroidism, was second. Photograph *F* (a healthy appearing man with minimal evidence of leprosy) was ranked seventh, and photograph *G* (a pair of hands with obvious acute and advanced chronic arthritic changes) was sixth. These observations suggest that gross facial evidence of the systemic and toxic manifestations is what Zinacanteco subjects respond to when judging seriousness, and that abnormalities not demonstrable in or linked directly to visages are less important.

Analysis of each group's ranking system. Keeping the groups separate, we again computed a mean rank for each of the seven photographs and by ranking the photographs in this way determined how each group as a whole judged severity. When we computed a Spearman rank correlation coefficient using each group's overall pattern of ranking we obtained a composite value of 0.96, which is significant at the .01 level. Thus, there is a statistically significant relationship between the way these two groups ordered the photographs. The results are shown in Table 12.

For purposes of comparison, we decided to conduct a similar study using persons familiar with biomedicine as our subjects. In the United States, we enlisted the cooperation of 14 Board-eligible or qualified North American academic physicians from diverse medical specialties and, using an equivalent instructional format, asked them to rank the

TABLE 12
Correlations of Severity Ranks on Seven Photographs

Category	H'ilol	Layman	Physician
H'ilol	1.00	0.96[a]	0.78[b]
Layman	0.96[a]	1.00	0.85[b]
Physician	0.78[b]	0.85[b]	1.00

[a] Correlation coefficient significant at .01 level.
[b] Correlation coefficient (r_s) significant at .05 level.

same seven photographs. The subjects at first viewed this task as difficult and problematic; but when they were told to rely on general and abstract notions of seriousness, they complied with the request and in fact behaved as if the task was appropriate. Little uncertainty and ambiguity was shown during their execution of the task. Conversations with subjects following the test suggested that seriousness was interpreted roughly as "life threatening." Following the method outlined above we constructed an average "specialist physician" rank ordering system. We then computed a Spearman rank correlation coefficient to measure the association that existed between physicians' judgments and those of the h'iloletik and laymen, obtaining values of 0.78 and 0.85, respectively, which are both significant at the .05 level.

H'ilol and lay judgments for each of the seven photographs were averaged, and for each photograph a measure of dispersion was computed. On the basis of these measures, the photographs were ordered to obtain a ranking system that indicated the degree of judgment variability. This procedure was done for each group separately. A photograph at the top of this rank, in effect, was one on which the particular group generally agreed about severity, whereas one at the bottom was viewed in a heterogeneous fashion by the group (i.e. there was general disagreement about how seriously ill the person depicted was).

In effect, this gave us two ranking schemes, one ordering the photographs on the basis of seriousness, and the other indicating the degree of consensus on the rank of each photograph. We then correlated each group's ranking scheme of seriousness with its corresponding ranking scheme of relative disagreement. The h'iloletik had a correlation of −0.75, which is significant at the .05 level. Apparently, h'iloletik tend to agree on photographs that they judge to represent relative nonseverity, whereas they tend to disagree as they judge more serious cases. When this procedure was applied to the physicians' ranks of seriousness and consensus, a correlation coefficient of −0.84 resulted, which is also significant at the .05 level. No such tendency was shown by the lay group.

Relationship between "seriousness" and folk notions of cause. Each Zinacanteco subject of Study C, it will be remembered, was asked to volunteer an opinion about the cause of the illness that affected each person depicted in the photographs, and did so when he judged that the person was ill. We will consider only those responses (the majority)

TABLE 13
Classification of Responses by Cause Category
on Seven Photographs

Response	H'iloletik	Laymen	All subjects
Division of total responses in each category:			
Natural	39%	61%	100%
Deities	63	37	100
Witches	49	51	100
Division of each group's responses among categories:			
Natural	32%	50%	42%
Deities	41	23	32
Witches	27	27	26

that could be classified as Natural (e.g., caused by food or cold wind), Deities (caused by punishment from the gods), and Witches (caused by witchcraft). Using cause as the classificatory variable, we constructed a contingency table (Table 13). Inspection of this table reveals that the two groups tend to differ in the frequency with which they use the various categories of cause. For instance, 61% of the explanations of illness that refer to naturalistic causes are made by laymen, compared to only 39% for h'iloletik. When the chi-square test is applied, this difference between the two groups is significant ($X^2 = 5.89$, p < .02). When one examines judgments involving deities, this time the laymen are underrepresented ($X^2 = 6.69$, p < .01). Viewed differently, 41% of all judgments of cause made by h'iloletik refer to the deities, whereas the corresponding figure for laymen is only 23%; one-half of lay judgments involve naturalistic elements, but only one-third of the h'iloletik judgments do.

To facilitate analysis of the association between nature of cause and degree of seriousness, we condensed the seven ranks of illness severity into three. Responses signifying each cause were then distributed into three severity groupings. For each group, we computed the percentage of responses of each cause category falling into each of the three severity rankings. This yielded the matrix shown in Table 14. There were two noticeable trends in the association between severity and cause: as the rating of severity increased, the proportion of witchcraft responses increased; and at the same time the proportion of naturalistic explanations grew smaller. This was the case for both h'iloletik and laymen.

TABLE 14
Association of Cause with Severity on Seven Photographs

Responses	H'iloletik			Laymen		
	Natural	Deities	Witches	Natural	Deities	Witches
Total number giving this cause	52	64	42	18	37	43
Severity ascribed to this cause:						
High	27%	39%	55%	27%	30%	51%
Medium	31	38	33	32	38	33
Low	42	23	12	41	32	16

Implications of Study C

Our photographs did not portray people in obvious acute distress or pain; hence the subjects did not have to consider this element while judging illness severity. The people shown, however, did evidence facial changes highly suggestive of weakness, malaise, and general debilitation, and some had disfiguring lesions—all indicators that can be associated with pain. Our analysis of the ranking scheme adopted by the subjects suggests that when Zinacantecos try to estimate illness, they are strongly influenced by general systemic conditions revealed in the human countenance. A person's skin coloration, the alertness of his glance, and his overall appearance of general debility are the important factors.

The fact that the judgments of both groups of Zinacantecos correlated positively and significantly suggests that within the constraints of the present study the occupational experiences of a h'ilol do not influence his overall judgment of illness severity. In other words, since both h'iloletik and laymen evaluated the photographs along similar lines, it is difficult to claim that the background experiences of practitioners affect their judgments of severity in any special way. The physicians' judgments that we obtained, if not prognostically valid, could at least be termed biomedically informed opinions about the "severity" of an illness that is viewed as life-threatening. From this perspective, the fact that each Zinacanteco group's ranking of seriousness correlated positively and significantly with that of the physicians suggests that all Zinacantecos may intuitively respond to the same underlying biomedical dimensions. Had the h'iloletik differed significantly from the laymen in their rankings of illness severity, and had they approximated the physicians more closely, we could find some support for the hypothesis that a h'ilol's experience will develop in him a greater sensitivity to the signs of disease. Our actual findings do not support this general hypothesis, although they do raise the possibility that all Zinacantecos are aware of and responsive to these signs.

One interpretation of our results would be that the unique experiences of nonliterate peoples with occurrences of disease are the basis for their "biologically" informed medical judgments. To these people, disease, disfigurement, and death are not abstract occurrences that can be separated from routine everyday affairs. In a nonliterate setting there are no ambulances, emergency rooms, or hospitals to isolate outbreaks of disease from the community. Instead, a man who shows signs of disease remains in the immediate setting of his daily life, where he and his immediate family attempt to meet the problem with the help of friends and relatives. As a result, all residents of the nonliterate community share in the events and processes tied to disease and thereby acquire knowledge of its manifestations and consequences. Our data, in short, suggest that from the standpoint of disease consequences (i.e. severity) the residents of a nonliterate community have a medical orientation that is relatively differentiated. In previous chapters of this book we have shown that when one considers formal knowledge about illness (i.e., taxonomy, classification, and theoretical explanation) there is much variability and some redundancy in native responses. Furthermore, at times we have noted apparent inconsistencies if one adopts a strict biomedical position, though alternative reasons for these "inconsistencies" were offered. However, at a general, impressionistic, and intuitive level it may be that knowledge about the strictly biological implications of disease is reasonably sensitive and accurate.

An altogether different interpretation of these results is possible, however. One could say that fundamental and cross-culturally shared perceptual traits are the basis of any evaluation of how seriously ill another person is. In other words, regardless of socialization experiences (broadly conceived), the judgment of sickness in another human rests on display rules and configurational features that are intuitively perceived by members of many cultures. From this theoretical perspective, intergroup agreement would follow "naturally"; and the notion that Zinacantecos may demonstrate a special sensitivity to biological implications reflecting severity becomes intellectually cumbersome (Ekman, 1969). Future re-

search is obviously needed to clarify this possibility that all persons intuitively recognize the biological implications of illness.

The association that was noted between a group's judgment of illness
severity and the extent of its consensus or agreement on this judgment
requires several comments. In the first place, if one group, compared to
another, shows high agreement across a range or series of instances that
are similarly organized conceptually, we can say that this higher agreement applies across the entire dimension or variable implicit in the domain. Specifically, if group A, while judging the extent of severity, had
manifested lower variability on each of the seven photographs than
group B, we could infer that group A was more certain of its judgment.
And if severity and group consensus had shown a positive correlation,
we could infer that the severity of illness is a kind of judgment that Zinacantecos make with greater certainty. Neither conclusion follows from
the present investigation. Instead, both h'iloletik and physicians show
a significant negative association between severity and consensus. That
is, these groups show relative agreement when judging that someone is
minimally ill but disagree about who is seriously ill.

Possibly the underlying features that lead h'iloletik and physicians to
judge minimal illness are to them salient, visible, and perhaps relatively
uncompounded. By implication, then, the factors that lead them to judge
someone seriously ill are less striking and evident, perhaps because they
are more complex and heterogeneous. The fact that both groups of
medical practitioners showed the negative association suggests that one
consequence of medical experience or socialization (broadly conceived)
is to render portions of the spectrum of illness severity differentially
salient. That is, experience in the practice of medicine tends to facilitate
a practitioner's identification of those who are minimally ill and at the
same time establishes differing parameters that enter into the determi-
nation of who is seriously ill. We feel that these questions need to be
examined and clarified in future ethnomedical investigations.

A general question underlying the present investigation was whether
h'iloletik are more likely to treat and get involved with patients whose
underlying disease process has a favorable prognosis. In the logic of
the present study, this position could be supported if one could demonstrate that folk practitioners (when compared to laymen) are in fact
sensitive to the correlates of illness that Western physicians associate

with severity, since we assume that to some extent these correlates reliably reflect the morbidity and potential outcome of the disease. But the hypothesis implicit in this question was not supported, and our overall results (i.e. those involving the ranking of severity *and* those involving degree of consensus) suggest a more general notion: namely, that as individuals folk practitioners, compared to laymen, may be differentially more sensitive to what specific illness occurrences and severity mean, and that this affected their judgment of our photographs.

Our results cast some doubt on the abstract culturological depictions of folk curing that regard biological or physical parameters of illness as irrelevant to the processes that transpire during curing. Of course, direct support for the formulation that folk practitioners are affected by physical or biomedical parameters of illness, from which we might infer that they tend to treat patients with more favorable prognoses, requires proof that the actual decisions demanded by the treatment process are consistently made on the basis of these parameters. Valid and context-specific medical evaluations would need to be systematically compared to native judgments of who is less seriously ill, and "seriously ill" must be precisely specified (in terms of the patient's likelihood of dying, incurability, and so on). As we shall see in Chapter 12, this is a very difficult problem to evaluate.

The fact that our Zinacanteco subjects show a positive association between the notion of how ill a person is and the causal interpretation that they place on the illness is relevant in several ways. First of all, it supports findings reviewed in the previous chapter. Furthermore, the nature of this association—that severe illness receives a supernatural marking—is likewise consistent with those earlier findings, which stemmed from altogether different methods of procedure. At another level, the results of Study C support the notion that the factors associated with the perception of severe illness are complex and variegated. At the very least, our results suggest that the interpretive correlates of this perception change as illness becomes more severe. Furthermore, the content of these correlates (e.g., that more serious illness stems from supernatural sources) confirms the impression of others that essentially emotive and moral dimensions attach to the interpretation of serious illness in folk settings. In other words, our findings tend to support the claim that to nonliterate peoples serious illness is a moral crisis implying misbehavior and consequent punishment, which probably associate highly with emotional concerns. This is the case because it is in supernatural terms (or "causes") that Zinacantecos frame the problematic and personally distressful dilemmas of everyday life.

The Classification of Skin Lesions (Study D)

In this study we tried to determine whether h'iloletik are sensitive to highly specific physical parameters of disease. This time we used photographs of the characteristic lesions of various types of dermatological disease. In contrast to Study C, in which subjects based their evaluation on faces or hands (both visible in everyday circumstances), this study examines the way isolated lesions confined to the skin are perceived and differentiated. The task we posed to the Zinacanteco test group, all of whom were h'iloletik, must be viewed in large part as a perceptual one. In a sense, then, we are trying to analyze the overall perceptual characteristics of shamans, characteristics that may underlie their evaluations of persons who are ill and who demonstrate physical evidence of disease in the form of discrete lesions.

Our sample included 35 male h'iloletik, each of whom evaluated 25 mat color photographs (5″ × 8″) of common skin lesions.* The test photographs, all taken at a distance of 10–12 inches, were arranged randomly on a large table. The subject was told that the photographs depicted skin illnesses of different types, and he was asked to group the lesions according to their similarity. He could form as few as one or as many as 25 groups, and each group could contain any number of photographs; the only criterion for categorization was that the lesions grouped together be viewed by him as similar.

Each subject was also administered, individually, a short version of

---

* The five main types of skin lesions were represented in the photographs as follows: five neoplastic lesions, five vesiculo-bulbous lesions, six papulo-squamous lesions, six infectious lesions, and three granulomatous lesions. Before the actual test, each subject was shown two sets of three photographs, which depicted skin lesions at different enlargements. First, the subject was shown a photograph of a male mestizo suffering from a generalized skin eruption; this had been taken from a distance of approximately four feet. The subject was then shown two closer views of the same skin lesion (one taken from around 30 inches and one from 10–12 inches); he was told that all three photographs depicted the same patient. The same pretesting procedure was repeated, but this time using similar photographs of another male patient with a different skin lesion. This procedure was followed to provide a perceptual context for the subject and to familiarize him with color photographs of skin lesions. During this preliminary "sensitizing" phase, the subject was told that the purpose of the study was to learn how he classified disorders affecting the skin.

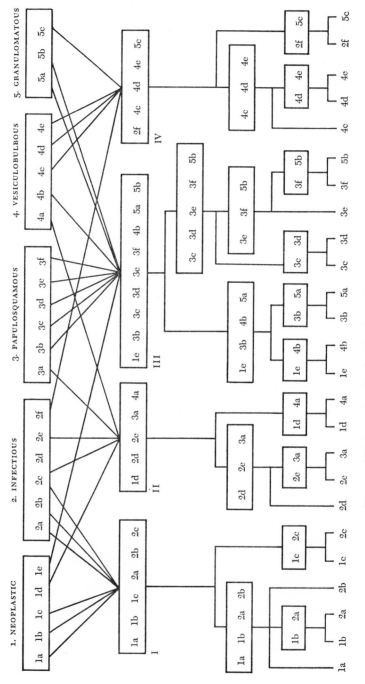

Figure 3. Western scientific classification and successive Zinacanteco categorizations of skin lesions.

Thurstone's Concealed Figures Test (CFT). This test, which resembles the Embedded Figures Test, requires that the subject determine whether simple geometric figures are concealed within more complex figures.* Scores derived from this test have in the past been used as indicators of the field articulation construct (Gardner and Moriarty, 1968; Gardner, Jackson, and Messick, 1960). The CFT scores, when ranked, allowed us to delineate two subgroups of h'iloletik differentiated by high field articulation (high CFT scores) and low field articulation (low CFT scores).

Background data involving the age and social prestige of the subjects was once again obtained by evaluating the cargo performance of each subject, and these measures were also ranked. In this study, we take a given position in this ranking as one sign of the individual h'ilol's intra-culturally assigned prestige and objective success; and we can again form two subgroups, this time differentiated by their "professional" competence. In subsequent analyses, we will refer to these subgroups as high-competence (*HC*) and low-competence (*LC*), and it is to be understood that intraculturally grounded indicators were used to arrive at this classification.

Modal classification scheme. Appendix C describes the mathematical procedure used to arrive at the scheme underlying the classifications of skin lesions by the h'iloletik. In general, we attempted to capture the fundamental associations that the subjects perceived between these lesions, and our procedure was designed to arrive at an approximation of the native classification groupings by placing minimal (external) constraints on the analysis of the data. In essence, we tried to establish the hypothetical classification scheme that guided each subject in executing the task we set him. It should be emphasized that the system of classification so developed is "constructed" empirically from overall similarities between skin lesions that the subjects themselves recognized. The classification is for this reason termed modal.

Our analysis yielded a hierarchically ordered array of skin lesions, and we assume that this array schematically represents the modal Zinacanteco classification of skin lesions. Since the task presented to each respondent was relatively unstructured, he could form any number of groups, depending on the degree of stricture or precision that he imposed on the

---

* The ease of administration and relative simplicity of the CFT were factors that contributed to our selection of this test. Instructions were communicated in Tzotzil, and each subject was supervised while he attempted three practice items. This was done in order to establish with certainty that the subject understood the requirements of the task.

categorization process. One subject might form five groups, another two, another nine, and so on. And presumably a subject who formed, say, nine groups might have applied his criteria more abstractly and formed fewer groups. Conversely, a partition that yielded three groups, we assume, could have produced seven groups; that is, the respondent might have formed seven groups instead of three had he been more restricted or precise in applying his criteria of similarity. The model employed to analyze our data thus assumes that the general criteria for classifying skin lesions are consistently applied by subjects, although the degree of stricture or abstraction that each individual may use varies; the stricture, however, we assume applies only within general categories.

The results of this analytic procedure are shown in Figure 3. At the top of the figure the various skin lesions portrayed are grouped in terms of Western biomedical typology. (Since the exact type of lesion in this typology, within broad categories, is of only marginal importance to us, we have simply numbered the pictures.) Below this are the initial and most abstract Zinacanteco categories. In the figure, we have indicated how the lesions that comprise a biomedically articulated cluster are parceled into the various Zinacanteco clusters.

It will be seen that each Zinacanteco category is composed of lesions representing several Western types. The lower levels of the chart show how the general Zinacanteco abstract categories were partitioned (a composite of all subjects' groupings). It can be seen that one of the segments branching from category III contains five lesions, and that four of these are classified as papulo-squamous. Similarly, the segment of three lesions branching from category IV is composed of vesiculo-bulbous lesions. These two branches, in essence, are the closest link between the two systems. Otherwise, the modal Zinacanteco classification scheme has no essential correspondence or overlap with the Western biomedical typology. We have no way of evaluating the degree of overlap that does exist.

Individual differences. The procedure described in Appendix C allowed us to estimate how closely the subjects resembled one another in their manner of classifying the skin lesions. The measures obtained are termed intersubject similarity scores and are used as measures of agreement between h'iloletik; the higher the score between two subjects, the closer their agreement on classification.

We next tried to determine whether subgroups of h'iloletik differentiated by other criteria also differed in their manner of classifying the skin lesions. First, we compared the h'iloletik in the high- and low-competence subgroups. The intersubject similarity scores of the *HC* group (18 h'iloletik and 153 intersubject similarity scores) were combined with those of the *LC* group (17 h'iloletik and 136 intersubject similarity scores), ordered in terms of diminishing size, and then compared by means of the median test. The value obtained was significant ($X^2 = 7.2$, $p < .01$), and the *HC* intersubject scores were overrepresented above the median. Thus, compared to *LC* h'iloletik, "competent" h'iloletik demonstrate closer agreement with each other in their manner of classifying the lesions. The same procedure was repeated, but this time performance on the CFT served as the basis for distinguishing between h'iloletik. The value obtained in this instance did not reach the level required for significance; thus field articulation ability is not associated with how closely h'iloletik resemble each other in their classification of the lesions.

Conformance with Western scientific classification. Each subject's grouping of skin lesions was also evaluated in terms of its correspondence to the Western system of classification. (The procedure used is also described in Appendix C.) In this manner we were able to measure the extent to which the lesions in each Western scientific type were grouped or separated in a subject's own classification scheme. Five scores were obtained for each subject, one score for each Western category; and each score measured the extent to which the subject's groupings dispersed a particular scientific category. A high score shows that the subject maintained a high conformance to the Western grouping.

The scores of the h'iloletik in the *HC* and *LC* subgroups were compared by means of the Student's *t* test. Five comparisons were undertaken, one for each of the five scientific categories. In none of these comparisons did the *t* value reach the level required for significance. Next, the scores of the h'iloletik in the high and low CFT score subgroups were compared in the same fashion. In two of the five instances, the *t* value was statistically significant; and in both of these the h'iloletik with higher CFT scores showed the higher mean score. Thus, professional competence (judged intraculturally) did not associate with conformance to the scientific manner of typing the 25 skin lesions. However, a measure of perceptual cognitive performance, namely field articulation, did bear a relation to this conformance (see Table 15).

TABLE 15
Comparison of Scores on Five Skin Lesion Categories
for High and Low Field Articulation Subgroups

Scientific categories	Field articulation group	
	Low ($N = 18$)	High ($N = 17$)
Neoplastic	.134	.142
Vesiculobulbous	.126	.143
Papulosquamous[a]	.126	.222
Infectious[a]	.104	.129
Granulomatous	.130	.125

[a] Difference in means significant at $p < .05$ for comparison of field articulation subgroups.

Implications of Study D

The findings of Study *D* confirm, substantially add to, and refine information generated by the earlier studies described in the previous chapter and in the earlier section of this one. Our general impression was that subjects identified the photographs as instances of skin eruptions, understood the task, and in fact found it interesting if not provocative. Initial analysis showed that the h'iloletik combined the various skin lesions in a manner that was clearly nonrandom, suggesting that their judgments were in some sense patterned. Since only the visible physical aspects of skin diseases appeared in the photographs we can tentatively hold that Zinacanteco folk practitioners may take into consideration this dimension of illness when they apply their native classification rules. As stated earlier, future studies of folk or native medicine should strive to clarify the influence that the organic-biological dimension of illness has in the process of medical diagnosis that is tied to treatment. We now have indirect evidence (Studies *C* and *D*) suggesting that biological factors of disease and their physical implications may influence judgments about illness. The question needing clarification is whether judgments of this type, in turn, actually influence practitioners during their efforts to diagnose and treat their clients.

In Study *D* culturally relevant criteria were used to distinguish between the professional competence of the h'iloletik. The results indicated that the Zinacanteco mode of determining healing competence was associated with how closely h'iloletik resembled each other in their manner of classifying skin lesions. Specifically, h'iloletik who enjoyed high prestige ratings in their sociocultural group tended to resemble each other more closely when they classified the photographs of skin lesions. These findings suggested that socioculturally determined competence is related in some way to the ability to consistently apply native medical criteria. This intracultural competence criterion for differentiating between h'iloletik, however, showed no association with a h'ilol's degree of conformance with the Western scientific typing of skin lesions. In general, the small overlap between the biomedical and Zinacanteco typologies supports our earlier conclusion that the two are effectively distinct. At what we could term the formal level of medical knowledge (taxonomy, diagnosis, etc.) there is little correspondence between the Zinacanteco and the biomedical frames of reference. This assertion does not contradict the results of Study C, for in that instance the implications of disease were in focus. That the Western biomedical classification of skin lesions itself bears an imperfect correlation with the long-range physiological and pathological consequences of the underlying disease is well known.

Criteria and principles associated with a Western biomedical framework (which, to repeat, is in this instance anatomical, structural, and tied to observation by the unaided eye) apparently have some influence among at least a subset of h'iloletik. We observed that a h'ilol's correspondence to the Western style of differentiating between skin lesions was related to his cognitive ability. Indeed, the task of distinguishing between lesions in this way would seem to draw on the testable cognitive ability that we used to differentiate the h'ilol subgroups. "Field articulation ability" is used to measure the capacity to differentiate elements of a perceptual stimulus. Those who score low on tests like the CFT are said to respond "globally" to a stimulus set: they respond to the overall, general features of the set but do not seem to differentiate its segments. By contrast, those who gain high scores on the tests by focusing on subsets or portions of the stimulus are considered more capable of regulating attention and information processing. Because the task posed requires the subject to systematically distinguish and relate segments of a complex stimulus field, the ability measured is termed field articulation.

To group skin lesions by Western criteria one must focus attention on each of the various structural properties of a lesion—elevation, border discreteness vs. border continuity, the apparent content or density of lesions, and associated changes in the surrounding skin. Since the ability to apply these criteria is formally related to that measured by the CFT, the h'iloletik with higher field articulation scores might be expected to adopt a Western classification method to some extent. The point requires further elaboration. All h'iloletik were asked to group skin lesions by Zinacanteco criteria of similarity; hence the composite of the criteria that we assume guided their execution of the classification task has been viewed implicitly here as the underlying Zinacanteco classification scheme. However, since each h'ilol was free to apply this scheme in a personalistic way, we can anticipate that his personal abilities will be reflected in the task of applying native criteria. And h'iloletik distinguished for their field articulation ability would thus be more likely to display this ability in performing the task given them. In this particular task, the ability is reflected by their greater conformance to the Western biomedical scheme of classifying skin lesions, a scheme that rests on physical criteria. It will be recalled that the group showing high CFT scores did not differ on the intersubject similarity measures. Thus, the influence of field articulation appears to be less important than the competence criterion in accounting for intergroup similarity.

This study and the preceding one (Study *C*) should be viewed as bearing on the concern that Vayda and Rappaport (1968) have termed ethnosystematics, which asks: What units and identities do subjects use as criteria in order to partition and structure their ecosystem in a manner that will allow adaptive efficiency? The folk-illness classification scheme in Zinacantan contains notions about etiology and directives regarding the treatment of the illness, and these "theoretical" notions are an inherent part of the scheme. We can assume, then, that the important process termed ethnoecology by Vayda and Rappaport (i.e. how and why the subjects act once they have segmented their world) is to some extent reflected in the Zinacanteco manner of grouping the skin lesions. We have seen that the Zinacanteco typology in general bears little relation to the Western scientific typology, which has allowed us a considerable control of diseases.

The biomedical typology of dermatological conditions is not a product or a direct expression of criteria involving treatment; instead, it rests on anatomic considerations and merely allows for the subsequent application of therapeutic criteria. And even if the biomedical framework were based on treatment considerations, the h'ilol's lack of conformance with this framework does not mean that his treatments are inefficacious. Determining the empirical usefulness of the native mode of treatment, of course, would require more direct investigation. We can merely conclude that its general orientation to skin disease does not conform to the Western system, which does form the basis for subsequent treatment plans that are relatively efficacious. The fact that cognitive factors involving the definition and interpretation of illness (factors having potential biological implications) are embedded in socially meaningful processes during the conduct of Zinacanteco healing will be illustrated in the next chapter.

Summary Comment

In this chapter we have reported on our attempts to evaluate a heretofore neglected aspect of ethnomedicine: that is, whether there are biological implications in the way nonliterate peoples regard medical problems. The answer to this question is a very tentative yes. Zinacantecos, in general, judge severity (i.e. "life threateningness") of illness in a way one could term "informed." H'iloletik, like physicians, show a greater consensus when judging "nonserious" illness, suggesting that to them serious illness is more complex and diverse. H'iloletik, in terms of cognitive ability, may attend more closely to biophysical features when they approach illness, although their success in Zinacanteco culture appears related to how consistently they apply native (and not biophysical) criteria. Finally, h'iloletik, as compared to laymen, tend to resort more frequently to supernatural explanations, though all male Zinacantecos who offer such explanations do so more frequently in the case of illnesses that they judge to be serious. Future work should aim at evaluating similar and related issues in actual instances of diagnosis and treatment.

Chapter nine

Dynamics of Medical Practice
in Zinacantan

IN CHAPTER 3 we emphasized that Zinacantecos have available several different sources of medical care. Here we will concentrate mainly on the characteristics of the h'ilol-patient relationship, since this is the most important medium for dispensing medical care in Zinacantan; but it should be understood that other care options are available and are used. It was mentioned that several of these options can be used concomitantly to effect a cure. Indeed, because of these characteristics of the setting, it is possible to say that a system of medical care delivery exists, and that the system has distinctive properties.

Zinacantecos, like members of other cultures, have a great deal of folk knowledge about ways of dealing with various illnesses and symptoms. We have seen (especially in Chapter 7) that the medical knowledge of laymen is very similar to that of h'iloletik. When ill, with recognizable symptoms, Zinacantecos may first resort to various self-contained measures, such as prayers, dietary restrictions, and/or household remedies— either treatments that have been repeatedly used by the patient himself or new ideas gained from friends and relatives. By traveling to San Cristóbal, the sufferer or a relative can also obtain advice from a commercial druggist. As we mentioned earlier, government restrictions on the sale of drugs are minimal, and it is very common for the local Indians who frequent these establishments to be sold inexpensive antibiotic or hormonal preparations after they have described their complaints.

In San Cristóbal there are also a large number of folk practitioners— spiritualistic mediums, midwives, owners of talking saints, herbalists, sorcerers, and witches. The sorcerers and witches may be Mayan or Ladino; some of them have achieved considerable renown in the region and are consulted regularly by Mayas of the surrounding municipios. The practitioners will on occasion make a visit to the home of the family to perform their cures.

Finally, when circumstances warrant it, licensed physicians in private practice or working in federal clinics may also be consulted; but the regimens they prescribe may not be followed if the necessary medications have not been purchased (usually because they are too expensive) or if the treatment plan has been poorly understood. Not infrequently, sick Zinacantecos travel to Tuxtla Gutiérrez, the capital of Chiapas, either to seek more sophisticated scientific medical care or to visit a spiritualist center that is located nearby.

All these ways of obtaining medical care should not be viewed as competing or disjunctional. They are usually followed concomitantly, and during the course of an illness the patient and his family may be involved in several of them at once. However, our experience suggests that although Zinacantecos may use several forms of medical care, they tend in both the long and the short run to remain relatively loyal to a single practitioner as long as they judge him to be helpful. Even in this very pluralistic setting, medical care is not a random or haphazard affair. A Zinacanteco may request medical care from a h'ilol, a druggist, and a physician within a short interval of time. For all intents and purposes, he is being treated for one set of symptoms by three different kinds of practitioners, and he sees no inconsistencies in this plan. He is less likely, however, to consult two h'iloletik at once, or two physicians at once.

In sum, Zinacantecos appear to draw general boundaries between categories of medical care and to shift from one curer to another within categories only when they judge that a healer has achieved no beneficial results. This strategy prevails only while actual treatment is being administered, and some shifting between h'iloletik does take place during the early, "diagnostic" stages of an illness.

The general system of medical care that prevails in the Chiapas highlands around San Cristóbal is thus an open one, with patients shifting readily between different forms of care. As in the Western system, any given strategy or plan of care is initiated by the consumer himself (or his representative). In Chiapas, however, the participants acknowledge differences in efficacy and suitability between various forms of care; and strategies that include different forms of care should be viewed as adaptive attempts to maximize potential benefits, not as signs of personal disloyalty or distrust of an individual curer. Trained physicians, of course, may condemn the Indian (or the lower-class Ladino) as ignorant and backward for distrusting scientific advice and espousing superstitions and magical beliefs. Nonetheless, physicians, folk medical practitioners, and consumers (Zinacantecos, other Mayas, and Ladinos) all anticipate and come to accept as modal the interconnectedness between the various curing options.

One could posit that since illness in Zinacantan is viewed as reflecting disturbances in various spheres of a person's life, and above all as highly uncertain and unpredictable in its consequences, the general rules designed to cope with its burdens would encourage the use of several kinds of healers and remedies. And it is because a patient's participation and involvement in healing are multibonded and ramified in this way that an investigator may have difficulty in delimiting the locus of healing responsibility. On the one hand, we can say that this heterogeneity appears to diffuse responsibility and thus protect the different practitioners, although the consumer may be perplexed and distraught when he sees his problems paralleled across the various components. On the other hand, this state of affairs sometimes seems to make each curer individually more vulnerable to criticism for the inefficiencies and failures that the system itself fosters. We cannot here detail further features of the highly diversified system of medical care existing in highland Chiapas (see Fabrega and Manning, 1973); but we shall see (Chapter 12) that special problems are created for those interested in evaluating the quality of care delivered.

The complex relationship between the various ways of obtaining medical care and the actual characteristics of an illness (namely, degree of discomfort, weakness, visibility of symptoms, duration, and presumed cause) is obviously an important problem; but its clarification was not possible during our fieldwork. However, it was apparent that even though alternatives existed, persistent and serious symptoms almost invariably led a Zinacanteco or his family to seek the advice and services of a h'ilol. In the following presentation, therefore, the h'ilol-patient relationship is conceptualized as the principal means by which Zinacantecos receive medical care; and we examine it as a series of stages or periods made up of decision strategies and behavioral options that are linked to native categories of meaning.

Some Initial Considerations

From our informants' descriptions of the h'ilol-patient encounter, it is clear that "what the blood says"—i.e. the curer's diagnosis—is final and unquestionable. In Zinacanteco theory, a patient's symptoms are frequently viewed as simply an illusory indication that some illness whose identity cannot be known by mere observation is present; hence the patient should not trust his own judgment but should defer to the h'ilol. In practice, many patients do become attached to their own theories of illness; and since they often know from experience the "styles" of several h'iloletik, the wish to obtain confirmation of their own opinions provides them with one motive for selecting a particular h'ilol.

Another consideration in choosing one's h'ilol is economic. Two factors must be calculated in estimating the cost of a curing ceremony. One is the magnitude of the ceremony itself—the quantities of ritual materials and food that must be bought. The other is the length of the postceremonial period of seclusion, during which the patient and those who care for him are unable to work. The second is easiest to assess, since each h'ilol has a fairly standard and generally known prescription for the taboo period. The cost of the actual ceremony is more variable, depending each time on the h'ilol's diagnosis, although some factors (e.g., the number of candles used at particular ceremonies) are known for each h'ilol and may affect the patient's choice. Less definable factors of reputation also come into play. Some h'iloletik, for example, seem predisposed to diagnose illnesses as witchcraft and to prescribe counteracting ceremonies, whereas others seem biased toward certain other causes. These tendencies are undoubtedly known to a curer's potential clientele, and may on occasion influence a patient's choice.

Another important factor in the selection of a h'ilol is his reputation for successful treatment. In general, a curer's reputation does not seem to extend much farther than the immediate environs of his own hamlet, where his identity as a curer becomes known through his participation in the public ceremonies. Outside the hamlet, unless his activities arouse unusual popular interest, he is likely to be known only to those with whom he has some sort of special tie, such as *compadrazgo*, previous acquaintance, or kinship. Beyond this, there seems to be an association between a curer's success and the extent of his reputation: h'iloletik who are considered *mas tsots* (more strong) or *p'ih* (spiritually alert) are widely known.

The quality of this reputation need not be entirely good. In fact, the h'iloletik who seem most famous (or perhaps notorious) in Zinacantan are those reputed to have extra powers and daring in treating witchcraft cases. Since the ability to treat witchcraft is generally taken as a sign of the curer's ability to practice it, a h'ilol who shows willingness to treat witchcraft cases is regarded with some suspicion. He is likely to be the subject of widespread gossip and scandalous allegation, but he also is sought by a large and eager clientele. This is, in a sense, a form of medical specialization—the only one we detected in Zinacantan. The respected h'iloletik who are not necessarily known for witchcraft generally enjoy widespread reputations simply because they have performed successful cures, or because they are thought to possess superior medical knowledge (as the result of special revelation).

The negative aspects of a h'ilol's reputation are three: age, incompetence, and lack of authenticity. Some informants say that very senior h'iloletik are less desirable than younger men, since years of ritual drinking may take their toll of a curer's mental faculties. Obviously, the h'ilol will be distrusted if his cures are chronically unsuccessful. And certain curers are not considered true h'iloletik at all: they merely pretend, it is said, to have received divine instruction in order to swindle their patients out of chickens and liquor. This reputation sometimes arises when the h'ilol in question becomes too intoxicated during curing ceremonies.

Our examination of a small sample of curing cases (about 130 cases involving the medical histories of 11 families) shows that when true illness is thought to be present the first source of therapy sought is typically a h'ilol who is either a compadre, a kinsman, or a neighbor of the patient (see Table 16). This pattern is especially characteristic of the outlying, more stable hamlets; it is less common in the valley of Hteklum, where the flux of temporary residents and the extraordinarily large number of h'iloletik creates an unusual situation. However, it seems to be a general rule that the first choice will be a h'ilol who is known to the patient personally.

Relations Between the H'ilol and the Sick

Initial contact. The decision to consult a h'ilol is reached when a person perceives himself to be chamel and believes that the illness will not

TABLE 16
Treatment in Representative Zinacanteco Curing Cases

Treatment	No. of cases
Treated by h'ilol at some point	102
H'ilol was a relative	32
H'ilol was a friend	67
H'ilol was a compadre	6
H'ilol was a "stranger"	2
H'ilol living nearer than 500 m, same hamlet	67
H'ilol living farther than 500 m, same hamlet	23
H'ilol living in another hamlet	11
Treated by another Indian curer	4
Treated by a Ladino physician or curer	21
Self-treated	12
Treated by more than one h'ilol or other curers in succession (av. 2.8 curers per illness)	15
When curing ceremony was performed:	
Held in patient's house only	60
Sacred mountains were visited	46

NOTE: The table considers 131 illnesses, occurring in 11 families (average 3.3 illnesses per person). The discrepancies in totals are caused by the many instances of multiple treatment.

improve and/or portends evil for him. Quite obviously, he is influenced by purely biological factors—hormone changes, chemical toxicity, physiological dysfunction, etc. These factors may be perceived owing to his prior belief that various punishments have been "sent," or their consequences as symptoms may merely be taken to indicate such punishment. In the broadest sense, then, the setting and context enveloping the patient are critically important. The status of a person's social ties becomes important, as do the obligations and responsibilities that he has or owes. The content of dreams by the patient or his family is even more important. Dreams reflect the activities of the ancestral gods and the migrations of the dreamer's soul, and are inextricably linked to the causation of chamel.

Events that may culminate in the dispensing of medical care by a h'ilol are set in motion when a representative of the sick person (usually a relative) speaks with the h'ilol and requests that he visit the patient. This initial meeting is accompanied by the ritual offering of a drink and lasts about one-half hour; usually, little information about the features of the illness or the patient's condition is exchanged. The meeting most often takes place in the h'ilol's home, but it may occur in the fields, the ceremonial center, or any other place the h'ilol happens to be. If the patient is not too sick and the distance involved is short, he himself may seek the h'ilol and request treatment. A diagnostic evaluation can then be performed on the spot.

This initial interaction usually ends when the h'ilol accepts the request to visit the patient's home and specifies a time when he can be expected —often later the same day. Not all requests for medical evaluation are promptly granted, however. If the initial request is made late in the day and the home of the patient is distant, for example, the healer may wait until the next morning rather than travel by night. Sometimes the h'ilol may not realistically be able to visit a patient immediately and will then suggest to the family that they consult another h'ilol. This occurs, for example, when he is actively preparing for another curing ceremony, when his own family requires his services, or when he has recently completed a ceremony and is in seclusion. Similarly, if his other activities (e.g., farming or selling his products at market) require his attention, he may not want to visit a patient. The patient and his family, of course, may be willing to wait, in which case the h'ilol may merely postpone the "diagnostic" visit. Thus, although h'iloletik clearly feel obliged to respond to requests for medical care, their personal duties often have a higher priority. This priority is always made explicit and seems to be inherent in the system of health care delivery in Zinacantan. It contrasts with what is observed in industrialized settings, where there is in principle a constantly available source of medical practitioners and facilities. One can say that physicians are (formally) expected to exercise their skill in times of need and crisis. But the h'ilol, it appears, has explicit options that protect him from involvement and allow him to express his personal choices and outright reservations regarding the decision to evaluate an instance of illness. From a sociopsychological standpoint, such options appear to the outsider as highly functional.

In almost all cases the requests for medical care come directly from persons who need and wish to be helped and who have no reason to harm the h'ilol's reputation (though there are exceptions; see below); and the h'iloletik consulted are those regarded as competent and most respected. A key symbolic element in the initial contact between practitioner and patient is the relative position of each on the dimension of evil and morality. If the request for medical evaluation is made by someone who has antagonized the h'ilol or his family in the past, the curer is likely to refuse his services. Similar refusals often occur when witchcraft is suspected. A h'ilol with a "good" reputation (that is, one who does not deal directly with malevolent agents or forces when healing) may refuse to get involved with someone who has antagonized a known witch, since the cure of an illness caused by witchcraft involves "wrestling" with evil and can lead to a personal confrontation with the witch. Even h'iloletik with "witch" reputations may refuse to be involved in cases where they suspect (or "know") that an especially powerful witch is operating. Essentially, h'iloletik will often decide against treating cases where strong antagonisms are associated with the people involved; antagonism involves witchcraft, and witchcraft may lead to personal danger for the h'ilol.

To summarize, the delivery of medical care in Zinacantan takes place in a setting where the dimensions of morality, evil, and friendship alliance are crucial, where informal and particularistic social relationships predominate, and where the "social distance" between the h'ilol, his potential patients, and other practitioners is small. This type of social environment and its rules regarding health-related behavior intimately affect the process of medical care delivery—promoting some healer-patient relationships, obstructing others, and constantly monitoring the course of treatment. The symbolic categories that structure and organize the interactions of a Western physician and his patient, classically described by Parsons (1951), are to be contrasted with these.

The diagnostic visit. This visit is made so that the h'ilol can determine the cause of the patient's illness and give suggestions and advice regarding treatment. The diagnosis is always accomplished by feeling the pulse of the patient and "listening" to his blood through the pulse. First, however, the h'ilol talks with the patient and his family, and it is during this conversation that he is introduced to the actual details of the illness —what the symptoms are, how long the patient has been sick, and whether he has already been treated by anyone for this or another illness. If the patient has received prior treatment, he will probably be asked the name of the curer, what diagnosis was offered, and what type of ceremony was performed. The patient usually remains fully clothed during the visit, and the h'ilol seems to confine his activity, other than feeling the pulse, to visual inspection.

The h'ilol then pulses the patient and prays that the illness be "handed over" or revealed to him; it is said that the gods speak to him through the blood, imparting a variety of information. On the basis of "what the blood says," the h'ilol diagnoses the illness and prescribes a cure. The cure is always implicit in the diagnosis: the blood not only tells the h'ilol the source of the illness, but also how many candles are wanted, what mountains and shrines must be visited, and so on. He also finds out how long the illness has really existed. What appears to the patient as a short, circumscribed condition may turn out to involve supernatural punishment or witchcraft that has been developing over a period of time unbeknown to the patient and his family. In any case, the blood will always give the h'ilol some basis for a diagnosis.

In Zinacantan, the reporting of an illness state and the subsequent request for the diagnostic services of a h'ilol are sufficient conditions for establishing that an illness exists, serious or not; the h'ilol merely confirms the illness by diagnosing it. One rarely observes a case in which the patient requests a diagnosis for a self-defined "illness" or problem and the h'ilol then announces that no illness is present. For all intents and purposes, there are no analogs in Zinacantan to situations in our own culture where a physician can comfortably tell someone who is not feeling well that he has no disease or that a "psychosomatic" problem (i.e. nonorganic or imaginary) prevails. On the other hand, a perceived *feeling* of illness is not a necessary condition for the judgment that chamel is present. The h'ilol may sometimes see someone purely for reasons we could term evaluative or preventive. That is, a request for the h'ilol's diagnostic services (and even curing ceremonies) can be motivated simply by a desire to exclude the possibility of illness or to protect the petitioner from potential evil. In this case the h'ilol's pulsing may or may not reveal illness. We can consequently say that both the consumer and the h'ilol have ultimate control over the amount of illness that prevails in Zinacantan.

After pulsing, the h'ilol announces his diagnosis, often discussing what the blood has told him with the household. This conversation, like the one before pulsing, may be brief; but both are important means of giving each party to the healing process a more intimate knowledge of the other. Sometimes, the h'ilol will arbitrarily inform the patient of what symptoms he must be suffering and why; whether or not this corresponds to the patient's own perceptions, he cannot properly challenge the curer's diagnosis. The h'ilol, for example, may say that the patient has certain symptoms because he has behaved disrespectfully toward the gods. The patient's response to this accusation reflects in part his degree of compliance and trust, as well as the extent to which he can be persuaded. Or the h'ilol may say that the illness stems from malevolent actions and inquire whom the patient has offended or antagonized—essentially forcing a confession to a past misdemeanor. This information is supposedly needed for a successful cure, and if the patient does not volunteer relevant information, he is viewed as lying about or denying aspects of his life. To the extent that in Zinacantan an illness state is held to be inseparable from its cause, he is also denying his illness.

During the diagnostic interview the topic of how the illness can be dealt with is discussed. The h'ilol may express his confidence that he can cure the illness and indicate a willingness to perform the ceremony. Or he may decide not to take on responsibility for the patient. If this is the case, he will state that the illness is difficult to cure, that it has no cure (he would tell this only to the patient's family), or that since he is inexperienced in dealing with this type of illness, another h'ilol should be consulted. The decision not to treat the patient is made when the h'ilol senses that the patient is moribund, when powerful witchcraft forces are suspected, or when the patient persists in his denial of past actions that the h'ilol believes are instrumental in having caused the illness. In some cases, the h'ilol may state that he is not available for a curing ceremony because of other commitments to his duties as h'ilol, family man, or farmer. Because the constraints that bind a h'ilol to a potential patient are rather loose and unstructured, h'iloletik are able to withdraw from those healing relationships that they judge for one reason or another not to be in their own best interests.

It should be emphasized that pulsing does not in itself commit the patient to perform a curing ceremony with the h'ilol who provides the diagnosis. In many cases (probably the majority) the patient does consult one h'ilol and has him perform whatever ceremony he prescribes. This is especially true when a Zinacanteco family maintains a long-term "family doctor" relationship with a single h'ilol, who is often a relative, close neighbor, or compadre. Not infrequently, however, the patient secures several diagnoses until he finds one that (a) conforms to his own preconceptions about the nature of his illness and/or (b) is consonant with the money and time he is willing to expend on the curing ceremony.

The objective reasons for a h'ilol's diagnosis are not completely understood at present; and the role that a patient's specific symptoms play is particularly unclear. We know, however, that the following considerations affect the diagnosis and treatment to some extent. First, the h'ilol can evaluate the general physical state of the patient, his degree of strength or weakness, and the toxicity and/or discomfort that is manifest. Second, the h'ilol learns the manner in which the illness has evolved or progressed. Symptoms that have evolved rapidly are designated by Tzotzil terms that differ from those used to designate symptoms that are slow and gradual in onset. Similarly, protracted illnesses (not improved despite previous treatment) and relapsing conditions seem to be attributed to malevolent sources and are denoted by still different terms. Finally, the h'ilol has information about the patient's social life. This can be derived from prior interactions with the patient, from hearsay and gossip, or from the content of dreams that the patient or h'ilol has recently experienced. The h'ilol's manner of presenting the diagnostic information appears to be influenced by his actual competence and experience, as well as by his interpersonal skills. He can either promote confidence or discourage the family's interest in using him in the ritual of treatment, and his attitude toward the patient and his family intimately affects the course of the treatment process.

The diagnostic visit lasts about half an hour. After talking with the patient and his family, the h'ilol may be asked to say a prayer for the patient and to suggest some herb that can be given to alleviate the symptoms; after this, he leaves. The patient and his family are left to think over the details and implications of what was discussed. The diagnostic session has involved both overt and covert activities of potential therapeutic significance, in the form of herbs, prayers, and various forms of sociopsychological persuasion; however, it is not considered a treatment in itself. The family must still decide whom to see or what to do for a cure. They have no obligation to use the same h'ilol for the actual cure; and they may in fact decide to ask another h'ilol for a new diagnosis, or go to San Cristóbal and consult a Ladino physician or druggist.

It is important to remember that ill health is one of the most critical events in the life of a Zinacanteco family. It can prompt many different actions, all aimed at gaining information and seeking protection. The choices that are made reflect not only the knowledge but also, and perhaps more importantly, the values of the patient and his family. The patient, for example, may improve spontaneously or as a result of medication prescribed by a physician or pharmacist. For all intents and purposes, he will then appear "normal" and be able to resume his usual duties and responsibilities. If he or his family attach meaning to traditional Zinacanteco medical practices, however, they will still seek a h'ilol to perform the recommended ceremony and complete the cure. For a Zinacanteco, "illness" is inseparably linked to its ultimate cause (usually supernatural), which can only be detected and cured by a h'ilol. Even though symptoms and signs disappear, the subjective sense of being sick persists as long as a ceremony is not performed.

If the family decides to ask the same h'ilol to treat the patient, they will send a representative to him within the next few days. After being offered a drink and talking with the visitor, the h'ilol is formally asked to perform a curing ceremony. (In some cases, this request is made during the actual diagnostic visit; however, we have no precise information on how frequently this occurs.) The h'ilol must now decide whether he wants to cure the patient. If he does, he gives the patient's family a list of items needed for the curing ceremony. Enumerating the types of curing ceremonies used in Zinacantan, and the preparations and requirements for each, is beyond the scope of this presentation. Suffice it to say that specific diagnoses of illness appear to be associated with distinct ceremonies, each ceremony requiring different preparations, expenses, and participants. The date chosen for the ceremony is usually only a few days away, depending on the h'ilol's current responsibilities, his judgment regarding the severity of the illness, and the family's finances.

After the ceremony. We will defer, for the moment, our description of an actual curing ceremony. The features that primitive curing ceremonies share with other specific therapeutic efforts (and with attempts at modifying behavior in general) have been reviewed in the literature (Frank, 1961; Kiev, 1964: 3–35). Holland (1963) has indicated that in the curing ceremonies of a related Maya group the healer takes an active, authoritarian role and manages to engage the patient emotionally. This process, as we shall see in Chapters 11 and 12, is substantially what one observes in Zinacantan. Using culturally sanctioned methods, the h'ilol often manages to restore the patient's sense of personal worth and change his psychosocial adjustment. When the ceremony ends, the family is left with instructions for the subsequent care of the patient: how he should be dressed, what food and medicine he should be given, how his activities should be restricted, and which ritual prayers have to be performed.

The h'ilol typically visits the family a few days after the ceremony to check on the condition of the patient. If this is unimproved or has worsened, the family may have asked the h'ilol to see the patient even earlier. At this follow-up visit, the h'ilol once again asks about the condition of the patient and offers new prayers. If necessary, he may perform a second pulsing and suggest a modification in the treatment plan (e.g., specific herbs or a new ceremony). The relationship between the h'ilol and the patient's family ends "naturally" when the patient recovers and is able to resume his usual duties; however, both parties are free to interrupt the relationship and the treatment contract at any period. If the patient's condition does not improve at all, either the h'ilol or the family is likely to suggest that a new treatment option be followed.

Pathophysiological processes with diverse long-range health consequences or prognostic implications may naturally underlie any particular cluster of symptoms for which help is sought. "Successful" ceremonies (in the sense that the patient feels relieved) are often applied to disease states that remain essentially unchanged biologically. Subsequent symptoms may then be defined as indications of a new illness; or they may reflect on the h'ilol's competence and induce the family to choose a new treatment option. The factors that associate with these differing interpretations are embedded in the interpersonal currents of the patient's transactions with the h'ilol, and in his relations with other Zinacantecos that he meets in his daily affairs. And the decision to continue with the same h'ilol under similar or changed premises also depends on essentially sociopsychological factors.

Implications of the Healing Process

We have viewed the process by which Zinacantecos receive treatment from h'iloletik as a series of graded transactions leading up to and receding from the curing ceremony. Each participant can interrupt the process at any stage, and Zinacantecos seem to make active use of this option. Both the patient's family and the h'ilol gain information about each other, and about the "illness" they are trying to cure, during each stage of the transactional process. The patient not only learns a particular perspective about his illness but also either gains or loses confidence in the ability of the h'ilol who is treating him; and at each stage the patient can be overtly or covertly encouraged or discouraged by the h'ilol. The h'ilol, in the meantime, has been gaining information about the illness itself and about the people with whom he has been dealing. In addition to intuitive judgments regarding prognosis, the patient's frankness, suggestibility, and morality play important roles in the h'ilol's decision to continue treatment.

Of course, the strictly medical tasks of the h'iloletik are only one dimension of their role in Zinacanteco society.* It has long been recognized that in folk or primitive communities the management of illness is accomplished in such a manner that other, and perhaps more important, social functions are also served (Ackerknecht, 1955; Fabrega and Metzger, 1968). In the case of the Chiapas highlanders the beliefs that explain illness, the social position of the practitioner, and the sanctions that he can use all enable him to modify and regulate the behavior of his clients in conformance with socially prescribed patterns (Fabrega et al., 1970). We will elaborate on this in Chapter 12. Here, we merely want to point out that it is possible, and to some extent valid, to say that the curing profession is one of several units involved in maintaining social control. (The increasing social disorganization of some Chiapas communities, which is reflected by a rising homicide rate, has been explained as stemming from the shamans' loss of power; this loss is believed to result from an increasing social awareness of alternative and better forms of medical care. See Nash, 1967.)

The salient characteristics of the manner in which medical care is traditionally delivered by h'iloletik in Zinacantan should be interpreted in the light of the broader functions that h'iloletik perform in the community. Medical care in Zinacantan is delivered through a series of particularistic social relationships, each of which is governed by reciprocally unstructured and fluid obligations. Such an open system of medical care delivery should not be interpreted merely as a result of the fact that medical functions are pursued in a context of inadequate or unsophisticated knowledge about disease. At this stage of our knowledge, the reasons for the existence of this particular system and the social functions that may be served by it cannot be precisely determined, but both probably involve strictly medical as well as nonmedical concerns. Generally speaking, just as this type of medical care can be seen as intrinsic to the type of social organization that has been classically associated with primitive communities, so it may also be viewed as a concomitant of the social changes that have taken place in Zinacantan as a result of contact with Spanish-Mexican culture.

The fact that Zinacantan, like other Maya communities in the region, has undergone substantial change as a result of continued contact with Spanish-Mexican culture is clearly reflected in the way many Zinacanteco

* For a point-by-point comparison of the h'ilol's actions and influences with those of a Western physician, see Chapter 12.

families use the traditional medical system. Medical information that the family obtains from the hʻilol is compared not only with similar types of information gained from other hʻiloletik (in the recent or remote past), but also with information obtained from spiritualists, pharmacists, friends, and in some cases Ladino physicians. It is likely that the patient and his family will be engaged in several of these medical transactions at the same time. The decision to continue treatment with a particular hʻilol depends on a continuous evaluation of his success in the light of these other transactions, as well as on the current resources of the family.

Chapter ten

Ceremonies Performed by H'iloletik

THE REGULARLY SCHEDULED public ceremonies performed by male h'iloletik, like the private curing ceremonies, are composed of certain basic ritual sequences, extended and expanded at each higher level of ceremonial complexity. These fundamental sequences are: the assembly, preparation, and sanctification of ritual materials; the performance of ceremonial music; the serving of ritual meals; the decoration of crosses; and the lighting of candles at crosses marking *ch'ul vinaheletik* (places of access to the Totilme'iletik). Each of these activities incorporates certain other pervasive ritual elements—the ceremonial drinking of rum, the firing of mortars and rockets to mark transitions from one phase of the ceremony to the next, ceremonial processions, and the like.

K'in Krus for the Sna and the Waterhole Group

The township ceremony of K'in Krus takes place twice a year, once in May around the time of the Catholic feast of Santa Cruz de Mayo, and again in October. At these times, smaller ceremonies of a very similar nature are held for snas and waterhole groups. Vogt (1965a) has described an ideal pattern in which each sna and each waterhole group holds a separate ceremony. But in many parts of Zinacantan only one ceremony takes place, usually on the level of the waterhole group. This will of course happen wherever the sna and waterhole group are coterminous. It appears to apply more generally in some hamlets. 'Apas, for example, has no K'in Krus ceremonies on the sna or waterhole-group level, but performs two hamlet-wide ceremonies a year. Paste', on the other hand, has no hamlet-level ceremonies but does have the sna and waterhole-group rites described by Vogt.

Meadow (1965) suggests that the differences between Paste' and 'Apas may be due to differences in size. The much greater size and territorial dispersion of Paste' increases the integrative value of localized sna and waterhole-group ceremonies. 'Apas, being small and compact, can encompass ceremonies at the communal level. Another factor may be a decrease in residential stability (evident in Hteklum), which tends to reduce the significance of the sna as a unit of social organization. In Navenchauk, finally, where K'in Krus ceremonies appear to be held only on the waterhole-group level, the very supply of water may be an important factor. Navenchauk is liberally supplied with natural and man-made wells, and no one waterhole is used by more than a few families; hence the sna and the waterhole group may tend to merge.

The situation, then, is quite variable. Some Zinacanteco families participate in four ceremonies annually (two each for their sna and their waterhole group), some in two, and some (e.g., residents of 'Apas) contribute financially to hamlet ceremonies but are unlikely to participate closely in them.

K'in Krus means "Fiesta of the Cross" and involves the ceremonial demarcation of the territories controlled by the members of the social unit sponsoring the ceremony. This is accomplished by conducting a ceremonial pilgrimage around the territory, visiting its sacred places— waterholes, mountains containing Totilme'iletik, and other shrines, each marked with a cross symbolizing an entrance to communication with the spirit world. The ceremony described below is that for a waterhole group; the sna and hamlet ceremonies, respectively, are simpler and more complicated versions of the same basic patterns.

The responsibility for providing the materials for the K'in Krus belongs to the *mayordomo,* a position that circulates in turn among all the male household heads in the waterhole group. The mayordomo also holds the first and final stages of the ceremony in his house. In some groups the expenses of the ceremony are shared at large, the mayordomo taking responsibility for collecting the money and purchasing the ritual items (candles, incense, skyrockets, rum, flowers, chickens, and corn to make tortillas). In other groups the expenses are borne primarily by the mayordomo himself. The system equalizes itself in the end, since the office rotates; but it may impose a heavy burden at any one time.*

---

* The expense can be illustrated by the actions of Domingo, one of the Harvard Chiapas Project's chief informants. In 1964 he suddenly dug a well in his sitio,

In ʻApas, where the ceremony is held only at the hamlet level, several elders, called *moletik*, manage all the fiestas and are in charge of levying a public subscription for each ceremony.

Whether or not he finances the fiesta himself, the mayordomo always devotes considerable time and effort to it. His wife, assisted by the other women of the group, undertakes the preparation of the food to be consumed in the course of the ceremony. The women start grinding corn for tortillas many hours—even days—before the event, prepare the special delicacies associated with Kʻin Krus (*atole*, a sweet thick beverage made from ground corn, sugar, and water; and *botil*, large red beans), and make ready the meat for the meals.

The initial stage of the fiesta takes place at the house of the mayordomo. If there are two mayordomos (as described by Vogt, 1964), this activity presumably takes place in the house of the senior one. In the ceremonies we observed, there was only one mayordomo.

The ceremony is conducted by either a group of hʻiloletik or a single hʻilol, depending on local practice. Whenever possible, the hʻilol is a member of the sponsoring group. Few groups are without a hʻilol (at least on the level of the waterhole group), but most undoubtedly perform the ceremony with only one. Besides the hʻilol and the incumbent mayordomo(s), the ceremony involves the mayordomo for the coming year and a variety of assistants and musicians. There are three musicians, playing the violin, the harp, and the guitar (always regarded and arranged in that order of ceremonial importance),* and set arrangements of musical passages are played at specified times throughout the cere-

---

having learned that he was to be named mayordomo of his waterhole two years later. He was thus prepared, when the time came for a deputation of neighbors to officially inform him of his appointment, to refuse on the grounds that he had his own waterhole and was no longer a member of the waterhole group. He successfully remained aloof from that year's Kʻin Krus; whether he can maintain his position indefinitely remains to be seen. The economic calculations behind the action were astute: the well, though expensive, was a one-shot operation, whereas Domingo could expect to be named mayordomo several times in his life; the immediate expense of the well was less than the long-term cost of remaining in the waterhole group.

* The native instruments bear a superficial resemblance to their Western counterparts but are very different musically. The violin, for example, has three pegs but only two strings. The harp is about the size of an Irish harp and has over forty pegs, but only half of these are strung. The music itself should be studied by an ethnomusicologist. To the untrained listener it sounds like the same short tune played over and over; to Zinacantecos, however, it is a series of distinct "songs" or passages arranged in definite patterns. (Vogt, 1969, reports that the ceremonies also involve a second group of musicians, who play flutes and drums.)

monial sequence. Other assistants perform the same functions as assistants at a curing ceremony. They carry the bulk of the ritual materials, attach pine boughs and flowers to the crosses, prepare the areas in front of the crosses with pine needles and rose petals, pour drinks, fire off powder charges and fireworks, etc. The role of women in the K'in Krus is limited to preparing the food, and they do not take part in the pilgrimage around the sacred places.

The ceremony has three phases: a ritual at the house of the mayordomo, a pilgrimage around the group's lands, and a final ritual at the mayordomo's.

The initial ceremonies. The participants assemble in the mayordomo's house, bringing with them the ritual materials. The h'ilol then prepares an altar by taking a low wooden table and orienting its long axis east-west. He covers the table with the *mantresh,* a woven ritual cloth; it is white with red stripes, which are also oriented east-west. The other ritual objects are arranged on and around the table. The candles are laid with wicks pointing east. Beside the table are a basket of red geraniums (*tsahal nichim*), a basket of incense wood (*te'el pom*) with a small paper of copal incense (*bek'tal pom*), and a smaller basket of pink roses.

The h'ilol seats himself on a low chair at the west end of the table and lights an incense burner, which he places on the floor near him. Around the edges of the room, on chairs or benches, sit the men of the group. Women, as always, sit on the floor, clustered around the grinding stones and fire, patting out tortillas, and chattering busily, apparently oblivious to the ceremony. Against the wall are seated the three musicians—from left to right, violin, harp, and guitar.

The h'ilol arranges several small bunches of red geraniums on top of the candles, censes them with the incense burner, and prays over them at length. Several of the key participants (in the ceremonies we observed, the incumbent and future mayordomos) then kneel at the west end of the table, cross themselves, and pray over the candles. Following the mayordomo's salutation of the candles (*nup kantela*), the h'ilol prepares the materials to be taken on the ceremonial circuit. He takes the requisite number of candles for each sacred place (usually three) and stands them upright in the center of the basket of red geraniums, naming the place for which each group is destined.

After arranging the candles and other materials, the h'ilol proceeds to the patio cross of the the household. The assistants decorate the cross with pine boughs and flowers, sprinkling the ground in front of it with pine needles and rose petals. The back and sides of the cross are protected with *petates* (woven mats) attached to poles driven in the ground. The h'ilol places candles before the cross, lights them, and prays. Drinks are served, fireworks are let off, and the men return to the house for a ritual meal.

Throughout this sequence of events that has been sketched certain ritual behavior recurs periodically. The most important is the ritual drinking of rum. (Drinking behavior is described in detail in Appendix D.) Rounds of drinks punctuate each of the curer's prayers (usually three rounds per prayer) and mark the beginning and end of each ritual sequence.

The firing of skyrockets and the *kamaro*, or mortar, also signals the completion of an important phase of the ceremony and/or the transition from one activity to the next. The skyrockets (*cohetes*), always of Ladino manufacture (see Goldberg, 1961), are cardboard tubes attached to long sticks. They are held in the hand and ignited with the end of a cigarette. The rocket shoots into the air with a characteristic hiss and explodes with a sharp pop. The kamaro is a small iron mortar 4–6 inches in length and perhaps 3 inches in diameter. It is filled with black powder and touched off through a small fuse-hole in the side. The firer holds the kamaro at arm's length, puts a finger in his ear, and awaits the shock, which can be truly formidable—especially when the mortar is fired in a narrow mountain gorge.

Finally, each segment of the K'in Krus is accompanied by the playing and singing (both done by the musicians) of ritual songs. This music is highly patterned, and the same set sequence of pieces is played at each event.

The ceremonial circuit. When the meal is over the ritual materials are loaded into nets to be carried on tumplines by assistants. The men line up in ceremonial order (h'ilol last, others in order of seniority with the most junior at the front), kneel at the table and hearth to cross themselves, and file out.

The ceremonial group proceeds counterclockwise around the lands belonging to the group, stopping at waterholes and other sacred localities marked with crosses. One party we observed, the waterhole group of Shun Vaskis of Navenchauk, stopped at about ten places—five of them crosses in the mountains and the rest waterholes. The hamlet of

'Apas has 33 sacred places (Meadow, 1965) that are visited during the communal ceremony. Sacred localities are believed to be doorways to the spirit world, either to the ancestral spirits within the mountains or to the demons underground. Typically, they are outstanding topographical features, especially caves, large extrusions of rock on mountainsides, and waterholes.

At each cross the ritual performed is virtually identical to that performed at the patio cross. The assistants prepare the crosses with pine boughs and red geraniums (sometimes this is done in advance), sprinkling the ground in front of them with pine needles and rose petals. The h'ilol kneels before the cross, places in front of him the incense burner (which has been carried by one of the assistants in the ceremonial procession), and prays. He lights candles in front of the cross, sometimes placing them in small pits to protect them from the wind. The lighting of the candles and the h'ilol's prayers are accompanied by music; after he finishes, the music ends, and then, after a brief pause, an entire musical sequence is repeated. Rounds of drinks are served throughout, and fireworks are let off. When the musicians finish, the party reforms in order of seniority and proceeds to the next cross.

The circuit terminates at the group's own waterhole, where the crosses are decorated and candles lit in the usual fashion. The procession then passes to the house of the entering mayordomo, and his patio cross is decorated. The party is entertained by the incoming mayordomo and his wife, and is given coffee mixed with rum to drink. The musicians play, and most of the men dance, shuffling from one foot to the other in time to the music.

After a period of dancing and informal relaxation, the party returns to the house of the incumbent mayordomo. Another meal is served, and the ceremony ends, the entire ritual sequence having taken some 6–8 hours.

Year Renewal Ceremonies for the Municipio and Hamlets

Ceremonies similar to the K'in Krus in form, although on a larger scale, are held to mark the beginning, middle, and end of the year. At *ach' habil, 'olol habil,* and *slaheb habil*—"new year," "midyear," and "year-end"—ceremonies are performed in Hteklum. These rites involve a ceremonial circuit of all the sacred places in and around the valley of

Hteklum—churches, sacred mountains, and sacred waterholes (the sacred places in Hteklum are described in Appendix D).

Besides sending representatives to Hteklum three times a year, the h'iloletik of the different hamlets mark the Year Renewal ceremonies themselves in various ways. In some hamlets all the h'iloletik join for a ceremony twice a year. A very few hamlets possibly hold no ceremony at all. The hamlet ceremony, too, consists of a ceremonial circuit of the major sacred places in Hteklum.

The Year Renewal ceremonies for the municipio are under the supervision of the Bankilal H'ilol of the valley of Hteklum, who initiates the preparations by approaching the authorities to secure an order for a public tax to underwrite the costs of the ceremony. An order is also sent to the Bankilal H'ilol of each hamlet, requesting him to send representatives to Hteklum on the appointed date. These representatives are usually the most junior h'iloletik in the hamlet.

A group of h'iloletik are sent to San Cristóbal to buy the materials for the ceremony—candles, fireworks, incense, and food. At the designated time the participants assemble at the house of the Muk'ta Alkalte, the highest official in the cargo hierarchy. The collaboration between the Bankilal H'ilol and the Muk'ta Alkalte in the management of these ceremonies, and the joint involvement in them of shamans and cargo holders, are the major points of contact between the two systems.

The ceremony itself closely resembles the K'in Krus. After preparations and a meal in the house of the Muk'ta Alkalte, the h'iloletik are divided into groups, each assigned to travel to particular sacred localities. At each shrine the crosses are decorated, candles lit, prayers said, and so on. The senior h'iloletik and cargo officials remain behind and spend the time praying in the house of the Muk'ta Alkalte and at Kalvario (see Appendix D). On the return of the junior h'iloletik more prayers are said, and the ceremony ends after the entire party has eaten another ritual meal.

Extraordinary Ceremonies

In addition to the regularly scheduled public ceremonies, there are occasional extraordinary ceremonies, directed either at the prevention of an epidemic or at the relief of drought.

If a h'ilol has a vision in which serious, contagious illness threatens the entire municipio or a part thereof, he has the right to approach the authorities and his fellow h'iloletik in the attempt to organize a public ceremony.* Such alarms do not occur frequently, but informants report them in the recent past. No set form seems to be prescribed for a mass curing ceremony, but it undoubtedly resembles the Year Renewal ceremonies. It is obvious that such a public endeavor, involving the services of many h'iloletik and financed by a public levy, can only be initiated by a h'ilol whose visionary powers are highly respected.

Rainmaking ceremonies are known to occur with some frequency (Vogt, 1965a), but they are not a regular part of the ceremonial calendar. Our informants state that this ceremony is the exclusive property of a single old h'ilol from Nachih and dates back some twenty years. At that time the h'ilol had a vision in which the Totilme'iletik instructed him to perform such a ceremony—involving a pilgrimage to the mountain 'Its'-inal Muk'ta Vits to the southeast of the town of Teopisca—in order to relieve a drought. Since then, he and a group of his associates have performed the ceremony, with the permission of the authorities, whenever necessary. It is not known whether this mountain, widely separated as it is from the other sacred localities of the Zinacantecos, had any ritual importance before the vision that initiated the rainmaking ceremony.

Curing Ceremonies

Any attempt at the systematic classification of Zinacanteco curing ceremonies founders on the same difficulties that we encountered in classifying illnesses: the great extent of variation in informants' responses; and the innate variability of the system, which makes it difficult for even a single informant to offer a rigorous classification.

This is not true of the public ceremonies performed by h'iloletik. These are named and clearly describable, and they generally take place without great variation (at least within the same hamlet; there are some important differences between hamlets). In this they resemble cargo rituals more than curing ceremonies. The lack of variability in these ceremonies is

* These visions of illness are perhaps one of the reasons for the Tzotzil term h'ilol, which literally means "one who sees." The vision is related to the kind of illness that threatens. A forest fire, for example, portends an onslaught of contagious fevers. Human figures in the vision, which often appear in the costumes of clowns like those who dance at Zinacanteco fiestas, are really *pukuhetik*, or demons. One of the most interesting of these is the Yahval Kuyel ("proprietor of smallpox"). This figure looks like the Ladino doctor who occasionally gives smallpox vaccinations in Zinacantan, and his appearance in a curer's dream is a warning of smallpox.

almost certainly related to their public nature: since many h'iloletik must cooperate in performing the ceremony, a fair degree of consensus on its form is necessary; and from the layman's point of view, the opportunity to observe many such ceremonies probably tends to develop stricter ideas of their proper form. The private ceremonies are subject to no such generally held notions of proper procedure.

Unlike the public ceremonies, whose form is entrusted to the body of h'iloletik on behalf of the general public, the private ceremonies are individually revealed to each h'ilol in his encounters with the Totilme'il-etik, and any variations he wishes to introduce can be attributed to divine revelation. This is all, of course, in the theory of the system. In practice, a number of factors limit variation. One is inertia—or more precisely, a general tendency toward regularity and conformity that we observe in Zinacantan and the Chiapas highlands in general. Another is the fact that this native system, like all ritual systems, is based on a set of concepts and symbols that are themselves relatively invariable. Any variation arises from the manipulation of ritual symbols and materials that are shared by all Zinacantecos. These are patterned according to certain principles of organization, which again are part of the underlying conceptual substratum. The ritual elements—e.g., lighting candles, bathing, and killing chickens—are the equivalent of a vocabulary, and the basic patterns of organization resemble a syntax. The ceremonial expressions that result from the interaction of the two are similar to the sentences of a language in their combination of patterning and variability.

Another limit on variation is acceptability. Each Zinacanteco, to be sure, has his own conception of the proper form of a curing ceremony, and he typically allows a certain latitude to the h'ilol. This is not boundless, however. Extremely deviant procedures are likely to be unacceptable to a curer's patients and may lose him his practice. The extent of acceptable variation depends heavily on factors of success and reputation; a h'ilol who is reputed to have strong antiwitchcraft powers can generally introduce greater variation into his procedures than the ordinary h'ilol.

The classification of private curing ceremonies, then, is vague and irregular. There are many more recognizable types of ceremonies than there are names, and there are many more distinct ceremonies actually performed than can either be assigned names or classified into types.

A list of eight general "curing sequences" has been published by Vogt (1965a). These are, in paraphrase:

(1) K'oplael. A brief ritual consisting of pulsing, prayer, and the administration of simple remedies. The name means "saying words."

(2) Lok'esel ta Balamil. "Extracting from the earth." The recovery of parts of the soul lost in the earth.

(3) Hok'nanehbail. "To arrange things." A ceremonial circuit in Hteklum, intended to restore good relationships between a family and the Totilme'iletik.

(4) Muk'ta 'Ilel or Muk'ta Nichim. "Big seeing" or "big flowers." A major ceremony involving pilgrimages to all the sacred mountains and churches in Hteklum. (See Chapter 11.)

(5) 'O'lol Nichim. "Half flower." The same as Muk'ta 'Ilel, but visiting only two mountains.

(6) Pertonal. "Pardon." An antiwitchcraft procedure designed to reconcile quarreling members of a family.

(7) Sa'el Hch'uleltik ta Balamil. "Searching for our *ch'ulel* in the earth." A ceremony in which the h'ilol visits caves and other places where he can communicate with Yahval Balamil and ransom a soul that has been sold to the earth.

(8) Chonel ta Balamil. "Selling to the earth." A "bad" ritual procedure involving the sale of someone else's soul to Yahval Balamil.

This list can be somewhat modified in the light of later fieldwork. On the basis of our own data, we would drop sequence 3, Hok'nanehbail, since we have not encountered the term in any of our own interviews. It may well be a legitimate Tzotzil term designating this kind of ceremony, but it is probably not in common use. We might most usefully regard all these ceremonies as a single general pattern, comprising visits to the mountains and churches in Hteklum, that can have various purposes—the treatment of illness, the reconciliation of quarreling kinsmen, or the improvement of a family's relations with the Totilme'iletik.

The final term, Chonel ta Balamil, must be discarded from any classification of curing ceremonies. It is clearly and unambiguously a maleficent witchcraft procedure that has no direct connection with curing ritual as such, except in those instances when a cure requires sending illness to others. Some Zinacantecos, to be sure, believe that only h'iloletik can perform this kind of witchcraft; but little purpose is served by grouping it with procedures that are otherwise therapeutic, since doing so violates the broad principles of classification that the informants themselves lay down.

Aside from a small number of terms that seem to be used by most Zinacantecos to designate recognizable complexes of ceremonial procedure, general rubrics and classifications differ from informant to informant. The terms on which there is little variation are *pik ch'ich'* (pulsing), Muk'ta 'Ilel, 'O'lol Nichim, K'oplael, and Lok'esel ta Balamil. Grouping these is a problem. The best that we can offer are the following statements, a combination of grouping and distinguishing principles advanced by a number of informants.

(1) The basic diagnostic procedure in all cases of illness is pulsing. This can be assumed as a feature of every ceremonial type; or, if one prefers to consider it a distinct ritual procedure, may stand outside the rest of the system.

(2) A basic distinction can be made between "good" and "bad" ceremonies. The term *alel vokol* ("asking pardon") is a general rubric for curing ceremonies, but seems restricted in its application to nonwitchcraft ceremonies, which are described as *tuk'il alel vokol* or *lekil alel vokol*. This class is opposed to a class of ceremonies involving witchcraft, but there is no term of equivalent status to describe the latter. The best that we were able to elicit was the phrase *skuenta 'ak' chamel*, meaning "on account of witchcraft." The division between the two classes is by no means sharp, and certain ceremonies can be purely innocent or may at times embody antiwitchcraft procedures that are of doubtful status. An example is the Pertonal sequence, which can be either good or bad. In the terminology advanced by Domingo de la Torre Pérez, one of our principal informants, it is necessary to classify Pertonal on the borderline when the ceremony involves a visit to Hteklum (Domingo calls it an *alel vokol* but indicates that it has suspicious elements); however, the ceremony of the same name that is held entirely in the house (also known as Valk'unel, "throwing back") is unequivocally witchcraft.

(3) The class of good ceremonies includes: K'oplael, consisting of simple prayers only; 'Och ta Svolim, a set of ceremonial variations involving the decoration of the patient's bed with flowers and a ceremonial circuit in Hteklum; and Solel Kantela, a set of procedures essentially the same as 'Och ta Svolim but without decoration of the patient's bed. 'Och ta Svolim can involve any number of mountains and churches. In its maximal extent, with four mountains and three churches, it is called

Muk'ta 'Ilel or Muk'ta Nichim. With two mountains and three churches it is sometimes called 'O'lol Nichim. The other variants seem to have no names. Solel Kantela can also involve any number of mountains and churches. Either 'Och ta Svolim or Solel Kantela can serve, with minor modifications, as a ceremony for the inauguration of a new h'ilol.

(4) The second major division of curing ceremonies incorporates all procedures that are "on account of witchcraft," and that are considered dangerous and evil because their antiwitchcraft procedures may involve turning illness on to others. There are three named procedures in this group that actually seem to occur (as opposed to witchcraft sequences for which we have descriptions but whose actual occurrence seems unlikely) and to follow some regular pattern. First, there are the two kinds of Pertonal, which we have already mentioned. Second, there is Sa'el Hch'uleltik ta Balamil, the recovery of a soul sold to Yahval Balamil by a witch.

In addition to these procedures, there are other, unnamed, ceremonies concocted by h'iloletik to meet various situations. As will become clear in Chapter 11, the formal description of named, standardized ceremonial types is only a beginning to describing what actually takes place in Zinacanteco curing.

Chapter eleven

The Private Ceremonies

ZINACANTECO CURING RITUALS are made up of constituent elements that are individually easier to name and describe with some degree of regularity than are the ceremonial patterns into which they are combined. This chapter, therefore, describes these elements as they occur in one of the major extended ceremonial patterns, Muk'ta 'Ilel. Other patterns are sketched with reference to Muk'ta 'Ilel as a prototypical curing ceremony.

It is the conceptual aspect—what Zinacanteco informants say about the proper form of these ceremonies—that is of primary interest here. The description of Muk'ta 'Ilel, therefore, has been taken from formal texts on curing ceremonies written by two informants: Mariano (Anselmo) Pérez, a young h'ilol, and Domingo de la Torre Pérez, a layman. We have augmented their accounts with our own observations of additional details that seem important for one reason or another. The informants' statements about the religious significance of various parts of the ceremony have been included wherever possible; these may represent the opinions of only a handful of informants, but we feel that the concepts we have included are in fact widely held in Zinacantan.

More detailed information on ritual materials and localities, including maps of sacred places and diagrams of the interiors of the churches, will be found in Appendix D, which also includes descriptions of certain basic ceremonial procedures, such as the ritual meal, that are common to most or all curing ceremonies but too lengthy to include in the already cumbersome description of Muk'ta 'Ilel. In Appendix E we offer the texts of typical prayers used in curing rituals.

Muk'ta 'Ilel

Of the ceremonies that can be classed under the rubric *tuk'il alel vokol* ("good" curing ceremony) and are performed for someone who is in a state of chamel, or illness, the largest is Muk'ta 'Ilel, the "Big Seeing." It is alternatively called Muk'ta Nichim, "Big Flowers." The entire class of ceremonies in which flowers are used to decorate the patient's bed can be referred to as 'Och ta Svolim, or Flower Ceremonies. Some Zinacantecos classify Muk'ta 'Ilel separately from Lok'esel ta Balamil, a sequence used to recover lost parts of the soul. Others consider Lok'esel ta Balamil an optional feature of Flower Ceremonies that can be performed or not according to necessity. In terms of the form of the ceremony, the sequence of events performed for a patient who has suffered soul-loss is basically a Flower Ceremony with the addition of certain clearly demarcated sequences.

To the observer, indeed, all Zinacanteco curing ceremonies look like variations on a theme; and it is possible to describe them in terms of a general ceremonial pattern into which certain optional procedures can be inserted at designated points to suit different diagnostic necessities. Zinacanteco informants, generally speaking, do not seem to apply this system of organization to the entire set of ceremonies, although some do to parts of it. For this reason, we have chosen not to compress the entire range of curing ceremonies into a single description. A reasonably detailed picture of Muk'ta 'Ilel will cover most, if not all, sequences of activity that occur in Zinacanteco curing ceremonies; our description of other ceremonies will be confined to showing how the elements already described in detail are rearranged and modified.

Our description includes both the informants' concepts of the proper form of the ceremony and our own observations of the actual forms followed in a sample of these ceremonies. Any statement in brackets is based on our own observations or on interviews with various informants. Statements without brackets are taken with little change from the formal texts on curing ceremonies volunteered by two informants. (Certain important sequences of behavior of particular interest are detailed in Appendix D.)

(1) *Finding a h'ilol*. The patient first seeks out a h'ilol, who pulses him to determine the nature of the illness and the steps necessary to cure it. The h'ilol tells the patient and his family how many mountains and

churches will be visited in the course of the ceremony and what quantities of the various ritual materials will be needed. The patient and the
h'ilol set a time for the ceremony and agree that someone will be sent
to fetch the h'ilol at the proper time.

(2) *Preparations.* [The patient and his family now prepare for the
ceremony, recruiting help and procuring the ritual materials. Four male
assistants (*hch'omiletik*) are recruited from the patient's immediate
family, or from more distant relatives, neighbors, and friends. Four or
more women are also sought to help prepare food and to wash the patient's clothing. These may be the wives of the male assistants, other
female relatives, neighbors, or friends. The assistants assemble at the
patient's house early on the morning of the ceremony.]

When the assistants arrive at the patient's house they immediately go
to collect the sacred water, one gourd full from each of seven waterholes.
[See Appendix D. The number of gourds of water used in the ceremony
and the waterholes from which they are drawn is a major point of variation among curers. In ceremonies we observed, the number ran from
four to seven. In all cases where less than seven waterholes are used,
however, the water is still drawn from some of the seven sacred waterholes.] Only the male assistants go to collect the water. On returning to
the house, they put the gourds of water in the corner of the house that
faces the head of the patient's bed. [In the ceremonies observed, and
in descriptions given by other h'iloletik, the gourds, as well as the black
chicken used as the patient's substitute, were kept under the bed until
they were needed in the ceremony. The bed itself, in this and other
ceremonies, has previously been enclosed with a rough wooden fence
about 5 feet high.]

After placing the gourds in the corner, the assistants eat a meal. When
they finish they get ready to go into the countryside. They take with
them two sacks for the flowers and pine needles, machetes, and a bottle
of rum to drink when they finish gathering the plants. They take *pozol*
(ground corn mixed with water) and tortillas to eat. The assistants
gather the following plants:

13 *krus 'ech'* (an air plant) for the crosses and bed
15 *ni ahan toh* (pine branch tips) to use in the mountains and at the
    patio cross
13 *ni ahan toh* to be used in the bed
13 *vohton 'ech'* (another air plant)

3 *ni bats'i toh* (tips of another kind of pine) to be used with the substitute at Kalvario

1 net of *tsis' 'uch* (laurel)

1 half-sack or more of pine needles

1 large bunch of *ahate'es* (myrtle)

1 small bunch of *vishob takil*, to be used in bathing the patient

13 *k'os*

13 *tilil*

[In addition one of the female assistants is sent to buy red geraniums (*tsahal nichim*), usually two baskets full. The *k'os* may either be sought in the mountains by the male assistants or purchased by the woman who buys the geraniums.]

The women remain in the house and grind corn for tortillas, except for three. One goes to purchase the geraniums. One or two others go to Ni Nab Chilo' [a waterhole near Kalvario] to wash the patient's clothing; these women are called *h'ukumaheletik*. They must be older women without infant children, for if one of them were to take an infant with her to Ni Nab Chilo', the child would be in grave danger of *mahbenal*, blows from the Totilme'iletik, because his blood is still too weak. [This belief seems to reflect a general association of danger with sacred situations. Contacting any supernatural forces is potentially dangerous to anyone whose vital forces are not fully developed or are weakened. Thus the patient, who is feeble both in body and soul, must take extraordinary precautions. In the curing ceremony, his contact with the spirit world begins with the arrival of the assistants and the commencement of preparations for the ceremony. From then until the end of the ceremonial taboo period some two weeks later he must avoid any activity that might attract the attention of the Totilme'iletik or of demons. He does not go outdoors alone; he talks little and in a subdued voice, and he is never left alone or in the dark, for fear of attack by demons. A child, whose soul is not firmly placed, is in particular danger, even if he is not the patient.]

The women wash a complete set of the patient's clothing, using *amole* [soap root] instead of soap. Amole is used because the odor of soap is offensive to the Totilme'iletik and would provoke them to punish the patient. In addition to the patient's clothing, the women take with them a gourd to bring home water for the patient's bath, food for their meals, and some rum. When the washing is finished, they eat eggs and tortillas and drink the rum. If they meet other h'ukumaheletik, each woman exchanges one egg, two tortillas, and a shot of rum with every other woman. After washing the clothing, the women return to the patient's house and hang the clothes to dry in the patio. While the women are washing, the patient must stay in the house and cannot go outdoors alone. He is susceptible to mahbenal because the gourds of sacred water are already in the house.

One or two men are sent to San Cristóbal to buy candles for the ceremony. If the patient has not been able to procure chickens for the ritual meals and pork is to be served instead, two men go, one to carry the candles and the other to carry the meat and the *kashlan vah* [Ladino bread] used at the ceremony. The number of candles bought depends on the h'ilol's dictates. Along with the candles the assistant usually buys the two kinds of incense used in the ceremony: *bek'tal pom*, the solidified resin of the incense tree, and *te'el pom*, chips of incense wood.

When the men return from looking for the flowers, they go to sweep the crosses. They prepare each shrine by removing the dried pine needles in front of the cross and replacing them with fresh needles. Four sweepers go to Hteklum, each taking care of one mountain. Each carries a cuarta of rum, which he drinks after changing the needles. If the sweepers encounter other sweepers or a curing party, toasts are exchanged with each person. When the sweepers and all the other assistants return to the patient's house they eat a meal.

[This completes the preparatory stage of the ceremony. In addition to the preparations made by the various assistants, some things will have been made ready by the patient's family beforehand. These include the purchase of two black chickens of the same sex as the patient, the construction of an enclosure around the patient's bed, and preparations for the ritual meals.]

(3) *Fetching the h'ilol.* When the group has finished eating, someone goes to fetch the h'ilol, taking a límete of rum [a bottle about four times the size of a small beer bottle] and two 20 ct. pieces of kashlan vah. Some people also take a bottle of coffee, and more kashlan vah. On entering the h'ilol's house, the messenger places the bottle of rum in front of the h'ilol. The h'ilol prays to the Totilme'iletik, and then he and the messenger drink the liquor. When they finish, the h'ilol prepares his things: the *bish*, his bamboo staff of office; and the *shakitail* or *bats'i chamaroil*, a red-trimmed black blanket that is worn poncho-style while

the h'ilol is praying. [This is the same as the blanket of a mayordomo in the cargo system.] A h'ilol uses a staff and robe only if he has participated with other h'iloletik in the Year Renewal ceremonies. He does not use them before that for fear that other h'iloletik will notice, accuse him of merely robbing other people of chickens to eat, and force him to participate in subsequent Year Renewal ceremonies.

The messenger and the h'ilol cross themselves at the h'ilol's patio cross and then go to the patient's house. Meanwhile, the assistants left at the house place a table with its long axis oriented east-west and place on it a bundle of all the candles, wicks pointing east. They split the pieces of incense wood. When the h'ilol is near, the messenger runs ahead to tell the household, at which point two incense burners are prepared. One is put in front of the patio, the other at the foot of the table.

(4) *Arrival of the h'ilol.* When the h'ilol arrives at the patient's house, he first stops at the patio cross and crosses himself. Then he speaks to the people and enters the house. [The h'ilol offers and receives the customary polite salutations when entering the house.] When he finishes greeting the people, he crosses himself at the table where the candles are, kneels there, and prays. Then he salutes the people. [He exchanges bowing and releasing gestures with everyone present. The junior individual always initiates the behavior by bowing his head and leaving it bent until released by touch from the back of the other person's hand. The Tzotzil term for bowing is *-nup k'obol,* "he bows," and *-nup -ba sk'ob,* "to release" (e.g., *snupbe sk'ob li vinike,* "he releases the man").] From the moment the h'ilol enters the house, the male attendants can no longer properly be called hch'omiletik; they are now *mayoletik.*

(5) *The h'ilol inspects the candles.* After the bowing and releasing, the h'ilol seats himself at the table and checks the candles and other materials. A round of drinks is served.

[The h'ilol puts a woven straw mat (*pop*) on the floor between the foot of the table and his chair and has the various ritual materials arranged on the mat, on the table, and at the sides of the table. The arrangement varies from curer to curer. The table is covered with the mantresh, a red-striped white cotton cloth, the stripes running east-west. The candles are always laid on top of the table parallel to the long axis and with their wicks pointing east. The incense burner stands at the foot of the table, usually close to the curer's right foot. The various plant materials are placed on the mat and around the table, in separate piles with the heads of the plants pointing east. The gourds of water are lined up on the floor at the sides of the table. The arrangement described by one informant is shown in Figure 4. The patio cross is then decorated and an incense burner placed there, if this has not been done on the h'ilol's approach to the house.

[After arranging the ritual materials, the h'ilol goes through a series of ritual sequences whose order seems to be somewhat variable. We give the sequence reported by our two chief informants, but have observed others. The censing of flowers and other materials always comes first; but the other procedures, up to the saluting of the candles, may come in any order. Each procedure, it should be noted, is punctuated with rounds of rum. The h'ilol's prayers are accompanied by rounds at the beginning, middle, and end of each; and for rounds during the course of the prayer the h'ilol interrupts his chanting to bless the liquor and to exchange bows with the members of the party as they down their drinks.

[Two kinds of behavior that are often observed should also be mentioned here. One is a complex series of bowing and releasing exchanges, accompanied by rapid ritualized speech, in which every member of the family engages every other in turn. It looks very much like the Pertonal sequence for conciliating domestic quarrels, without the toasting and exchange of bottles of liquor, and may be a minor conciliatory sequence introduced at the h'ilol's behest. The second behavior occurs when the

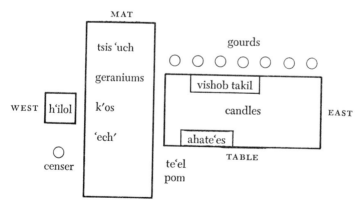

Figure 4. Arrangement of candles and plants for a
curing ceremony.

candles are saluted. As the h'ilol is about to begin his prayer he engages in bowing and releasing exchanges with each member of the party. He says, "I am going to salute the candles," and is answered, "Salute the candles!" The same exchange goes on between all members of the party when it is time for each person to salute the candles.]

(6) *The h'ilol prepares the plants and the bed.* The h'ilol assembles the bunches of plants, using one or a few of each kind of plant. These are tied together with strips of palm leaf by one of the mayoletik and are held by another. The bundles for the bed are composed of pine tips, laurel, and red geraniums. Twelve other bunches are put together, using air plants and laurel; these are for the sacred places. The h'ilol places bunches of flowers around the inside edge of the patient's bed, and the mayoletik construct an arch at its entrance.

[The preparation of the bunches and the arch is preceded by the censing of the plants. The h'ilol takes the incense burner in his hand and moves it in circles (three counterclockwise passes, in the cases we observed) over the materials. The inside of the bed is similarly censed after the bunches of plants have been placed there. The composition and number of bunches vary greatly. In some cases, all the bunches are put together in the same fashion: the curer simply takes a few of each kind of plant until all the piles are exhausted. A certain number are set aside for the shrines and the rest are placed in the bed. Three bunches per sacred place seems to be the usual complement. The arch over the patient's bed is made by fastening one substantial pine bough to each of the posts forming the sides of the entrance to the enclosure. The tops are then bent over and tied together, forming an arch. Clusters of red geraniums are attached across the top and partway down the sides of the arch.]

(7) *Preparation of the bath.* The h'ilol calls for a large earthenware jar and puts into it a small quantity of each kind of plant, along with water from each of the seven gourds. The jar is then put by the fire to heat.

(8) *Praying over and saluting the candles.* The h'ilol prays over the candles (*nup kantela*). The words he speaks are received by the Totil-me'iletik and Kahvaltik ta Vinahel (our lord in heaven) at the moment he utters them. The parts of the ceremony received by the gods are: the h'ilol's words, the rum, the gift given to the h'ilol at the end of the ceremony, the meals eaten in the house and at Kalvario, and the

candles. When the h'ilol finishes praying over the candles, he calls forward the members of the curing party, either singly or in pairs, to salute the candles. They kneel before the table, cross themselves, and pray briefly.

(9) *The bath*. The h'ilol bathes the patient in water from the jar that has been heating. The bathing is accompanied by three rounds of rum in the *muk'ta pis* ["big glass," holding about three times the volume of the usual small shot glass].

[The h'ilol has the bathwater brought forward and placed near the table. The patient seats himself on a small chair in front of the curer. In most cases, where the patient is an adult and will disrobe completely, a mat is held up by several mayoletik to shield the h'ilol and the patient from the rest of the house. The h'ilol pours some of the water into a flat gourd. Dipping with his hand, he washes the patient's head, arms (stroking down toward the hands and fingertips), and finally the rest of the body. While the bathing is going on, women are censing the patient's clean clothing—the set washed at Ni Nab Chilo'. A large wicker basket is upended over an incense burner; the clothes are laid on this and suffused with the aromatic smoke. When the h'ilol is finished bathing the patient (if the patient is an infant, one of the parents is bathed as well), the patient dons the censed clothing.]

(10) *The h'ilol bathes the substitute*. A black chicken of the same sex as the patient is then bathed in the same water. When the chicken has been bathed, its throat is cut and about a cupful of blood drained into a bowl. The patient drinks the blood in order to gain the strength possessed by the chicken. [When the h'ilol drains the blood from the chicken, he daubs some of it on the patient's forehead and cheeks (probably in the sign of the cross), then gives the bowl to the patient to drink. The wound in the chicken's neck is sewn up to prevent further bleeding, and the bird is placed, still alive, on a layer of pine needles in a basin or plate. More pine needles are laid on top and around and the whole is wrapped in a mantresh. This chicken is the substitute (k'esholil) that will be taken to Kalvario and left in the patient's place as an offering to the Totilme'iletik, in the hope that they will consume the chicken instead of the patient's soul.

[After the chicken is disposed of, the h'ilol prepares the other ritual materials to go to Hteklum. The candles are placed upright in the middle of the basket of red geraniums. The h'ilol takes the three or four candles for each sacred place, states the name of the shrine for which they are destined, and places them in the basket. The basket is then placed in a large net for carrying. The pine boughs, pine needles, and bunches of plants are similarly loaded in nets, along with the substitute, bottles of rum, food for the ritual meal and for snacks, firewood, and *ocote* (pitch pine, used for kindling and for making torches at night). These preparations may either precede or follow the ritual meal.]

(11) *The ritual meal.* The participants at the table are the h'ilol, the patient, the mayoletik, and the h'ukumahel. [The complete ritual is detailed in Appendix D.]

(12) *The curing party leaves the house and goes to Hteklum.* At the end of the meal everyone rinses his mouth and washes his hands. Then the curer asks for a bottle of rum, which is left on the table for those who remain behind in the house. Those who remain in the house are the women. If there is an old man in the family, he will also remain. If the party is going to four mountains a límete will be left; if only two mountains, a media is left. The bottle is to ensure that those remaining in the house will not sleep while the others are gone.

[We have heard this bottle referred to as a *totilme'il*, and have seen one left on the hearth as well as the table; neither is consumed until the curing party returns. The occupants of the house must protect the patient, whose illness puts him in special danger. By remaining awake they guard against the entrance of demons, and against the general danger of incurring divine displeasure because there are sacred objects (e.g., the gourds of water) in the house. The full symbolism of alcohol in Zinacantan is still obscure, but the contexts in which it is used seem to suggest that it is seen as establishing contact between men and gods; certainly, no sacred occasion can take place without the consumption of rum. The open bottle left on the table apparently maintains the line of communication between the household and the Totilme'iletik while the curing party is absent, and symbolizes either the actual presence or at least the watchful awareness of the Totilme'iletik. For this reason, its presence acts as a powerful sanction against sleeping in the house while the curing party is gone.]

After the bottle is placed on the table, the things are loaded to be carried to Hteklum. One mayol carries the candles and the k'esholil. The others carry the other materials. When all have adjusted their loads they bow to the h'ilol and then line up in order [with the h'ilol at the rear, the patient next to him, and the other participants in front in descending order of seniority, the most junior assistant leading the procession]. They kneel and cross themselves at the table and then at the hearth, and salute all who remain in the house. Then they line up outside and kneel at the patio cross, after which they assemble in proper order and march to Kishtoval Vits.

[The order in which the party visits the mountains and churches in Hteklum is variable, as is the choice of additional sacred places to be visited. The order may be determined by the direction from which the curing party enters Hteklum. In all the ceremonies that we observed, the first place visited was the upper shrine on Mushul Vits; but this seems to be a result of the curing party's approaching by car rather than by foot. Kishtoval Vits is probably the most usual starting point for parties coming on foot from outside the valley.

[The ordinary ceremonial pattern involves visits to the top of Kishtoval Vits, the foot of Sisil Vits, the top and foot of Mushul Vits, Kalvario, the church of San Sebastian, the church of San Lorenzo, and the chapel of Esquipulas. To these may be added various other visits, as the h'ilol prescribes, among them Ni Nab Chilo' and the top of Sisil Vits. The k'esholil is usually left at Kalvario, where there is a special niche for its deposit; but we also saw it buried at Ni Nab Chilo', and at the top or foot of Sisil Vits (when smoke arising over Kalvario indicated to the curing party at Sisil Vits that there was already another party at Kalvario). Various lesser shrines and waterholes may be briefly visited en route, or a mayol may be sent to leave flowers or a candle at them. Among these are Mishik Balamil ("the navel of the world") and Vo'ch'ohvo'. The sacred places are described in Appendix D.]

When they arrive at Kishtoval Vits, the mayoletik and then the patient and h'ilol cross themselves at the cross and remain there in a kneeling position. When the patient and h'ilol have finished crossing themselves, the h'ilol sends the mayoletik to tie the flowers to the crosses. The mayol who is carying the basket of flowers leaves it at the foot of the crosses, along with the k'esholil. The h'ilol picks out the flowers and gives them to the mayoletik to attach to the crosses. Then they may withdraw and rest, after sprinkling pine needles in front of the crosses. When everything is ready the h'ilol lights the candles, large or small ones according to his custom. At the base of the candles he places three pine tips [*ni 'ahan toh*] that are called *mak kantela* ["fastener of the candles"].

He also places three small bunches of red geraniums. The h'ilol and the patient pray. When they finish praying, everyone drinks a shot of rum; then all bow to each other, cross themselves, and go on to Mushul Vits.

[As the curing party makes its way along the trails it is preceded by one of the mayoletik carrying burning incense, either in an incense burner or in a bucket. Some of this is taken out and put into another burner, which is then set in front of the crosses at each shrine. The sequence of behavior is identical at each mountain, with the addition at Kalvario of the burial of the k'esholil. The basic pattern is the following: the mayoletik prepare the crosses, which may include attaching fresh pine boughs; the h'ilol prays; the h'ilol lights candles; the h'ilol and patient pray together. Rounds of rum are served throughout the sequence. The basic elements may be augmented by other procedures, depending on the kind of ceremony and the tastes of the h'ilol. In a Pertonal sequence, for example, exchanges of liquor among the members of the curing party take place at each mountain. If witchcraft is involved in the illness, the h'ilol may light small candles of many colors in addition to the large white ones that are customary for Muk'ta 'Ilel. Chickens may be left in more than one place, in which case the ritual for their deposit is the same as that described below.]

The curing party visits the churches: Muk'ta Ekleshya [the church of San Lorenzo], Martil [the church of San Sebastian], and Iskipula [the chapel of Esquipulas]. They light candles and pray.

[The order of visiting the churches is variable. San Lorenzo and Esquipulas are side by side and are usually visited together, Esquipulas first. San Sebastian is some distance away, and can be visited either before or after the other two. (See Appendix D; a detailed description of the churches appears in Early, 1965.)

[Procedure on visiting the churches is quite standardized. Before the entrance to San Sebastian and in the enclosed plaza on which San Lorenzo and Esquipulas both face are sets of large wooden crosses set in cement bases, which are saluted by the curing party. These shrines seem analogous to the patio crosses outside the dwelling, which the party also salutes in passing. The salutation is the same in both cases: each person touches his hand to the base of the cross, brings it to his face, and crosses himself.

[The curing party then assembles at the door of the church, where another round of drinks is served. As the party prepares to enter, the junior members bow to the senior, and everyone bows to the hʻilol, saying *chibat,* "I am going." He responds *batan,* "Go!" as he releases them. The party enters the building in ceremonial order and just inside the door lines up facing the altar; everyone kneels, crosses himself, and prays. The process is repeated at a point halfway between the door and the altar, and again directly in front of the altar. The hʻilol and his patient remain on their knees, while the assistants rise and make the necessary preparations. The incense burner is set before the altar, a round of drinks is served, and the hʻilol proceeds to light candles and pray, accompanied by the patient and possibly the patient's spouse. The prayers, as always, are punctuated with rounds of drinks, and the customary spitting is carried on as freely inside the church as elsewhere. The assistants are called upon to light candles and place small bunches of geraniums before the saints' images and other religious objects apart from the main altar. When the prayers are completed, the party makes a circuit of the church, genuflecting at each image; and the three entering genuflections are repeated as the party moves to the door. Once outside, another round of drinks is served. The curing party reforms in ceremonial order and marches to the next church or mountain.

[The size and number of the candles lit to the various saints are determined by the hʻilol. Large candles are generally lit for the major saints on the main altar, and smaller ones for the others.

[In some cases the ceremonial circuit will be interrupted for a brief meal after the curing party finishes praying in San Sebastian. This meal is informal and includes hard-boiled eggs, tortillas, and coffee. It seems to be no part of the curing ritual itself, but rather a necessary break when when the curing circuit is extremely long.]

The curing party goes to Kalvario and prays before the crosses. Everything is done as at the other sacred places. Then the hʻilol and the mayoletik go to deposit the kʻesholil, while the patient and his parents or spouse remain kneeling before the cross. [The chicken is left at the side of the knoll on which the crosses are located, in a small stone-lined offertory chamber that is kept sealed with loose stones.] The hʻilol goes to the place where the kʻesholil is left and places it inside with its head pointing east. The head is pointed east because this is the direction from which Kahvaltik ta Vinahel [the Sun] will rise and come to receive the offering. A 20 ct. candle is lit and left in the hole also; then the chamber is closed up.

One must always use a chicken of the same sex as the patient. [And it must be black.] Although pork can be substituted for chicken in the ritual meals of the curing ceremony, it cannot be used for the k'esholil because it is always bought in San Cristóbal and has no ch'ulel for the Totilme'iletik to receive. If the patient can find only one black chicken to serve as a k'esholil, it will be left in the house to be used when the patient enters his bed, and only the 20 ct. candle will be left at Kalvario.

The k'esholil is received by the Totilme'iletik and Kahvaltik ta Vinahel, who arrive when the h'ilol begins praying at Kalvario. The actual place where the Totilme'iletik gather is not at the Kalvario crosses themselves but at the very top of the hill; the crosses are merely the doorway to the Totilme'iletik. The mayoletik of the Totilme'iletik do not sit in the same place. It is like the cabildo, where the authorities sit on the bench to hear cases and the mayoletik are sent here and there to carry out their orders.

The chicken left at Kalvario disappears in various ways. It may be kept by the next h'ilol who comes along, it may be eaten by animals, or it may be stolen by boys who live nearby. It appears that the Totilme'iletik do not strike a thief with mahbenal. If the chicken is alive when left, it may get out by itself and join the flock of some nearby house.

The h'ilol and the mayoletik take a límete of rum with them when they go to leave the k'esholil. Some curers stay to finish off the whole bottle; others merely have three drinks with their assistants. Then the h'ilol himself returns to the crosses, and he and the patient finish praying there. The incense that has been carried with the curing party during the circuit is left in a burner kept for that purpose at Kalvario.

When all this is finished, the curing party eats a meal, either chicken or pork [sometimes eggs]. Then they return to the patient's house.

(13) *The party returns to the patient's patio.* When the curing party returns, candles are lit at the patio cross, and fire is brought from the house to light new incense in the burner. Three rounds of rum are drunk.

[Sometimes the candles used here are left on the ritual table while the party is in Hteklum and are fetched by one of the mayoletik as the party approaches the house. The candle-lighting sequence is often quite lengthy and elaborate, embodying procedures connected with special aspects of the ceremony, such as recovering a soul or fending off a witch.

A simple Muk'ta 'Ilel involving no antiwitchcraft procedures would ordinarily require three or four candles at this stage, as at the other crosses. If witchcraft is involved, the curer may use many small, colored candles in addition to the large white ones, lining up rows of little candles and then dousing them with kerosene or rum, cutting them with a knife, and/or burning them upside down.

[Before the candles are lit, the patio cross is walled off behind and on the other side by a screen of mats tied to posts (often hoes or digging sticks). In some cases, the cross is completely enclosed with a roof and walls, forming a small chamber in which the h'ilol and his patient pray and perform various secret rites. When we saw this done, the later presence of small, mutilated candles indicated that the h'ilol was performing some witchcraft rite, probably *valk'unel.*]

(14) *The curing party reenters the house.* When the party finish praying at the patio cross, they line up in order and enter the house, where they first cross themselves at the table and hearth and then formally greet all the people in the house. The h'ilol then washes the hands and feet of the patient with the same water he used for the first bath. Then the patient gets into bed.

[According to Domingo's text, the hands and feet are the only parts of the body that are bathed, nor are there any rounds of drinks served. In the ceremonies we observed, however, the patient's entire body was bathed in many cases; in others only the arms, legs, and head were washed, but in all cases rounds of drinks punctuated the bathing. The second k'esholil is usually bathed at this time as well.]

After the patient enters the bed, the h'ilol takes the incense burner and makes three circular passes over the patient. He prays to the Totilme'iletik to come and watch over the patient. Then he kills the k'esholil and tosses it onto the patient to see how it performs. If it performs well —that is, jumps around a lot while dying—the patient will get better. If the patient is going to live, the chicken's head will fall to the east; and if the patient is to die, the head will fall to the west. If the chicken's head falls to the west, the h'ilol turns it to the east and puts it next to the patient's head. The Totilme'iletik are said to arrive to inspect the patient at the moment the h'ilol prays over the bed.

The chicken remains for one day [usually hung head down from a hook on the outside of the bed enclosure] and then is eaten by the patient.

(15) *A ritual meal.* When the bed ceremonies are finished, a ritual

meal is eaten. The h'ilol, the mayoletik, and the h'ukumaheletik eat at the table; the patient eats in his bed. When they finish drinking the ceremonial coffee, they drink the bottle of rum that has been on the table. This bottle is called *ya'lel mesha* ["the table's water"]. The h'ilol does not finish his meal, but hands his plate to someone; later it will be taken to his house. The others finish their meals.

When they finish the meal, the h'ilol goes home, accompanied by a mayol who carries the curing gift. The gift includes four bottles of rum, four [dead] chickens, 80 tortillas, and $2 worth of kashlan vah. These gifts are received both by the h'ilol and by the Totilme'iletik and the Sun. When the h'ilol receives the things, he prays to these gods, asking them to come and receive their gifts. Sometimes the h'ilol drinks some of the rum with the mayol who has escorted him home.

(16) *Postceremonial care.* The various assistants go home. If the family is large enough to keep someone always in the house, they will care for the patient themselves. If there are not enough of them, they look for a widow to care for the patient. This may be a sister, grandmother, or aunt of the patient; or, if there is no available relative, she may be anyone the family knows. The amount of time she looks after the patient depends on the h'ilol's prescription. She must not weave or do any other work, but only watch over the patient. If there are two guardians, one will sleep while the other watches. Someone must always be watching to make sure that the patient does not suffer mahbenal from the Totilme'iletik, and that he is not attacked by demons. At night the woman who is watching may sleep, but only if the light is not extinguished.

Neither cabbage nor black beans may be eaten in the house during this period; the patient will suffer mahbenal if they are. Only white beans, eggs, pork, and chicken may be eaten [besides maize]. These prohibitions last until the flowers have been removed from the bed. After that the watchers can eat whatever they wish. The patient, however, must wait four or five days after the flowers are removed before he can eat what he wishes. The patient takes two or three days to finish eating the k'esholil. He collects the bones in a pot and saves them to be taken by the h'ilol when the flowers are removed. The same is done with the feathers.

During this period the patient stays in his bed and cannot talk to the watchers. No visitor can enter the house. When the patient goes outdoors to relieve himself someone must accompany him, and another person must sit in front of his empty bed to guard against demons. Sometime during the period of seclusion the Totilme'iletik and their mayoletik come to look at the patient. Their arrival is marked by their appearance in the dreams of the patient or the watchers—whoever is more *p'ih*—and the arrival of the mayoletik alone is signaled by the singing of a sparrow. Demons come also, but they are kept from bothering the patient because the watchers are awake in the daytime and the light is burning at night.

(17) *Removing the flowers from the bed.* The day before the flowers are to be removed someone goes in the afternoon to ask the h'ilol if he will come the next day. This messenger brings a bottle of rum as a gift for the h'ilol. The h'ilol comes alone the next morning at about 5 o'clock. Of the assistants, only two men and two women need be present. When the h'ilol arrives he first crosses himself at the patio cross, before which an incense burner will already have been placed. Then he enters the house and crosses himself at the hearth. He greets the household, and a round of drinks is served.

The h'ilol then takes an incense burner and stands before the patient's bed. He prays and censes the bed with three circuits of the burner. When he is finished, he takes the flowers and rubs the patient with them. Then he takes all the flowers and pine needles from the bed, puts them in a sack, and sends the two male assistants to leave the flowers in the branches of a tree at Kalvario. The assistants take with them a cuarta of rum to offer toasts to anyone they encounter.

The h'ilol also removes the gourds of sacred water and the potfull of water left from the patient's bath. When the assistants return from Kalvario, they help him bury the bones and feathers of the k'esholil in a hole, about 60 centimeters deep, that they dig behind the patio cross. Then they all eat a meal of chicken or pork. They eat at a table, but only a media of rum is placed on the table, and ceremonial coffee is not served. After this meal the ceremony is over, and the h'ilol returns home. He receives no further gifts.

(18) *Further restrictions on the patient.* Two or three days after the flowers have been removed, the patient can get out of bed for short intervals to warm himself at the fire. He still cannot be left alone in the house. His bed need not be watched while he is warming himself at the fire, but three ears of corn are left in it as a substitute and a protection against demons. After the flowers have been removed the watchers can weave, but only with black wool, since white objects attract mahbenal.

The patient cannot be left alone in the house until he has taken a sweat bath. He uses his own bathhouse, if he has one; otherwise, he borrows a neighbor's. The patient can only enter the sweat bath in the morning: it is believed that the sun is young in the morning and will give youth to the patient's body; but if he bathes in the afternoon, when the sun is old, his body will rapidly age. The bath-fire is kindled by the patient's wife, or if he has none, by his mother. He is accompanied in the sweat bath by his wife or mother and cannot be left there alone. He bathes in boiled laurel water. [Meanwhile, his bed in the house is watched.]

After the first bath the patient can stay alone in the house, but he still cannot go outdoors alone. Three days after the first bath he takes another, the same as the first, and after this he can go outside to warm himself in the sun and can stay there alone. In order to prevent mahbenal he rubs salt on his veins before going out. Three days after the second bath the patient takes a third. This time no one watches his bed while he bathes, and after this he can go out by himself. The first day he stays in his own sitio. After that he gradually goes farther and farther, until he is going about as usual. This ends the cure.

[The postceremonial procedures are subject to much variation and depend heavily on the idiosyncracies of the h'ilol. The length of time a h'ilol is known to prescribe for postceremonial seclusion is often an important factor in the patient's choice of a curer.

[Informants occasionally describe a smaller-scale version of Muk'ta 'Ilel under the term 'O'lol Nichim, "half flower." This sequence is identical to Muk'ta 'Ilel but involves visits to only two of the mountains in Hteklum, with a corresponding reduction in the quantities of ritual materials and number of assistants.]

The Lok'esel ta Balamil Sequence

[If the Lok'esel ta Balamil sequence is used, it occurs at a point in the main ceremony when the curing party has reentered the patient's house but before the ritual meal is eaten. This sequence is performed to recall lost parts of the patient's ch'ulel.]

The h'ilol prepares three pine tips, some oak branches, and some corn grains for the purpose of calling the patient's ch'ulel. White salt is dissolved in water, which is then placed in two little gourds. One gourd is played by a mayol during the calling [by blowing over the opening he makes a shrill whistling sound that is supposed to attract the errant soul]; into the other the h'ilol places grains of corn. [The usual number of grains is 52—13 of each of the colors white, yellow, black, and red. The symbolism of this is obscure. The usual number of parts in a ch'ulel is said to be 13, but there is no ready explanation for their being represented in multiples of four, nor for the colors. The descriptions given of how this divination is performed are vague; and since it is done by flickering firelight in a dark hut, when the participants are already in an advanced stage of inebriation, it seems to allow great leeway for the h'ilol to improvise.] The little gourds used in this ceremony are called 'ik'ob bail tsu [summoner gourds]; and the pine and oak bundle is called *mahobil* [striker] because it is struck on the ground while the h'ilol is calling the patient's soul.

The h'ilol finishes his preparations and goes outside to the patio cross. He prays, calling the soul toward the place where the patient lost it. He lights candles of the 20 ct. size, two tallow and one wax. If the patient was frightened out of his soul right there in the sitio, they call the soul there. If the loss took place far away, it may be necessary to go to the spot; but first they try recovering the soul by calling it from a distance.

The h'ilol prays to the Totilme'iletik to send their mayoletik and fetch the soul from wherever it was lost. He also prays to the Yahval Balamil to free the soul, since it has not stolen anything [see Appendix E]. The mayoletik of the Totilme'iletik arrive while the h'ilol is praying before the patio cross. There are six of them, and they all go together to fetch the soul. The mayol plays on the gourd while the h'ilol is praying. The h'ilol strikes the mahobil on the ground. He holds a bottle of rum in his hand, from which he fills his mouth and sprays on the ground.

The h'ilol can see when and where the patient suffered soul-loss when he puts the grains of corn in the gourd of salt water. If the grains float on top of the water, the patient has lost his soul in water or in the river. If the grains are lying on their side, the parts of the soul are also lying on their side, at the place where the patient was frightened. If the grains are leaning to one side, the patient was in this position when he fell and suffered soul-loss. If the patient's ch'ulel is well and no parts are missing, all the grains will be "seated" [i.e. upright] in the cup. Each grain represents one of the 13 parts of the soul.

Some curers call the soul only in front of the cross. Others make three circuits around the cross, accompanied by the mayol playing on the gourd. The h'ilol places 'ech' [a flower] in front of the cross and then enters the house to call the soul. When the h'ilol and the mayol, still playing on the gourd, enter the house, the women also begin to call the patient's name. The h'ilol rubs the patient with the oak and pine tips and places them in his pillow. The ears of corn from which the grains were taken for the divination are placed beside the patient's head, along with a little salt. These are to protect the patient, and if they were not there he would suffer mahbenal. The little gourds are also placed beside the patient's head. All these things remain in the bed for three days. At the end of that time the h'ilol comes in the morning to take them away. He first censes the patient and rubs him with the branches to draw the illness out of the body. Then the branches are taken outside and put on top of a tree in the sitio. The gourds are returned to whoever owns them, but the grains of corn are fried on the *comal* [clay griddle] and ground up to be eaten by the patient.

[In the Lok'esel ta Balamil ceremony that we observed, the divination with corn grains was supplemented by information from the patient about the possible location of parts of his soul. A chain of mayoletik passed the information from the patient in his bed to the h'ilol, who was praying in front of the patio cross. The patient recounted incidents in which he had been frightened or startled, had fallen down, etc., and gave their locations. The h'ilol then went through a calling sequence for each incident, calling, praying, beating the ground with the mahobil, and spraying rum from his mouth, while the mayol blew shrill whistles on the gourd. The number of incidents recounted was substantial (perhaps 20–25), and the sequence lasted an hour or more.]

Other "Good" Curing Ceremonies

The sequence of ritual described for Muk'ta 'Ilel is merely the maximal extension of a ceremonial pattern that can be carried out on any scale and with visits to any number of mountains and churches, from a single mountain to the four mountains and three churches described in the ideal pattern. Only the four-mountain/three-church and two-mountain/three-church versions are named, but any other variant is equally possible. Some minor variations follow the change in scale. When less than four mountains are visited, for example, the patient's bathwater is likely to be drawn from fewer than seven waterholes.

Informants describe virtually the same set of procedures, but without the placing of flowers in the patient's bed, under the term Ta Solel Kantela, of "candles alone." The same features of extensibility and variability apply here as to 'Och ta Svolim, the major difference being the omission of the decoration and censing of the patient's bed. Smaller quantities of plants are obtained, and they are used only for the crosses and the patient's bath.

A very similar pattern of ritual sequences is described as constituting Tsva'an sba H'iloletik, the debut ceremony for new h'iloletik. The major omission in this case is the sacrifice of chickens at Kalvario and in the house. Sometimes, however, a new h'ilol may be ill, his illness being a sign of divine election to the h'ilol role; thus the ceremony may be both a debut and a curing ceremony, and a k'esholil may be used. The debut ceremony visits all the sacred places that the new h'ilol will use in his practice, since part of the purpose of the ceremony is to introduce him to them.

Ceremonies to ward off illness. A ceremony can also be held for prophylactic purposes—that is, to ward off illness from a family. The procedure is the same as that for Muk'ta 'Ilel, but without the decoration of the bed and without a k'esholil. All the persons on whose behalf the ceremony is being performed are bathed and change their clothes. They all observe a period of postceremonial seclusion, but do not remain in their beds. The number of mountains visited is determined by the h'ilol.

Ceremonies without candles. Finally, in the class of ceremonies that can be described under the rubric tuk'il alel vokol ("good curing ceremony"), the only procedure carried out without candles and without visits to sacred places is K'oplael, "saying words." The basic procedure is prayer, often accompanied by the administration of some remedy, usually herbal. The K'oplael is ordinarily preceded by pulsing and is usually performed on the spot by the h'ilol if his diagnosis reveals that nothing more complicated is required. Sometimes a meal is served.

Skuenta 'Ak' Chamel

The second broad category of curing procedures comprises those whose purpose is the treatment—and occasionally the use—of witchcraft. No such ceremony can be described as tuk'il alel vokol; any connection with witchcraft, even if the patient is an innocent victim, excludes the ceremony from the class of "good" procedures. The criterion seems to be less the personal motive of the patient and/or h'ilol than the nature of the supernatural forces that are believed to be involved in the illness and to whom the ceremony is directed. The "good" ceremonies are directed to the Totilme'iletik, the Sun, and the saints. The witchcraft ceremonies involve the Yahval Balamiletik, demons, and other malevolent supernaturals, as well as the Totilme'iletik in their aspect as punishers and senders of witchcraft. This aspect of the Totilme'iletik seems somewhat inconsistent with their role as guardians of morality and protectors of Zinacantecos. Some informants report, nonetheless, that the Totilme'iletik can be appealed to by witches to send illness against their victims—with indications, however, that the victims of such illnesses are always in some way deserving of them. The idea manifests itself in the Pertonal sequence, where the victim apologizes to the possible senders of illness in his family for whatever transgressions might have incurred their hostility. Although this conciliatory aspect of the ceremony seems innocuous, it is often accompanied by the burning of small candles and other antiwitchcraft procedures, putting it in the class of skuenta 'ak' chamel.

Pertonal. There are two kinds of Pertonal sequence, one involving a trip to the mountains, the other occurring only within the house. The first type closely follows the form of Muk'ta 'Ilel, with the following changes and additions (the numbers refer to stages in our description of Muk'ta 'Ilel).

(1) The quantities of flowers procured for the ceremony are less than those for 'Och ta Svolim.

(6) No flowers are placed in the patient's bed.

(8) After the h'ilol has prepared the patient's bath and finished praying over the candles he calls for as many bottles of rum (either cuartas or límetes) as there are people in the household. These are arranged on the table at equal intervals along both long edges. The rum will be used by the members of the household to beg pardon of each other if they have quarreled; when their difficulties are terminated, the patient will be restored to health.

When the h'ilol has arranged the bottles on the table he prays over them and the candles. In the middle of the prayer he calls on the patient and all those in the household, who come forward and kneel before the table. First they cross themselves; then the h'ilol hands each person one bottle of rum. They speak to each other, measuring out shots of rum and exchanging toasts, so that they may be in harmony once again. After all members of the household have toasted one another, they may offer rum to the assistants. Some h'iloletik include the assistants in the Pertonal because they, too, may have quarreled with the patient. It is necessary that the participants drink up all the rum, even if they become drunk, since only in this way will their difficulties be resolved. Their affairs will be put in order by the Totilme'iletik, who arrive when the h'ilol begins to pray at the table. The rum consumed by the participants is also received by the Totilme'iletik.

(9) The h'ilol bathes the patient and whoever is going to accompany him to the mountains, usually his wife or mother. Three rounds of rum accompany the bathing.

(12) The curing party usually visits two or three mountains in Hteklum. The procedure is essentially the same as 'Och ta Svolim, with the following additions. The h'ilol lights both big and small candles, and the small candles are placed outside the enclosure at the foot of the cross where the larger ones are lit, in order to shield the large ones from the demons. Some h'iloletik again give the patient and whoever is accompanying him conciliatory bottles of rum to drink at this point. The h'ilol fills the bottles before he begins to pray, and they stay in front of the cross until the middle of the prayer, when he hands them to the patient. They are then measured out and served to everyone. The mountain in question receives only the odor of the rum; and the Totilme'iletik set the patient's affairs in order, forgiving his sins.

When the h'ilol finishes praying, he makes a circuit on his knees, facing in each direction and praying to all the Totilme'iletik and the saints in the churches. The party then proceeds to the other mountains, ending at Kalvario. Here the mayoletik attach the pine branches and flowers as before; the h'ilol lines up the bottles of rum, lights his candles, and begins to pray. When he finishes praying he strikes the patient three hard blows with a leather tumpline. He must strike so hard that the patient begins to cry and implore the Sun to absolve him of sins; if the patient does not weep, he will not recover. After this, the bottles of rum are drunk. Then the patient remains praying before the crosses while the h'ilol and the mayoletik go to leave the k'esholil. All then eat a meal of pork, rum, and coffee. Everything must be finished, for mahbenal would result if they returned to the house with the coffee and rum.

(13) The return to the house is the same as before, with a ceremony at the patio cross. During the ritual meal, the patient eats at the table

with the rest of the party. After the meal the h'ilol goes home, accompanied by a mayol who carries the gift. The patient maintains three to six days of seclusion, watched over by his brothers or other members of the household group. He may take two or three steam baths during this time, but it is not imperative. On the first day he cannot eat green vegetables; after that he may eat whatever he likes. On the third or fourth day he can go out into the streets. The h'ilol makes no further visits.

A Pertonal ceremony can also be held in the house without traveling to Hteklum. This is clearly a witchcraft procedure, however, since it involves returning the illness to the sender. The procedure is often referred to as *valk'unel* or *sutp'inel*, "throwing back" or "returning." The ceremony takes place entirely in the house at night, and with only family members as assistants in order to maintain secrecy.

The h'ilol arrives in the early evening and prays at the patio cross, borrowing incense from within the house. Then he enters and crosses himself at hearth and table. He greets the people, and inspects and blesses the candles. Then the h'ilol and the patient go into the patio, where a Pertonal sequence is held with all members of the family participating. When they return indoors, the h'ilol sets up a small pinewood cross against one of the interior walls of the house and sticks three pine boughs in the ground in front of it. He next lines up his candles in front of the cross, along with bottles of rum for a second Pertonal sequence. The candles he uses are of several sizes and include all seven ritual colors.

According to the nature of the illness, the h'ilol may light the candles in various ways. He may light them only once during the night, or three times; he may line them up in one or more rows; and if he is trying to return the illness to its sender, he may cut the candles into three pieces and then throw gasoline and kerosene on them before lighting them. Some h'iloletik light the candles upside down with the point buried in the ground. If these things are done, the illness may be thrown back, and the person from whom it came will begin to suffer pricking pains in his body, since it is his soul that is represented by the candles that are cut and burned. Soon he will begin to feel as if his body is burning. Some h'iloletik prick the candles with a needle, and the victim feels the same pricks in his own body.

In the middle of the curer's prayer, after he lights the candles, he again calls the members of the family forward for another Pertonal sequence. Then a meal is served, but a simpler one than would appear in a major ceremony. The food may not be chicken, since this is not a "good" ceremony, or beef, which is never used in curing ceremonies. Pork may be served or, depending on the dictates of the h'ilol, such special foods as bull's liver, tripe, or fish (all especially associated with witchcraft). If any of these are served, the meal may be eaten without a table. Ceremonial coffee is not served, and the patient eats with everyone else.

After the meal the patient gets into his bed, which has not been prepared in any fashion, such preparations being reserved for "good" ceremonies. The bottles and glasses are left lined up in front of the little cross, to be taken away three days later by either the h'ilol or the owner of the house. The pine boughs are placed in the branches of a tree in the patio. The patient remains secluded for three days, but he can eat anything and his bed need not be guarded. After the first day, the woman who is watching can do a little work. After the third day the patient can go outside, putting salt on his veins to avert mahbenal. He does not take any sweat baths, and can go out in the streets after the fifth day.

Sa'el Hch'uleltik ta Balamil. There is one other witchcraft procedure that is named and described by Zinacanteco h'iloletik and laymen: the ceremony performed to recover a soul that has been sold by a witch to the Yahval Balamil. This is called Sa'el Hch'uleltik ta Balamil, "looking for our soul in the earth," or sometimes Conbil ta Balamil, "sold to the earth." It is a highly dangerous procedure, and possessing the ability to recover a soul is the same as being a witch oneself. Many informants, indeed, state emphatically that only a h'ilol who has sold souls to the earth knows how to get them back, and say that a patient will often go to the h'ilol he suspects of responsibility for his illness and pay him to reclaim the soul. Few informants will talk about the ceremony, and very few h'iloletik will admit that they can perform it. Only one of our informants, Lol Pérez Komyosh (who is indeed known as a powerful but dangerous h'ilol), admitted to performing the ceremony. It involves visiting caves, where the h'ilol communicates with the earth and lights small candles of the seven sacred colors. The same is done at the patio cross.

Variant Ceremonial Forms

The foregoing descriptions are a set of ideal patterns of curing ceremonies that are named in Tzotzil or are otherwise discussed and described with reasonable regularity in Zinacantan. But, as might be expected from the generally loose classification of curing ceremonies and the wide latitude of variation built into the system, the actual practices of h'iloletik include a much wider range of variant ceremonial forms—even taking into account the expected and delimited areas of variability that we have mentioned. We cannot adequately describe the entire range of variant ceremonial manifestations, dependent as they are on idiosyncratic decisions by individual h'iloletik, to which the system gives full rein. From our sample of some 130 curing cases (see Chapter 9), it can be said that major ceremonies on the complete model of Muk'ta 'Ilel constitute only a small proportion of the typical family's medical experiences. Many cases, for example, were treated with ceremonies that took place in the house only but were more complicated than K'oplael. Very few of them adhered exactly to the patterns described above, but most seemed to be composed of elements contained in the ideal patterns. The arrangements of these elements into variant ceremonial forms tends to respond in part to the nature of the illness, as well as to a variety of individual characteristics of the h'iloletik.

Other Ceremonies

Two kinds of private ceremonies are performed by h'iloletik in a non-medical setting: agricultural rituals, and the ceremony for the dedication of a new house. The agricultural ceremonies are performed in the lowland fields two or three times during the growing season and resemble K'in Krus in form (Vogt, 1965a). They are performed entirely by male h'iloletik (since women do not ordinarily accompany the men to hot country) on behalf of a family or farming group. Not all Zinacantecos continue to practice these ceremonies, and they are never performed for lands in cold country. We have no direct information on the ceremonies, but a description is among the unpublished reports of the Harvard Chiapas Project (Stauder, 1961).

The new house ceremony is performed for every new dwelling that is constructed. There are some indications that it can also be performed to rededicate an older house, but it is not clear in what circumstances this takes place. The following description, provided by the h'ilol Mariano Anselmo Pérez, is more elaborate than the reports of some other informants, in that it incorporates a ceremonial circuit of Hteklum as well as a ritual in the new house.

The owner of a new house first approaches a h'ilol with a gift of rum and asks him to dedicate the house; they decide on a date for the ceremony. The h'ilol inquires if the owner wants to go to the mountains, and if the answer is affirmative, he gives instructions for the purchase of candles, washing of the patient's clothing, etc. All preparations are made as for Muk'ta 'Ilel, with the owner treated as a patient.

On arriving at the new house, the h'ilol advises the owner on the location of the patio cross. When it has been set up, he crosses himself at it, then enters the house and makes his obeisance at the table. He checks the candles, prays over them and the plants, prepares the water for the bath, and places it in the fire. He then prays over the candles and calls all the company to do the same. The water is brought from the fire and the h'ilol bathes the owner of the house, his wife, and his children. The bath water is then thrown into the corners of the room. A ritual meal is eaten.

After the meal, the party leaves for Hteklum, where they pray at the mountains and churches for the protection of the new house. The procedure is essentially identical to Muk'ta 'Ilel. On returning to the house, they salute the patio cross and the table and greet those who remained behind. The h'ilol seats himself and calls for the rooster that has been stored in a basket. The rooster is killed and hung from a beam in the center of the house. The assistants open a hole in the floor below and the fowl is buried. Then the h'ilol lights candles in each corner of the room and in the center of the house. A ritual meal is eaten. Following the meal, the musicians (harp, guitar, violin) play, and the men dance. The dancing concludes the ceremony.

(Vogt, 1969, reports that there may, in some cases, be two such ceremonies—one at the midpoint of construction and one at the end.)

Chapter twelve

The H'ilol in Zinacanteco Society

IN THIS CHAPTER we will examine several important aspects of the h'ilol's position in Zinacantan. First, there are the societal functions served by the h'ilol in everyday social relations. Though he is manifestly concerned with the spiritual and supernatural aspects of Zinacanteco life, his influence is most strongly felt and most easily observed in the context of the interpersonal relations that envelop his patients. Secondly, we will examine general attitudes held about the h'ilol in Zinacantan. This will be followed by a brief analysis of the corporate relations between the h'iloletik and the judicial authorities. Fourthly, in keeping with the fundamentally comparative orientation of our study, we will attempt to analyze the strictly biomedical functions served by the h'ilol. In order to articulate this problem, it will be necessary to review current opinions in medicine and behavioral science about the problems of medical care and behavioral change. The chapter ends with a general summary of the position and role of the h'ilol in Zinacantan, and with a comparative analysis of the Zinacanteco system of medical care.

The H'ilol's Activities as Adjustive Mechanisms

The most important function of the curing ceremonies and other shamanistic activities, from a sociological point of view, is to mediate disputes and resolve the conflicts arising in daily Zinacanteco life.* These

---

* The mediatory aspect of shamanism is not unique to Zinacantan, and the literature abounds with illustrations that this dimension of curing is significant in many settings. Bunzel (1952) describes a case in Chichicastenango in which the patient's confession of his sins and his begging pardon of members of the domestic group were prominent features of a curing ceremony. The other factors that contribute to the mediatory potential of shamanistic curing are also present in Chichicastenango—unverifiable divination, witchcraft and supernatural sanctions as causes of illness, and

are generally conflicts within the domestic group, between close kinsmen or other inhabitants of the patient's immediate social and physical surroundings—that is, between the very people who are most likely to be participants in a curing ceremony. One ceremonial type, the Pertonal sequence, is in fact explicitly intended to reconcile the quarreling members of a household. In the house and at the shrines the members of the family, often with friends, neighbors, and kinsmen who are involved in the dissension, exchange bottles of rum. Bowing and toasting each other, they ritually beg pardon for their transgressions, apologize to each other, and are reconciled through the actions of the Totilme'iletik.

This particular ceremony is quite obviously meant to be adjustive; but the mediating function of curing seems to extend to the entire range of possible ritual activities. Zinacanteco curing, in brief, puts a potent, albeit informal, power of mediation in the hands of the h'ilol. The framework for his exercise of this power is built on three factors. First, he has complete control over the actual diagnosis and interpretation of an illness, including both cause and cure, and he speaks with supernatural authority. His method of divination cannot in principle be verified by the patient. Second, the h'ilol is likely, especially in remote hamlets, to be familiar with his patient's social and family affairs, and is thus in a position to know about any dissension within the domestic group and the neighborhood. Finally, Zinacanteco beliefs about the causes of illness are well adapted to the mediatory role of the h'ilol. Most illnesses are ascribed either to witchcraft, which stems from some social disturbance, or to divine punishment for the patient's transgressions, which include both social and domestic concerns.

Men and gods are linked, in Zinacanteco thought, in a triangular relationship, and the conflicts of social life are believed to manifest themselves in illness. Illness can arise from interpersonal tensions in three ways. One party to a dispute may take direct action against his antagonist through witchcraft. The gods may take direct action to punish someone for socially reproved behavior to others (quarreling with his family, excessive drinking, etc.). Or an aggrieved Zinacanteco may actively solicit divine punishment for his enemies through the medium of *'ok'itabil*

---

the curer's membership in the local group. Among the Eskimo (Rassmussen, 1929), to take another example, the shaman and all the inhabitants of the village join together in a ceremony to secure the confession of the patient's sins and publicly announce communal forgiveness for them. (The reader who wishes more examples of this nature may consult Kiev, 1964, and Fabrega, 1972.)

chamel, "illness sought through weeping." This borders on witchcraft, but may be considered a legitimate practice when the complainant's case is just.

Illness, more generally, can be seen as an expression of the individual's standing in the community. A Zinacanteco who suffers an illness like *ta skuenta*—i.e., who is afflicted because he has failed to maintain a properly respectful attitude to the Totilme'iletik, as manifested by the occasional performance of public social obligations or private curing ceremonies—is supposedly in conflict with the gods. In fact, he is likely to be in conflict with the community, since failure to commit a reasonable amount of one's resources and energy to propitiating the gods is not only an offense against heaven but also an offense against the basic values of Zinacanteco life. Religious expenditure is the most highly approved way of dealing with excess income, and a Zinacanteco's neighbors usually have an envious but accurate picture of exactly how much excess income he has. (We found that several of our informants could unhesitatingly give complete figures on the economic activities of a very large number of neighboring households.) A man who fails to dispose of his earnings in a socially approved fashion undoubtedly hears the verdict of the community in the curer's declaration that his illness stems from divine displeasure. The elaborate ceremony that ensues serves to dissipate excess wealth and to demonstrate the patient's adherence to community values. In many cases, the circumstances compellingly support many observers' inferences that the illness itself is occasioned by the patient's feelings of guilt and his perception of communal disapproval.

These social and psychological factors no doubt influence and shape the behavior of Zinacantecos regardless of whether a structural or demonstrable physiological disturbance is present. Many illnesses that are traceable to underlying biological processes, in other words, can fortuitously provide concrete instances for the curer's manipulation of concurrent stresses and strains in the social fabric. At the same time, in a society where illness is conceptualized as reflecting the status of one's interpersonal relationships, it can safely be assumed that many instances of illness are the result of what one could term psychosocial crises.

When the label of illness is applied to his condition, a Zinacanteco puts a heavy demand on his social environment that cannot ordinarily be denied. If he has been subjected to severe pressure from others, his illness may be a means of retreating and of demanding sympathy and support. But at the same time, he is assuming responsibility for whatever allegations the curer's diagnosis may make about his own behavior. In the case of suspected witchcraft, illness provides the patient with a socially approved and psychologically unambivalent opportunity for voicing his personal suspicions and hostilities, which at the very least must be assumed to provide some cathartic relief; and believing that one is a victim of witchcraft may also reflect a perception of one's social dislocation. An illness, which is composed of psychological and/or bodily symptoms, when tied to this perception of one's social displacement, thus calls forth the adjustive mechanism implicit in the curing ceremony and the h'ilol's activities.

Many actual witchcraft cases show similar mediatory patterns. The h'ilol is in a position to know the domestic affairs of his patient and to attribute hostility accordingly to various members of the household or local group. The ceremony is likely to include the other parties to any quarrel; and pressure toward the resolution of their differences is exerted, either through a Pertonal type of sequence or indirectly through the investment of time and energy involved in the ceremony. (According to some informants, a Muk'ta 'Ilel type of ceremony can be held to straighten out affairs within a dissension-ridden family, one member assuming the role of patient for the purpose. It is not clear if this really differs from the Pertonal ceremony.) Two aspects of curing are of special importance in this context. First, most patients tend, at least at the first appearance of an illness, to use a h'ilol who is either a relative or a close neighbor; and, particularly in the outlying hamlets, they maintain a relatively stable relationship with one or more h'iloletik to whom they bring all cases of illness. Second, witchcraft is considered to be the cause of many (according to some informants, virtually all) illnesses in Zinacantan, placing them squarely in the area of interpersonal relations.

These facts emerge very clearly from curers' accounts of their practices. Telesh Gomis Rodrigo, a successful and much-sought h'ilol in Paste', gave witchcraft as the cause of every illness he had cured during a period of about three months before he was interviewed, and said all the patients lived in his own sna. Although he claimed not to have made open accusations against the persons guilty of witchcraft, he stated he had clear knowledge in each case of the culprit and of the reasons lying behind the casting of the illness—invariably quarrels within the domestic group or immediate households. In some cases a Pertonal sequence was used to bring about a reconciliation. In others, antiwitchcraft procedures were used, apparently to frighten or chasten the witch into withdrawing his witchcraft. In every case the suspected witch was included in the curing ceremony.

One observes, then, that a curing ceremony acts to promote social organization and to control the interpersonal relationships of the participants. The services of ritual assistants, for example, can usefully be seen as part of a set of reciprocal exchanges that define and maintain certain social relationships, such as those between kinsmen, compadres, and friends. Assistance in the curing ceremony is a service the patient most often procures from someone obligated to him, and it is usually reciprocated in some fashion—rarely (except in the case of compadres) by the same kind of service, but always by some exchange of social or economic worth. (For a general and theoretical statement of the role and implications of this type of reciprocal social arrangement in the functioning of social systems, see Gouldner, 1960.)

This view of ceremonies as involving duties, obligations, and payments, of course, is an observer's analysis of the situation. Zinacantecos themselves do not talk about the recruitment of ritual personnel in terms of an exchange of services, but the principles of selection strongly suggest it. The ideal order is the following. First one recruits from among one's sons. If the patient has too few sons to complete the complement of assistants, he recruits from his younger brothers, then from older brothers, brothers-in-law, compadres, neighbors, and friends, in that order of preference. If the patient is entirely without anyone who will care for him, he must "borrow" the house of a friend or neighbor, who takes responsibility for the ceremony (sometimes in return for being made the patient's heir) and recruits assistants from his own family and friends in the same order of preference. The recruitment of female assistants follows the same general line; they may be the wives of the male assistants, or they may be recruited separately from the patient's daughters, sisters, etc. (Although we have never seen a man acting as assistant for his son or grandson, it is not unusual to have a woman do so—especially since the role of h'ukumahel requires an elderly woman.)

It is clear that ideally the assistants should always be junior to the patient and as closely related as possible. It seems, then, that this service is part of a set of obligations owed to one's elders and reciprocated by other kinds of obligations (economic support, etc.). On a less imperative and possibly contingent basis, curing assistance enters into the expected relations between in-laws, compadres, and friends. As one moves down the scale, the contingent quality of the obligation probably increases, so that a Zinacanteco has a legitimate claim on the services of a compadre, for example, only after he has exhausted all possibilities among his relatives.

One function of the exchange of services involved in the curing ceremony is undoubtedly to strengthen the social relations involved. A participant in the ceremony invests a considerable amount of effort and attention in the patient's well-being. In the process, he both reinforces his commitment to the patient and communicates this commitment to the patient. The patient, in turn, is placed under an obligation that reinforces his own interest in the relationship. Similar effects occur between all the participants.

A lesser but related aspect of Zinacanteco curing ceremonies is that they provide one of the few legitimate outlets outside the cargo system for expending excess income. They are also one of the few events on the household level in which anything out of the ordinary, daily routine can be expected to happen. In short, they have entertainment value. This function should not be discounted in a culture that has no provision for a gathering of people bent only on entertainment (this applies to the household only; there are gatherings of men in cantinas, etc., that have enjoyment as their only ostensible purpose). The few religious fiestas are the only regular opportunities for pleasurable gatherings on the family level. Aside from these, curing ceremonies, weddings, and baptisms are the only events where a family and its friends can legitimately indulge in such delicacies as chicken, atole, and the like at a time and place of its own choosing. Where the ceremony is prompted by severe illness, of course, these considerations are minor. It is clear, however, that some wealthy families indulge in a great many curing ceremonies unconnected with major illness. Here, entertainment and conspicuous consumption seem almost as important as curing.

The use of surplus income above basic subsistence needs in Zinacantan is severely limited by social pressures that militate against the outward manifestation of differences in wealth. These are maintained by gossip and accusations directed against the wealthy, and by the fear that socially disapproved consumption will incur envy and witchcraft. The only legitimate avenues of expenditure are the cargo system, limited reinvestment in agricultural enterprise, and necessary living expenses, which include curing ceremonies. Within reasonable bounds, curing ceremonies can be held without a serious event of illness, since it is believed that they help in maintaining a family's relations with the Totil-me'iletik, and insure that these deities will not be tempted to send an illness in order to extort chickens and other ritual offerings from the victim. Ceremonies can also be conducted to reconcile family quarrels or to ask for protection on a journey. Any of these can provide a socially acceptable occasion for the outlay of large amounts of money and effort. Not only do the participants enjoy the sensual and dramatic pleasures of the ceremony, but they indicate to the rest of the world their economic status in a fashion that cannot properly be censured.

Attitudes Toward the H'iloletik

The h'iloletik are the only channel of communication from the supernatural world to the municipio, a fact of great importance. The cargo holder, the Catholic priest, and the individual Zinacanteco when he performs religious ceremonies, direct communications to the gods in the form of prayers, sacrifices, and gifts of ritual materials. Only the h'iloletik, however, are capable of receiving divine communications as well as offering them. In a culture where the intentions of the gods are of outstanding importance to both public and private endeavors, this function has great social significance.

Drought and epidemic disease are the two major afflictions that can be directed by the gods against the community as a whole. The prediction, prevention, and curing of both is the job of the h'iloletik. In the private sphere, illness and various other misfortunes (such as the death of livestock, which is usually thought to be caused by witchcraft) are supernatural manifestations and are handled by a h'ilol. The monopoly that the h'ilol still enjoys, then, concerns central issues of Zinacanteco life.

Corporately, the h'iloletik conduct public ceremonies, performed on behalf of local groups or the municipio as a whole, that are independent of but complementary to those performed by the cargoholders. In a sense, we can see Zinacanteco religion as simultaneously a cult of the saints, whose functionaries are the cargoholders, and a cult of the Totil-me'iletik practiced by the h'iloletik. The first has its locus in the churches and chapels, the latter at the *ch'ul vinaheletik*. This is, of course, an oversimplification, since the curing ceremonies and public rituals of the h'iloletik include visits to the churches and since the activities of the cargoholders are not directed only at the saints. There is a segregation of function, nonetheless, which can be seen in terms of each group's primary emphasis. The distinction is clearly related to geography and level of social organization: the cargo cult is centered in Hteklum and exists on behalf of the entire municipio; the public ceremonies of the h'iloletik express the identity of snas, waterhole groups, and hamlets, and tend to be located outside Hteklum. The link between the two systems comes precisely at the point where the activities of the h'iloletik are undertaken on behalf of the entire municipio.

By virtue of their public religious function, in no way subordinate to that of the cargoholders, the h'iloletik as a body (at least the male h'iloletik) enjoy the general respect of the community. However, this prestige attaches itself differentially to the h'iloletik as individuals. It seems to pertain most to the senior h'iloletik in the various hamlets who are responsible for the organization and direction of the public ceremonies or who have ratified their status through frequent participation. It extends itself least to the undeclared h'iloletik who avoid their public service. And it presumably does not at all affect the status of female h'iloletik (which is still likely to be higher than that of ordinary women).

In addition to their public functions, of course, the h'iloletik derive considerable prestige from their specialized medical abilities. A Zinacanteco interprets the improved well-being that may result from a curing ceremony as a consequence of the h'ilol's intervention; the cultural meaning of illness and the group's definition of the h'ilol's actions contribute to and reinforce this conviction. An evaluation of the general position of the h'ilol in Zinacantan, then, must include an awareness of the strictly medical implications of his role. The positive aspects of this dimension of the h'ilol's position, of course, are counterbalanced by the liability that he incurs in being held accountable for the lack of improvement or actual deterioration of health that a patient may experience even after repeated ceremonies.

This leads to our earlier observation that the unambivalent respect accorded the h'iloletik as a group is accompanied by a strong component of suspicion, resentment, and fear on the individual level. The amount of suspicion depends in each case on the curer's reputation for possible witchcraft and/or his insincerity of motive. The resentment may result from an inadequate cure, from the performance of an improper ceremony (at either the personal or the social level), or from a felt conviction that illness has actually been generated by the h'ilol. Fear, of course, varies directly with the degree of awe attached to a particular h'ilol. All these emotions may be felt by other h'iloletik as well as by laymen; and they are often manifested in conflicts whose outcomes run from court cases to assassination.

Relations with the Judicial System

Since there is such a clearly developed mediatory function attached to shamanistic curing, one wonders how this curing fits into the general structure of social control in Zinacantan. Zinacantan does not present as clear-cut a case as societies (e.g., the Eskimo) where the shamanistic role appears to be the only specialized leadership role in the community and the shamanistic performance the only communal activity suited to mediatory functions. Nor is it like societies where institutions of superordinate social control are nonexistent or ineffective and shamanistic curing assumes their function. Zinacantan has a well-developed institution of adjudication and social control, the civil government. It is provided with powerful sanctions such as fines and imprisonment, and with a native police force to actualize its authority. Mediatory curing does not exist, therefore, to perform an otherwise vacant function. Rather, there seem to be a division of functions between the two—or perhaps more accurately, a point beyond which the formal system of adjudication is not suited to act but where a need for superordinate mediation exists.

Although serious domestic difficulties are sometimes taken to the native court in Hteklum, most problems are not given such a hearing. From the outlying hamlets it is a considerable trip to Hteklum, and one must present the usual gifts to the Presidente Municipal and perhaps to other officials before the case is heard. One, and often several, trips must be made, often with witnesses and supporters, so that time is lost and expense incurred by many people. Moreover, the litigants all run the risk of fines, imprisonment, lengthy delays, occasional capricious and/or extortionate behavior on the part of the civil authorities, and so on. The gravity of the case, in short, must be weighed against the disadvantages of taking it to Hteklum. Many domestic upsets, of course, do not manifest themselves in any overt fact of sufficient importance to warrant litigation, although they may be nonetheless real and upsetting. Indeed cases of unresolved tension for which no outlet can properly be sought in the courts seem most likely to contribute to the behavior of some of those carrying the label of illness.

Allegations of witchcraft occasionally come before the court in Hteklum, especially in cases where the suspected witch is a h'ilol. Usually these are cases where fraud is involved, where there has been considerable property damage or a long string of illnesses and misfortune, or where there is some public danger (as when someone is suspected of having sent a highly contagious illness). Barring a situation where the supposed victim can bring corroborating witnesses or some sort of material evidence, however, little is gained by bringing vague allegations against one's neighbors and relatives to the court. These complaints are better objectified through illness and handled informally by a h'ilol.

Conflict in Zinacantan thus seems to fall into two spheres. In one are the major problems that warrant formal adjudication, because of their importance to the people involved or the society as a whole. In the other are less significant domestic or localized tensions, often inchoate or submerged, whose mediation by some superordinate institution is necessary to the stability of a family or local unit but whose nature makes them inappropriate for referral to Hteklum. If it is correct to see the dividing line (at least in part) as a matter of weighing the costs of court action against the possible advantages to be gained, then propinquity to the cabildo in Hteklum should be a factor. Such evidence as we have does indeed suggest that the factors supporting the mediatory role of the h'ilol—a stable patient-h'ilol relationship, the h'ilol's knowledge of the local situation—are less prevalent in the valley of Hteklum than elsewhere in the municipio. Not enough evidence is available, however, to test the hypothesis satisfactorily.

As we stated earlier, the h'iloletik appear to occupy a somewhat controversial position in Zinacanteco society. As a group they are both feared and respected for their supernatural powers. These earn them an indispensable and often prestigeful role in society but at the same time label them as potential witches. H'iloletik operate with great independence in some areas but against strong judicial opposition in others, specifically wherever there is a question of misuse of the curer's powers or of witchcraft. Their position mainly complements that of the civil officials in the area of social control, but it is in many ways a competing role. We suspect that in this particular domain one can observe the

beginnings of a social erosion of shamanistic powers, a process that is
in many ways inevitable, given the colonial origin and persisting influence of the civil system. The complete unity that may have characterized the ancient Maya life in the realm of illness, well-being, and social
process—what one could term a psychological and sociosomatic view
of illness—no longer prevails (see Chapter 7), and it can be hypothe-
sized that the colonial influences are partly responsible.

The municipal authorities, even so, play an important role in maintaining the system of shamanistic curing, and their relations with the
h'iloletik are by and large cooperative. The h'iloletik are in charge of the
planning and execution of the public K'in Krus and Year Renewal ceremonies (and sometimes of public curing or rainmaking ceremonies);
but the authorization of the civil authorities is necessary in order to
collect funds for the costs of these rites. In the hamlets this procedure
seems to be informal and variable. In 'Apas, for example, there is a group
of elders who have acquired local authority over such matters as the
collection and disbursement of public funds. Such groups may include
the senior h'iloletik, but their composition is not prescribed by any formal pattern of organization. In other hamlets it appears that the h'iloletik
themselves are able to collect public subscriptions for the ceremonies.

On an individual level, by contrast, the relations between h'iloletik
and the Zinacanteco authorities tend to be coercive. It is through the
judicial system, for example, that a new h'ilol who is practicing surreptitiously is unmasked and forced to fulfill his public duties. It seems
clearly implicit in Zinacanteco thinking about h'iloletik, and in the actions of the authorities, that the curing role benefits the practitioner and
establishes his responsibility to use his powers for public as well as private welfare. Failure to participate in the public ceremonies is thus an
offense against the public good, as well as against the other h'iloletik,
whose own burdens are increased by another's default. The h'iloletik
have no power to discipline one of their own number however; and it
is the court that hears such cases and applies judicial sanctions.

A second major occasion for judicial proceedings against a h'ilol is the
complaint of a dissatisfied client, usually an accusation of witchcraft
(see J. Collier, 1973). Such cases are fairly frequent (although we lack
sufficient data to accurately estimate the frequency of any class of law
cases in Zinacantan). Typically, the h'ilol will promise to cure a patient
in some unorthodox fashion (such as using a talking saint) in return
for money. When the promised cure is not effected, the patient, failing

to get his money back on demand, takes the h'ilol to court. The complaints usually center on the misrepresentation involved, since the patient shares the stigma of whatever illicit or witchcraft procedures he has solicited from the h'ilol and so finds it safer to complain about his loss of money than about the h'ilol's methods per se. The authorities, however, tend to focus on the method involved, especially where talking saints or witchcraft are in question.

Besides suffering the complaints of dissatisfied customers, h'iloletik may be accused of witchcraft by kinsmen, neighbors, or supposed victims. Such accusations are most likely when the afflictions of the victim are particularly severe, or when the witchcraft is a public menace, as in the case of an epidemic. According to informants, there have been several threatened instances of the latter in recent years, which have been averted only by arresting the culprit and forcing him to withdraw the disease. Not all witchcraft cases involve h'iloletik; but many do, since h'iloletik are more likely than other Zinacantecos to be witches (according to some informants, all witches are h'iloletik).*

Biomedical Implications of the H'ilol's Activities

The classic studies of Ackerknecht (1942–47), which led to the development of important insights in the study of ethnomedicine, are a convenient reference point in evaluating Zinacanteco medicine and treatment. These early contributions must in many ways be regarded as transitional: they were the first attempts to critically review and analyze a large body of information (much of it anecdotal, impressionistic, and highly biased) that had been accumulating about the medical practices of nonliterate people. Researchers like Clements (1932), Evans-Pritchard (1937), and Rivers (1924) had dealt with the conceptual styles of "primitives" in a variety of contexts, with considerable focus on medical concerns. Ackerknecht reviewed their assumptions, clarified their logic, and developed a perspective that is still valuable today, despite its limitations. (For subsequent developments of this theme, see Erasmus, 1952; Simmons, 1955; Frake, 1961; Scotch, 1963; Fabrega and Metzger, 1968; and Fabrega, 1972 and in press.)

---

* It should be mentioned as a possible hazard of the h'ilol role that the assassination of witches, either by their putative victims or by vigilante mobs, has been a frequent occurrence in the past. These homicides appear to be infrequent at present. The reasons for the decrease are not clear, but may include the fact that a local political boss, Mariano Zarate, was prosecuted by Ladino authorities and imprisoned for allegedly authorizing the killing of witches.

What Ackerknecht first pointed out was the need to attend to the premises and the assumptions underlying primitive medical beliefs and practices. He emphasized the imprecision and ambiguity associated with the attempt to distinguish the concept of supernatural causes (causes attributed to sorcery, witchcraft, deities, etc.) from that of natural causes (e.g., old age, exposure to cold or heat). Elaborations of the "natural" usually contain supernatural premises; conversely, probing for explanations of the "supernatural" often involves an appeal to events or interpretations that could be labeled naturalistic. In an attempt to resolve this intellectual dilemma, Ackerknecht suggested that what had often appeared to be natural in an explanation or conceptual style may merely have been habitual—that is, there had simply been an absence of urgency and an "automatic" character to the way in which the medical explanations described as "natural" had been offered. He noted that natives most often used these "natural" causes to explain illnesses that were non-problematic, highly visible, and very common.

The critical limitation in Ackerknecht's early work is his confusion about what constitutes rationality in a medical explanation (a legacy from the earlier, biased impressions of others). At times he equates this with the Western or the valid, at other times with the "natural," and usually by implication with the desirable or modern in a native's mode of thinking. Quite obviously, the explanation that a person offers may be considered "rational" if it follows the rules of logic, regardless of the epistemological status of its premises. The confusion, in part, stems from thus confounding the structure or logic of explanations with the presumed status of their premises.

We will not further detail the relevance of Ackerknecht's early contributions, but we wish to make several points regarding his intentions. The utility or purpose of classifying and differentiating medical explanations (e.g., whether they are "supernatural" as opposed to natural or rational) is clear when one's goal is to assess the medical value or "correctness" of native practices and beliefs—that is, when the investigator, assuming Western medical principles to be valid, tries to determine the degree to which native beliefs and practices approximate the Western ones. But this can only be accomplished when the knowledge and methods of the biological sciences can be used to simultaneously analyze and interpret what appears to take place, within this Western framework, in the particular setting where "primitive" medicine is being practiced.

Ackerknecht's accomplishment was to sensitize observers to the distinction between evaluating what actually transpires in these primitive medical transactions (contrasting the efficacious or medicinal with the useless) and determining what the natives believe or surmise has taken place. In other words, he distinguished the instrumental value of a belief or action in a particular setting from the interpretation placed on it by the subjects themselves. From the interpretive standpoint, one value in differentiating the natural from the supernatural (assuming this distinction can be agreed on) may be the usefulness of the distinction in explaining the behavior that attends differing native interpretations. There are, of course, any number of reasons for differentiating or typing the nature of the premises used in a medical explanation, depending on the analytic intentions of the investigator.

In line with the distinctions drawn by Ackerknecht, we wish to make two points about medical concerns in Zinacantan. First, we must emphasize once again that Zinacantecos (including h'iloletik) do not view the body as an interrelated system whose functioning determines or affects an individual's state of health. The value of herbs, poultices, and other physical remedies is always explained on spiritual grounds and ultimately involves the notion of revelation. We cannot determine to what extent trial-and-error testing and evaluation have contributed to the use of particular remedies, although recent literature in medical anthropology suggests that this may sometimes be a significant factor in ethnomedical practices (Laughlin, 1963; Alland, 1971). The second point we wish to make is that we did not address ourselves to this empirical and essentially ecological issue; consequently, we have no information on the physiological effects of the various herbs and preparations used in curing ceremonies.

The ideas of Jerome Frank (1961) must also be considered in assessing the medical value of curing ceremonies in preliterate settings. He emphasizes the critical importance of the emotional states accompanying a condition of disability that rests on or is principally "caused" by underlying biomedical processes. (The contemporary literature in psychosomatic medicine, of course, is replete with observations that urge us to adopt such a unified perspective toward disease—see Engel, 1960; Lipowski, 1969; Fabrega and Manning, 1973.) The emotions invariably linked with an occurrence of disease are analogous to those we label as hopelessness, despair, and anxiety. The consequences of these emotions for the sick person are negative: probably through the hormonal imbalances they are associated with, they contribute to the deterioration of his physical status; at the same time, their behavioral correlates can interfere with proper rest, hydration, and nutrition, which aid the body in its attempts to ward off the effects of the disease process.

Frank emphasizes the strong social and psychological effects that nonliterate curing ceremonies can have. A ceremony draws the key personal contacts of the patient together, and enhances his self-esteem by promoting the sympathy and good intentions of his friends even as he is expiating past sins. Moreover, these sociopsychological effects occur in a culturally meaningful context that generates hope and the anticipation of help and improved well-being. Thus the negative emotional correlates of disease, which can retard improvement, are counteracted, and are replaced by feelings that have a beneficial effect. The patient gains confidence and hope that others, including spiritual agents, are working on his behalf through the mediation of the curer. These factors, Frank implies, may even affect the disease process itself by altering hormonal balances and promoting the body's natural recuperative powers; previously withdrawn and isolated individuals will begin to show an interest in food, activity, and their social environment generally as a result of the enhanced self-value bestowed by the ceremony.

Frank's approach, then, is aimed at explaining the beneficial effects of curing ceremonies on those who are suffering from morbid pathophysiological processes. If to his list of potentially beneficial factors we add the possibility that an undefined subset of patients improve simply because the purely social definition of their illness is eliminated by the curing ceremony, we complete the picture of how curing ceremonies can promote healing in Zinacantan as in other nonliterate settings. Several previous reports have drawn attention to the role that purely social factors can play in generating illness conditions (see Rubel, 1960; O'Nell and Selby, 1968), and we have already reviewed related considerations in Zinacantan. Many people no doubt experience distress and are labeled as ill by themselves and their associates even when they have no physiological problems. Whether they only adopt the "sick role" (Parsons, 1951) for socially expedient reasons, to what extent this decision is rationally or consciously determined, and which concomitant bodily sensations and biological processes lead them to choose the role are difficult questions to answer. They require a type of analysis that we did not regard as productive at this stage of our knowledge, given the nature of the existing constraints in Zinacantan. The point we wish to stress is that a ceremony can have concrete curative properties insofar as the illness episode is tied entirely to social circumstances, since the crises that generated the illness behavior are often resolved by the ceremony. In other words, the *label* of illness is removed as a consequence of the curing.

Many reports in the literature, both in Latin America and elsewhere, claim to validate the actual efficacy of native curing practices and have generally offered support for Frank's formulation (e.g., Gillin, 1948; Holland and Tharp, 1964; Madsen, 1955). However, the impression one gains from these reports is that the investigators have not focused on the patient's illness longitudinally. By this we mean that we are given no data on the long-term consequences of ceremonies, in the sense of detailed and multidimensional analyses (i.e. from both the biomedical and the cultural perspective) of the careers of sick persons in preliterate settings.

In our work in Zinacantan it was not possible to carry out such analyses. First of all, obtaining permission to merely observe ceremonies is quite problematic, since they are, above all, highly private affairs. Similarly, the tenuous moral, social, and biological status of a patient following a ceremony renders visits and interviews with even his family equally problematic. We also found it difficult to obtain information about who was thought to be developing illness in a hamlet, and hence were not able to determine early in the "career" of sick persons the nature of the symptoms and signs present. Zinacantecos are reticent about their private and moral concerns; and quite often the label of illness (accompanied by the decision to seek treatment) is applied rather abruptly, being determined by social and private contingencies as well as by the subjective magnitude of the patient's discomfort. Interviews with our informants indicate that an illness state is sometimes perceived when minimal objective evidence is present; but more often the perception appears at a stage that a Western physician would judge to be late indeed.

A final, and crucial, impediment to the critical medical evaluation (from the Western standpoint) of a patient treated within the Zinacanteco system is the difficulty of obtaining consent for a physical examination. This consent, if it is ever obtained, is usually given to Ladino physicians in San Cristóbal, and it most often comes at a very late stage of the illness. The patients examined in this way quite understandably tend to be seriously ill, and are usually those who have experienced no benefit from traditional shamanistic treatments.

One final comment should be made about the strictly biomedical implications of the h'ilol's activities. As we have seen (Chapters 3 and 9), Zinacantecos and other residents of the region have ready access to various pharmaceutical products that are sold commercially in San Cristóbal. These products range from the pharmacologically active (e.g., antibiotics and steroid preparations) to the (apparently) physiologically innocuous; and a Zinacanteco patient very often uses several of these commercial remedies in addition to the more "traditional" cures prescribed by the h'ilol. This exposure to multiple sources of influence creates an additional and somewhat formidable obstacle to any systematic empirical evaluation of the h'ilol's activities.

In sum, the attempt to critically examine the medical value of the h'ilol's activities is a difficult undertaking. One must accurately and repeatedly evaluate the physiological status of the patient, the pharmacological value of the native remedies that he uses, the unique sociopsychological consequences of the ceremony, and the therapeutic contribution of other practitioners and medications from San Cristóbal. It was the existence of considerations such as these that led us to restrict the focus of our inquiry and to adopt an essentially ethnomedical framework in evaluating the activities of the h'iloletik.

The reader should be aware that similar attempts to evaluate the actual quality or effectiveness of medical care in Western settings are also quite problematic (Kerr and Trantow, 1968; Last, 1965; Weinerman, 1966). The developing literature in this field of medicine has pointed to the many unresolved conceptual issues that exist. We must define concepts such as health and illness. And we must establish an operational measure of quality. (Should it be, for example, improved well-being, exposure to competently trained physicians, or the administration of medical procedures judged to be scientifically optimal or acceptable?) The methodological difficulties are equally impressive (Donabedian, 1966).

General Statement Regarding H'iloletik and Medical Care in Zinacantan

H'iloletik are the average Zinacanteco's chief link with the spiritual forces that guide and supervise his worldly activities; and this function is most evident during illness and curing. Because he "sees" the ideal world peopled by the gods, the h'ilol can petition these beings on behalf of the sick persons who seek his services. Similarly, by praying to the earth owner or by entering into direct contact with various malevolent agents, he can undo harm and retrieve the patient's soul, thereby restoring health.

We have seen that illness in Zinacantan, which is signaled by a variety of psychobiologic changes and infirmities, elicits a characteristic pattern of actions on the part of the sick person and his family. If the illness is persistent and seriously disabling, of course, the family will call the h'ilol in for a "diagnostic" visit. Often, however, it is the social context of the illness that proves decisive in the decision to seek a h'ilol. As we saw in Chapter 9, intercurrent social events (such as rivalries and tensions) or the occurrence of personally inciting experiences such as dreams (which are believed to portend or reflect "supernatural" happenings) frequently provide the motivating reasons for this action. For it must be emphasized that to a Zinacanteco illness represents a state of moral and spiritual discord—an individual's displacement or disarticulation from his regular position in the scheme of things. The h'ilol who visits a patient and takes on the responsibility for his cure is thus quite literally restoring that person's sense of belonging to an ordered and meaningfully structured world that connects with the one beyond.

The h'ilol's other duties, though less dramatic, are equally characteristic of his role as mediator between the earthly and spiritual worlds. New house ceremonies compensate Yahval Balamil, the earth owner, for the materials used in building the house. The K'in Krus ceremony, when performed at the level of the sna, reaffirms the ties that the sna has with its patrilineal ancestors, spiritually uniting the group members as common worshipers and upholders of traditional customs and beliefs. When performed for a waterhole group, the same ceremony would appear to symbolize the rights and obligations that the members share in drawing water. And at the hamlet level, K'in Krus symbolizes the connection that Zinacantecos see between their respective ties to their group, their physical environment, and their bodily and spiritual well-being. Rain-making ceremonies, too, would appear to reflect the h'ilol's vital role in linking Zinacantecos' physical needs to the affairs of their gods. Finally, in the Year Renewal ceremonies, the h'iloletik symbolically affirm the spiritual ties between all Zinacanteco hamlets and the ancestral tribal gods of Hteklum.

The h'ilol's duties and responsibilities, then, reflect the unity or holism that Zinacantecos see in the forces that maintain the individual and his group in a balanced state of optimal functioning. Illness and health are only transitory stages in man's perpetual struggle to sustain himself physically and spiritually. The isomorphism that Zinacantecos, like other Mayas, see between earthly and otherworldly happenings is mirrored in their beliefs about illness, in their curing practices, and in the myriad of social and spiritual functions performed by the h'iloletik. In societies like our own, medical activities are secularized and separated from other activities that reflect the workings of presumably independent "institutions." In Zinacantan, one can still observe the integrated nature of folk life, wherein physical survival, spiritual communion, social cohesion, and psychobiologic well-being appear to be fused and all-expressive of man's position in the world. It is this essential unity that the h'ilol is empowered to control and restore.

The material reviewed in Chapter 4 suggests that socially, despite the demands of their role, h'iloletik do fairly well in the cargo-ranking system of Zinacantan. From a remunerative standpoint they may achieve fewer economic returns for their efforts; but they cannot, on the average, be said to earn less than Zinacantecos who are full-time agriculturalists or part-time workers in Ladino-dominated enterprises. Psychologically, there is little to link those who become h'iloletik with psychopathology or psychiatric disorder. Indeed, the projective responses to our tests indicate that h'iloletik may be less restrained and constricted in their relations with others and in their private reminiscences or fantasies. One way of interpreting many of these responses, we observed, was to see in them time-related correlates of occupying a position that requires delving into the socially and psychologically uncomfortable matters that we associated with chamel. The essentially conservative and traditional social posture of the h'ilol, demonstrated in the same chapter, is in keeping with the socially sanctioned functions that involve him with the time-honored spiritual traditions of the group. H'iloletik, almost by definition as well as empirically, are essential yet very modern representatives of the sacred ways of the Maya.

The information reviewed in Chapters 7 and 8 indirectly corroborates the fundamental social and spiritual sanctions that validate the h'ilol as a medical practitioner. Definite and rather interesting response tendencies, some with far-reaching implications for our understanding of ethnomedical systems, characterized the h'iloletik when they were questioned about their knowledge of illness and curing. However, what must be termed their conservative view of illness was also prominent. In a region where Western biomedical notions of disease (i.e. a naturalistic orientation to causation and treatment) are slowly eroding indigenous and colonial orientations (Aguirre-Beltran, 1963), h'iloletik maintain a supernaturalistic and essentially restricted view of illness. This was evident when they were confronted with photographs of obviously diseased persons and asked to scale the severity and name the sources of the illnesses involved. Furthermore, we observed that with regard to the meaning of illness, whether defined denotatively (i.e. in terms of bodily mechanisms and actual physiological manifestations) or connotatively (i.e. in terms of affective dimensions), no qualitatively distinct view prevailed among the representative group of h'iloletik we studied.

In the domain of illness and curing, then, a h'ilol's specialized knowledge of bodily mechanisms or manifestations of illness is not important. Rather, it is the spiritualistic power he owns that appears to sanction and confirm his actions in the medical sphere. The implicit rules that seem to underlie and govern this ethnomedical system of care were outlined in Chapter 9. We also noted the interesting premises that sustain this mode of medical care delivery and appear to protect the h'ilol in his precarious and vulnerable enterprise of wrestling with supernatural, malevolent, and potentially life-destructive cosmic forces.

In Chapters 10 and 11 we reviewed the intricate ritualistic duties that h'iloletik perform in Zinacantan. As we saw earlier in this chapter, it is in these duties and actions that the essential influences and functions of the h'iloletik inhere. For it is in performing the various public and private ceremonies amidst the social and interpersonal affairs of men that the h'ilol displays the time-honored powers linked to his role. His mediatory ritualistic acts seem designed to bind earthly man in his everyday social world to the deliberations of ancestral and other supernatural beings, and they display for us the h'ilol's supporting and unifying functions in the culture.

In this book we have tried to analyze illness and medical care in Zinacantan while preserving as much as possible the native view and perspective. At the same time, we have adopted a comparative orientation to this analysis, and ideas from the social sciences and from biomedicine have been used to explain and understand the Zinacanteco approach to illness and medical care. We believe that in many ways the Zinacanteco approach can be used as a paradigm of how certain simple folk societies are oriented to disease, and that consequently a comparative analysis will be informative insofar as it makes explicit the changes and modifications brought about by complex processes such as urbanization and technological development. Illness or disease, in short, is universal; and all groups, regardless of their culture, are in some way forced to cope with its burdens. By concentrating on an institutional domain like medicine, therefore, one can highlight many fundamental properties of a social system's functioning and psychosocial orientation.

As a way of summing up certain points made in this and other chapters, it seems useful here to offer an overall comparison of the Zinacanteco system of medical care with the system that prevails in more complex societies like our own. This we do by offering a set of summary propositions that appear to underlie and guide the curing process in each setting.

Western Biomedical System	Zinacanteco System
1. The body is understood as a complex biological machine, and its structure and function are partitioned logically into specific parts and systems. Each of these is evaluated by its level of function, and interdependence among systems is differentiated in a relatively precise manner.	1. The body is seen as a holistic, integrated aspect of both the person and his social relations, which are vulnerable and may be easily affected by gods, by malevolent agents or spirits, by other people, by passions, and by natural forces. Categories referring to the body are unrefined, and the body as an anatomical and physiological entity is only generally partitioned. A simple view of function, extension, and meaning of parts is held.
2. In general, character types and personality styles are only minimally significant in the diagnosis and treatment of disease. Such labels as "moody," "insensitive," and "silly" exist and are socially relevant but not biologically so; disease is given a reality apart from these modes of self-presentation.	2. "Character types" and "self-presentation" are intrinsic parts of how social relations are judged; and social relations bear on the cause, type, diagnosis, and cure of illness; illness is not given a reality independent of the individual, his relatives, and his social relations.
3. Disease is universal in form, progress, and content; and it can in fact be logically divided into stages, each with a beginning and end point.	3. Illness, to a significant extent, is idiosyncratic in form, progress, and content; and it can only be understood in the context of the individual and his relations with others, including in particular the ancestral gods.

Western	Zinacanteco
4. The consequences of disease are seen intersystematically and organically.	4. The consequences of illness may be seen in virtually every facet of a person's social transactions, activities, and concerns, as well as in his relations with supernatural beings.
5. Disease and behavior are logically separated.	5. Illness and behavior are linked both logically and empirically.
6. Time and mechanical forces govern the progress of disease; the unfolding of disease is inexorable in the absence of medical intervention.	6. Spirits, evil forces, and other people govern the progress of illness; the unfolding of an illness depends on its cause, which also determines the requisite curing options.
7. Specific, identifiable causal processes of disease are known, and are identified by accumulated chemical and biological evidence. There is a separation between the causes, which are specified in a technical form, and social relations.	7. Generalized categories of illness cause exist, but they lack technical bases and precise delimitation. Categories of cause reflect and are reflected in social relations.
8. The role of the curer is highly differentiated, segmented, and profes-sionalized: (a) full-time occupa-tion; (b) extensive formal training; (c) high specialization; (d) high technical skill; (e) complex, ex-tensive knowledge base, which dis-tinguishes curer from clients; (f) strong social and political control of access to the profession; (g) legal title validates role.	8. The role of the h'ilol is not fully differentiated: (a) part-time occupation; (b) little or no "formal" training; (c) relatively little speciali-zation: (d) low technical skill; (e) limited knowledge base, and this base does not distinguish him from lay comembers; (f) almost "open" access to curing role; (g) revelation, spirituality, and social sanctions validate role.
9. Medical specialization is based on precisely defined knowledge, tech-niques, and procedures, all of which are discontinuous from ordinary social processes.	9. Specialization in cures is based on types of cause: illness resulting from witchcraft must be treated by a witch, bodily malfunction due to nonmalevolent forces by a "good" h'ilol, etc. The rationale for under-standing and affecting these pro-cesses is continuous with ordinary social processes of everyday life.
10. Disease is seen as an abstract entity with specifiable properties and a recurring identity. It can be treated anywhere and anytime, provided the necessary technical prerequisites are present.	10. Illness is personalized, idio-syncratic, and mysterious, involving complex forms and processes. It must be treated in special locations at highly "critical" times, using many symbolic and multivalued elements.

Western	Zinacanteco

11. The relationship between physician and patient is highly patterned and based on formal, almost contractual, role prescriptions that are discontinuous from everyday situations. It is instrumentally oriented, universalistic, neutralistic, and focused.

12. Confidence or trust in a healer is to a considerable extent pre-established or "legislated" by formal means: titles, credentials, certification of legal right (license), and membership in professional organizations, all of which are supported by an appeal to scientific knowledge.

13. The presentation of one's self and the presentation of one's body are separated for all practical purposes, and the treatment relationship is directed to either, depending on the type of disease.

14. The basis of the curer's power and authority over patients is scientific knowledge.

15. The treatment relationship is characterized by distance, coolness, formal relations, and the use of abstract concepts (jargon).

16. The responsibility of the practitioner appears to be principally to the patient; the scientific and legal-judicial communities implement this.

11. The relationship between h'ilol and patient is informal, diffuse, non-contractual, and semicontinuous with everyday situations. It is expressively oriented, particularistic, affective, and diffuse.

12. Confidence or trust in a h'ilol is transactional, and it must be situationally legitimized by the way the h'ilol and patient are seen to relate to each other. Trust varies with time, place, person, day, and symbols used, and is highly affected by the course and outcome of the transaction itself, as well as by intercurrent social happenings. Because the course of illness affects trust and reflects on the morality of h'ilol and patient, it may be viewed as more changeable.

13. Body and self are seen as presented together, and the treatment relationship is directed to both, in the context of various spiritual and social factors.

14. The basis of the h'ilol's power and authority over patients is personal charisma and/or spiritual revelation, as conveyed by repute, authenticity of recruitment, appearance, and past curing performance.

15. The treatment relationship is symbolized by closeness, shared meaning, warmth, informality, and the use of everyday language.

16. The responsibility of the h'ilol is to the patient, to his family, to the community, and ultimately to the ancestral gods; legal-judicial systems as well as supernatural agents implement this. Patient is but one instanciation of a series of duties and functions that the h'ilol performs for gods and for his people.

Western	*Zinacanteco*
17. The responsibility and aim of the practitioner is principally to remove disease (biomedically defined), but also to alleviate discomfort.	17. The immediate responsibility and aim of the h'ilol is principally to undo the harm, punishment, or evil that has caused illness, but also to alleviate discomfort. Ultimately, he is to please the gods and further the continuation of the group.
18. Except in limited instances (e.g., mental illness), the practitioner's decisions, actions, and judgments do not directly affect the workings of the social system.	18. The h'ilol's decisions, actions, and judgments intimately act on, reflect, and feed back to workings of the social system. Illness is taken as evidence of social wrongdoing, leads to the implementation of social sanctions, and thus becomes an element in the articulation of social policy. What the h'ilol judges and believes about illness leads to social action.
19. The practitioner is geared to probe an impersonal entity (i.e. disease), using abstract and technological "language."	19. The h'ilol is constantly assessing morality, guilt, and "character" as his basis for deciding to treat and choosing a mode of treatment, and he uses the language of social relations.
20. The practitioner may acknowledge his inability to cure by specifying the nature and extent of the "pathology" of a disease, but is always obligated to render help.	20. The h'ilol may acknowledge his inability to cure and render care by specifying the nature and strength of the evil influences causing the illness, or by claiming preexisting social or economic commitments.
21. The practitioner, in principle, is obligated to help and continue to give help when consulted.	21. The h'ilol has the option of noninterference when consulted, since a primary responsibility is to his family as agriculturalist and supporter.
22. The physician influences a patient's actions (i.e. compliance) by invoking his biomedical knowledge of disease processes to sanction the validity of his advice. He does not appeal to moral considerations.	22. The h'ilol influences a patient's actions by invoking his spiritual knowledge of illness and his own capacity to directly aggravate illness. He appeals to moral considerations to shape behavior of patient.
23. The patient does not, in principle, fear the practitioner's retaliation for any past or present slight.	23. The patient always fears the h'ilol's retaliation for any slight.

Western

24. The risk a practitioner may incur by accepting responsibility for the treatment of an illness is *collectively distributed* by: (a) legal systems; (b) professional associations; (c) insurance; (d) the referral system (horizontal); (e) specialization (vertical); (f) collective "business" organizations such as group practice, partnerships, and hospitals.

25. Referral is highly patterned, rationalized, differentiated horizontally and vertically, and rule-oriented.

26. Curing time is purchased in discrete units and is contractually shared. The clock governs the availability of the physician, and the day is highly segmented—15-minute time units, 8-hour day, 6-day week, and 11-month year of practice.

27. Treatment procedures are universal, formal, learned, and impersonal; they are not altered significantly by the time and place of treatment or the personality of the physician.

28. Treatment is frequently seen as mechanical and impersonal, and only for "mental illness" does the curing process involve self-expressive, self-modifying components.

29. Curing tools and procedures are specialized, discontinuous from, and unavailable to a person in everyday life—e.g., otoscopes, X-rays, and lab analysis techniques.

Zinacanteco

24. The risk a h'ilol may incur by accepting responsibility for the treatment of an illness is individualized and *personal*: (a) a person's being is his most significant possession and cannot be protected by formal means; (b) legal controls on the provision of health care are minimal or nonexistent; (c) no professional associations or collective means of distributing risk exist; (d) there is relatively little referral from one h'ilol to another.

25. Referral is "unpatterned," i.e., personalized, idiosyncratic, localistic, and lay-dominated. It is nonhierarchical and undifferentiated.

26. Time is judged analogically, jointly owned and shared, and partitioned complexly: e.g., "moral" or "intersubjective" time, time since the event "causing" the illness, and general time of day for appointments. The day is segmented into relatively few units.

27. Treatment procedures are personalized and idiosyncratic; they are based on the particulars of the transaction, have an interpersonal basis, and are ultimately validated by the presumed spiritual insights and gifts of the h'ilol.

28. For all illnesses, the curing process makes use of emotionally charged symbols tied to the patient's body and person; and it involves culturally defined moments or situations that include significant associates of the patient as well as the relevant supernatural agents.

29. Curing tools and procedures are not specialized, but are continuous with and available to a person in everyday life—e.g., candles, flowers, and rum.

Western	Zinacanteco
30. Curing procedures are aimed at revealing, probing, and adjusting a mechanical entity, the body.	30. Curing procedures are intrinsic to social relations, are consistent with other symbolizations of social relations, and directly implicate supernatural agents.
31. Curing settings are specialized and segregated—home vs. office or clinic.	31. Curing settings are multipurpose. The basic curing setting is both the patient's home and a religious place. Ceremonial cures also take place in public settings that have varied and complex religious functions in the group.
32. Treatment settings are rationally rule-governed. A specific staff with special roles is employed. Paperwork dominates the procedures, which are hierarchical and authoritative—i.e., a bureaucracy governs appointments, treatment, and billing.	32. In the treatment setting, diffuse, overlapping, and socially diverse transactions take place. No special "staff" exists, and family members or relatives help in the ceremony. No paperwork. The healer has limited formal authority over his helpers. Family structure is replicated in the organization of treatment.
33. Curing resources are technological and "scientific," purchased in a market economy, manufactured and complex. They are available in complex systems, e.g., hospitals.	33. Curing resources are proximal, and many are available naturally. Some are purchased, others (drink, herbs) are made or grown. There are many simple and a few specialized systems for obtaining curing resources.

Epilogue: The Relevance and Future of Ethnomedicine

Ethnomedical inquiries afford the analyst an opportunity of uncovering basic premises about illness, disease, and medical care that have often been concealed within the general medical orientation he has developed while "learning" his own culture. Few experiences provide so vivid a context for studying fundamental biocultural traits as do those relating to illness and disease. The relative nature of even these highly personalized experiences is graphically set forth when native patterns of disposition and behavior are examined cross-culturally. At the same time, as we have tried to show in this book, the set of categories, rules, and plans that cultures "offer" their members as a means of explaining and coping with illness are not only highly patterned but also embedded in fundamental premises about the nature of reality and social relations.

Ethnomedical studies, then, can enrich the fields of both social and psychosomatic medicine, since, by unmasking ethnocentric assumptions about disease and medical care, they can lead us to a more refined and rational understanding of how man in general responds to and copes with disease. (See Fabrega, 1971, 1972, and in press.)

In our estimation, anthropological studies can also benefit from the cross-cultural evaluation of illness and medical care. However, mostly because fundamental conceptual issues have not been clarified, work in ethnomedicine has not progressed to the stage where this benefit can be fully realized. As we have indicated, the analytic approaches so far employed have not managed to clarify the basic relations between disease and the workings of a social system. Anthropology requires the examination of paradigmatic assumptions and frameworks, and often the development of new ones when particular problem areas do not lend themselves to resolution. However, rather than bringing this stratagem to bear on the study of medical problems, anthropologists have by and large opted for the biomedical-epidemiological framework, which is designed to answer altogether different types of questions—namely, those aimed at understanding the causes of disease in order to control it effectively. And when a cultural framework has been adopted in studying medical problems, the orientation adopted has usually failed to clarify the basic concepts that are needed for cross-cultural analyses. The usual anthropological orientation, in short, has produced findings that make generalizations and comparisons difficult; hence the basic requirements for theory-building in ethnomedicine have not been met.

Our claim is that to a large extent anthropologists who study medical problems have stopped short of critically addressing themselves to the fundamental problem: that is, explaining how man and his unique human institution, culture, affect the expression of disease and in turn are affected by disease occurrences. When anthropologists have studied the mutual interactions between culture and disease, they have used rather abstract formulations, which leave the process of social life out of focus. Such studies involve general, long-range consequences of disease and are germane to the fields of population biology and cultural evolution; they do not focus on the social consequences of discrete disease occurrences, and consequently cannot deal with the detailed elements of social organizations and change that are influenced by disease. We believe that medical-anthropological studies can and should deal with these detailed questions, and furthermore, that a framework allowing for the comparative analysis of these issues is possible.

In this context, our book represents an initial effort aimed at providing the type of basic information needed to develop an ethnomedical framework that may eventually allow comparative analyses. Hopefully, the material presented will stimulate others to work on just such a task. Our own work in Zinacantan and our involvement in the field of ethnomedicine have convinced us that the primary requirements for this work are suitable medical concepts—that is, concepts that allow one to organize the basic native ("emic") concepts in an accurate manner. With regard to medical issues, what is needed is an initial enumeration of the basic concepts that are assumed to have cross-cultural extensions (e.g., "disease," medical practitioner, and medical procedure), as well as a framework allowing for the accurate definition of these concepts in a form suitable for cross-cultural analysis.

In other words, the ethnomedical analyst must first of all establish a language that can be used to describe and compare important processes in the medical experiences of various peoples. This language, we maintain, should be so articulated that it will automatically lead one to examine the functioning of social and cultural systems. The empirical use of such a language in various cultural settings should yield a pool of information that will achieve certain basic aims: (1) the accurate description of medically related expectations, practices, procedures, and behaviors; (2) the "placement" of these various features in specific sociocultural units whose demography, patterns, values, potential for change, and ecological setting are already known or can be adequately described. Once both aims are realized it should be possible to develop a body of propositions about the interrelations of culture, society, and medicine that can be incorporated within a more general theory and science of man.

Our work in Zinacantan prompts us to suggest that the language we need to describe illness may have to address phenomenologic and social matters. We also believe that suitable indicators of illness can be developed by concentrating on altered behavior. Cultural anthropologists, like other social scientists, easily see the value of focusing directly on human behavior, for it is in this domain that the set of rules or expectations subsumed under the term culture are most accessible. The accurate depiction of illness in a behavioral framework thus accomplishes two things: it focuses on processes that reflect both cultural rules and cultural changes; and it allows for more static (or structural) analyses insofar as the components of medical behavior can be mapped or coded in some abstract way. Both are fundamental to a truly social approach to illness and medical care.

Another reason to regard "illness" as the concept most needing precise articulation in a cross-cultural analysis is that any given illness episode is the central fact around which other medical forms and activities are organized. Illness occurrences interrupt social processes, cause alarm, require attention, can initiate changes in the organization of a group, and can alter relations between groups. They are the focus of all medical activities, and everything that is medically relevant in a social group is brought to bear on them directly or indirectly.

To recapitulate, then, it would seem that anthropologists, in studying activities that can be called medical, are presented with material essential to the development of theories about human behavior and its underlying cultural rules. A fundamental imperative of all social groups is that of dealing with the problems of illness; and medical activities, because they reflect so many basic aspects of sociocultural functioning, can offer the anthropologist a fruitful area of study. First, however, he must establish precise definitions and descriptions of the fundamental elements in medical activities. In particular, since the problems posed by actual illness are in many ways the foci of all medical activities, a suitable set of concepts about illness would seem to be a basic requirement for cross-cultural comparative medical studies. Furthermore, since actual illness occurrences also reveal many structural, processual, and functional aspects of a cultural system, concepts of illness that facilitate the description and analysis of these occurrences will in turn allow one to deal with theoretical questions about culture in general.

The material presented in this book suggests that certain biological aspects of illness (e.g., severity or degree of disability) may be arranged in terms of phenomenologic and moral categories, and that these categories, in turn, affect the way illnesses are treated and handled socially. Such categories may have to be incorporated in any language of illness suitable for cross-cultural use. Intercurrent social events differentially mark an occurrence of illness and can contribute to the way members of the group respond to the occurrence; we may also need some way of marking and retrieving these events. The comparative orientation we have used in Zinacantan has yielded a series of related observations and generalizations that must still be tested and refined by further empirical work. But even such generalizations can ultimately contribute to the development of sociomedical theory.

Attributes and Dimensions of Illness

THIS APPENDIX lists and describes the various dimensions and attributes (e.g., cause, severity) that Zinacantecos employ to classify and interpret illness. Most of the dimensions reviewed here, and all of the terms denoting illnesses that are listed in Appendix B, were the basis of our questionnaire on medical knowledge in Zinacantan (see Chapter 7). This questionnaire, at a later stage of our work in the field, was administered to a representative sample of male h'iloletik and male laymen. For each of the 76 illness terms separately, subjects were asked to assign the illness a value on each dimension. The purpose of this study was to evaluate in a more or less controlled fashion the role of medical knowledge in a h'ilol's practice. By consulting Appendix B the reader may learn how Zinacantecos interpreted each illness in terms of the dimensions we outline here.

Cause

Our informants were asked to volunteer potential causes or sources of illness (see Fabrega, Metzger, and Williams, 1970), and the list that follows includes any concept or term mentioned by at least one informant. No single informant mentioned all of the causes on the list; nor were all causes mentioned equally often. Some terms subsume others but are listed separately because at least one informant insisted on the distinction. In general, the informants' level of abstraction was low, and we found it hard to combine various causes into more general categories.

An observer would find it most convenient to class all Zinacanteco concepts of cause into three general categories, based on the ultimate origin of the illness: (a) illnesses sent by the gods; (b) illnesses originating in hostile human action; (c) illnesses caused by "natural" events. This level of abstraction, however, is somewhat foreign to Zinacanteco concepts. The closest approach made to it is the occasional grouping of all illnesses caused by malevolent human action under the rubric *ta uts ta kolo'* ("witchcraft") or *skuenta krischano* ("due to people"). This classing can be properly expressed in a Tzotzil sentence like *'Oy htos chamel ta skuenta krischano*—"There is a kind of illness caused by people." This large class appears to include a number of other classes that can each be expressed independently: for example, "There is a kind of illness caused by people who sell souls to the earth." This pattern of classification is not maintained when it comes to the other causes of illness, and we have been able to elicit no overall term for "supernatural causes," or "natural causes." Some informants go so far as to lump the Totilme'iletik and the Sun together under the term Kahvaltik (Lords or Gods) as a source of illness. But not even this degree of grouping applies to "natural" causes of illness, each of which appears to be maintained as a separate category.

An illustrative set of statements discriminating illnesses by the attribute of cause is the following, collected from Lol Arias of Navenchauk:

1. There is a kind of illness caused by the ancestral gods.
2. There is a kind of illness caused by the gods in heaven.
3. There is a kind of illness caused by the earth.
4. There is a kind of illness caused by evil people.
5. There is a kind of illness caused by demons from hell.
6. There is a kind of illness caused by the wind.
7. There is a kind of illness caused by cold.
8. There is a kind of illness caused by water.
9. There is a kind of illness that comes by itself.

This classification is typical of those offered by many informants. To a limited extent, the distinctions made among illnesses on the basis of cause seem to correspond to methods of curing. Each of the last four classes, for example, implies a different curative approach. Similarly, the approach taken to an illness caused by evil people is radically different from the cure for one caused by the ancestral gods or by demons. However, although most informants insist strongly on the distinction between illnesses caused by the ancestral gods and those caused by the gods in heaven, there are no major distinctions in the curative procedures taken; most curing ceremonies, in fact, are directed at both kinds of deities. The correspondence, then, is not perfect; but it is salient enough to at least reinforce other indications that concepts of cause and cure are intimately bound up with one another in Zinacanteco medical beliefs.

The list of all factors mentioned by informants as causes of illness is as follows:

1. *Kahvaltik ta Vinahel* (Our lords in heaven). Some confusion arises over the number and nature of the heavenly deities. It seems fairly certain that the principal deity is the Sun, Totik K'ak'al, who may be identified in some Zinacantecos' minds with the Catholic figure of God the Father. This deity is the foremost heavenly source of illness, which he sends as a punishment for transgressions of divinely sanctioned morality or for failure to exhibit proper respect to the gods. There are three major types of heavenly visitation mentioned by informants. One is the "direct blow," described below. The others are indirect visitations. In one, the illness is sent to a particular individual as a punishment for his acts. In the other, it is let loose against the entire human race as a general punishment or admonition.

Some informants locate Hesukristu among the heavenly deities, but no illnesses are attributed to him. Another deity is Hch'ul Me'tik, the Moon. Her role also seems limited. A possible exception is the illness *chlok' hch'ul me'tik ta sat* ("the moon appears in the eye," probably cataracts), which occurs when one looks at the moon. Some informants consider this a punishment from god in heaven because of the divine status of the moon, but others see it as merely a natural occurrence.

According to some informants, finally, the souls of the saints also reside in heaven, although others believe that they live in the churches. It is said that the saints can strike one with illness for failure to pay them proper respect—especially in the case of a cargoholder who does not properly discharge his duties. No informant, however, has attributed any given illness to this cause, even as a possibility.

2. *Smantal htotik hme'tik* (illnesses sent by the ancestral gods). Illnesses are inflicted by the Totilme'iletik in three ways. One is by the "direct blow" (see No. 4 below). The second is by sending an illness directly to punish the victim, as the god in heaven does; apparently, illnesses sent in this way are always aimed at a particular individual. The third way the ancestral gods cause illness is by mistreating the victim's *chanul* (animal spirit or soul), which is in their custody. Any injury incurred by the chanul is also felt by its human companion, since the two share the same soul. In order to punish a Zinacanteco, then, the Totilme'iletik can injure his chanul in various ways: by directly beating it; by failing to feed it; by inflicting illness on it; or by releasing it from its corral to wander the mountainsides and risk injury or death. If the chanul dies, death is inevitable for its human companion. Some informants express the belief that a person may have three or four chanuletik, so that the death of one does not automatically kill him. Some h'iloletik are reputed to be able to cure by replacing a patient's chanul within the short time between its death and that of its human counterpart.

Illness caused by the Totilme'iletik, through whichever mechanism, is always seen as divine punishment. There are two aspects to avoiding this punishment: one must live in accordance with divinely sanctioned concepts of morality; and one must maintain a proper relationship with the Totilme'iletik through the occasional performance of curing ceremonies. Even if a Zinacanteco is fortunate enough to escape illness over a long period of time, he is supposed to show his respect for the Totilme'iletik by holding a preventive curing ceremony, and there is a special ceremonial form for this purpose. If he fails to hold the ceremony, he may suffer illness because the Totilme'iletik "want" him; that is, they demand either his soul or the sacrifices and signs of respect offered in a ceremony.

3. *Smantal pukuh* (illness sent by demons). Despite their importance as agents of illness, the nature of the *pukuhetik*, or demons, is curiously vague in Zinacanteco mythology. In versions that seem strongly influenced by Catholicism, informants state that the pukuhetik serve a deity named Impierno, who presides over the fiery hell of K'atin Bak. To some, demons are the souls of deceased sinners; to others, they are a separate class of beings. The belief

that seems most widely held is that the pukuhetik are a completely distinct class of supernatural being, unconnected with hell, but possibly under the command of the ancestral and heavenly gods.

A few informants talk of demons as messengers of the gods, and say that two of them are always following each Zinacanteco, awaiting the divine word to strike him with illness. It seems more commonly believed, however, that the demons themselves can initiate illness, either by striking the individual directly (mahbenal) or by sending an illness. The illness can apparently be warded off by divine protection or by various precautions (for example, by the postceremonial restrictions described in Chapter 11). The demons occasionally appear in human form, especially in the dreams of h'iloletik, where their appearance is taken as a portent of illness. Their actions in striking men with illness seem motivated by general malevolence, and they are particularly liable to strike when the victim is in a weakened condition from some other illness.

4. *Smahben kahvaltik* (direct blows from the gods in heaven). Illness caused by direct blows is often lumped into a single category, mahbenal; but some informants distinguish between blows inflicted by heavenly gods, ancestral gods, and demons. The symptoms are the same in all three cases. The victim feels the physical sensations of being beaten and suffers aftereffects like aches, pains, and fever. If he is already ill, the mahbenal may aggravate his condition.

5. *Smahben htotik hme'tik.* Direct blows from the Totilme'iletik.

6. *Smahben pukuh.* Direct blows from demons.

7. *Komel ta balamil* or *shi'el* ("remaining in the earth" or "fright"). This is the widespread Middle American phenomenon of *espanto*, or soul-loss. In Zinacanteco belief the ch'ulel, or immanent soul, has thirteen parts, and any or all of these can leave the body under various circumstances. The entire soul leaves the body during sleep, encountering experiences that the individual sees and remembers through dreams. The soul can also leave the body when a person is frightened; and it can be separated from the body by witchcraft. (See Foster, 1953; and Rubel, 1964.)

Parts of the soul that leave the body because of fright pass into the ground at the point of shi'el. There they fall into the custody of a Yahval Balamil, or earth owner, who uses them as household laborers and beasts of burden. The mistreatment suffered by parts of the soul in the underworld is communicated to the remaining parts and their body in the world above. (One feature of this concept is the belief that earth owners assume the form of fat, rich Ladinos and turn captured souls into mules to carry their enormous riches. The Ladino-driven mule trains that are a common sight in San Cristóbal are, for Zinacantecos, objects of suspicion. One never knows if the hard-bitten muleteer is not really a sinister Yahval Balamil herding the captive souls of his Zinacanteco victims.)

Soul-loss can be occasioned by any sort of frightening experience. The most common is falling down, which almost inevitably leads to shi'el (perhaps because it combines fright and physical contact with the earth). If one dreams of a frightening or painful experience, the soul can also be lost. In this case the victim may see it in dreams, laboring for the earth owners. Such dreams can help a h'ilol diagnose the illness and locate the proper site for a recovery ceremony.

8. *Chonbil ta balamil* ("selling to the earth"). The soul can also pass into the possession of an earth owner through witchcraft. The witch speaks to the subterranean world in a cave or swamp,* asking the Yahval Balamil to take the victim's soul and inflict illness on him. This may be accompanied by other witchcraft procedures designed to cause illness, such as the burning of many small candles of the seven magic colors (white, red, black, green, yellow, gold, tallow). These are cut into small pieces, burned upside down, pricked with needles, doused with gasoline, kerosene, and rum, or buried in the ground; all these manipulations are believed to transmit pain to the victim. If brooms and fish are hung by nooses in the cave, the victim will suffer sensations of choking. And if a piece of meat is left in a cave or river to rot, the decomposition will also manifest itself in the victim's body. Witches are also believed to change themselves into animals, in which shape they wander the trails at night, frightening and attacking their victims.

9. *Ak'bil chamel* ("thrown" or "given" illness). This, the second kind of witchcraft illness, is sent directly by the witch without recourse to a supernatural intermediary. The procedures used are often those described above. At other times, the illness is sent by placing foreign objects in the victim's food or drink, often in a glass of rum that the witch offers him in a spuriously friendly fashion.

10. *Kuybalal chamel.* This is a rather rare form of witchcraft. Some informants regard it as a single illness, others as a cause that can lie behind several different kinds of illness. Kuybalal chamel is a virulent epidemic that can be sent only by the inhabitants of two Ladino towns in Chiapas, Totolapa and Simojovel. A malevolent Zinacanteco may solicit it from one of these towns; or, if a Zinacanteco incurs the displeasure of someone from the town, the illness may be sent directly. The origin of this belief is unknown. Totolapa and Simojovel are widely separated towns, one to the north and the other to the south of Zinacantan.

11. *Ok'itabil chamel* ("illness sought by weeping"). Illness may be called down by appealing directly to the gods. This procedure is said to be used by an injured victim against an aggressor, but some informants see it as a form of witchcraft. Occasionally, according to a few informants, an individual may cry to the gods to end his own life, or to send an illness severe enough to win him sympathy from his family and friends.

12. *Sat k'ak'al* ("hot eye"). Certain illnesses, especially those of children,

---

* A list of caves where the soul may be sold was obtained from the h'ilol Lol Pérez Komyosh, who claims to know the ceremony for recovering a soul. He includes: 'Isak'tik (hamlet of 'At'sam); Nakleb 'Ok ('At'sam); Lach Chikin ('At'sam); Na Hoh (Hteklum); Pat Toh (Hteklum); Hoyo Ch'en (Pat'osil); Toch' (Nachih); K'uk' Ch'en (Sekemtik). Other informants mention Buro Vo' and Avan Ch'en, near Paste'.

are caused by the gaze of another person, who may be completely unconscious of his power. The glance of a pregnant woman, for example, may be dangerous to young children. Or someone may fall ill when subjected to the gaze of a large number of people, as when walking past a crowd or addressing a public meeting.

13. *Ta 'ik' nosh* ("because of wind alone"). Some illnesses are caused purely by the action of winds, especially cold winds. Some informants use the term *ta 'ik' ta sik,* "because of wind and cold."

14. *Ta sik nosh* ("because of cold"). Some illnesses stem purely from the effects of cold.

15. *'Ipah yech nosh stuk* ("fell ill solely alone"). Some illnesses just occur, without any exterior cause.

16. *Ta k'ok' nosh* ("purely due to heat"). Some illnesses are caused entirely by the effects of heat.

17. *Smantal hve'eltik nosh* ("due solely to our food"). Some illnesses stem purely from the ingestion of bad food.

18. *Ch'ambalal chamel,* or *ta skuenta vo'nosh* ("because of water only"). Some illnesses are encountered through contact with water.

19. *Minor causes.* There are several causes of illness that are either specific to a single illness or are mentioned by only a few informants. Some are : (a) excessive consumption of trago; (b) hunger; (c) hot country, that is, the Chiapas lowlands; (d) sunstroke; (e) *Sok' ch'ich'el,* or "spoiled blood"; (f) one illness is caused by slugs; (g) one illness is caused by the moon; (h) shame; (i) sadness; (j) fatigue; (k) strain from carrying heavy loads.

Other Illness Dimensions

Chamel. The general Tzotzil term for illness is chamel, which can be used as either adjective or noun. The defining characteristics of a state of chamel are not completely clear, but they seem to include pain, impairment of bodily function, lack of desire to work, and loss of appetite. (The problem of illness components is analyzed in Chapters 6 and 7.)

It is also difficult to determine the limits of applicability of the noun chamel, since not all terms that are descriptive of pain, impairment, etc., can be described under this rubric. The test we used was a frame sentence *'Oy htos chamel .... sbi,* "There is a kind of illness whose name is ...." (The word *htos,* meaning "kind" or "class," is actually a numeral classifier consisting of a root, *–tos,* with the approximate meaning of "a separate kind" and a number-marking affix *h–,* "one.") Our subjects were asked to substitute each of 76 possible illness terms in the frame, and were then asked about the correctness of the resulting Tzotzil sentence. The results of this procedure are discussed in Chapter 7.

Here we would like to offer a few observations on the properties of the concept labeled as chamel. Insofar as any common features emerge from the analysis of this term, it appears that the underlying characters are these. (1) A chamel is not an innate characteristic of the victim (or, in most cases, one acquired very early in life), such as a birth defect. Thus congenital conditions are frequently excluded from chamel. (2) An operative factor seems to be duration. Many informants do not apply the term chamel to a medical condition that lacks sharply defined boundaries in time such that it is marked as an event in one's life rather than an ongoing condition. (3) Impairments resulting from natural events, such as an accidentally broken bone (although a bone broken in one's dreams, i.e. on the level of the soul, is a chamel), or minor and universal ailments, such as gas pains, acne, and some rashes, tend not to be considered chamel.

This minimal definition of chamel, then, would include only illnesses of marked duration (including incurable illnesses that are fatal) and of relatively infrequent occurrence (i.e. not a normal part of ordinary life) whose cause is other than the ordinary physical hazards of daily life. A broader definition is implied by some informants, who apply the term to any pain or impairment regardless of its duration or mode of onset.

Magnitude. Another dimension of discrimination between illnesses is magnitude. Illnesses can be classified as major (*muk'ta chamel*) or minor (*bik'it chamel*). The distinction is not entirely clear, and informants offer different configurations of discrimination. In general, major illnesses are incapacitating and often incurable, whereas minor ones pass. Major illnesses can be fatal; minor ones are not ordinarily fatal. Major illnesses affect many people, minor ones just a few. Major illnesses are difficult to cure, minor ones easy. Sometimes magnitude depends on cause: major illnesses come from witchcraft or the gods, minor ones from other causes.

Some informants insist on an intermediate category, *lek no'osh*, in which an illness is neither major nor minor. Still another category must be included for informants who state that a particular illness has no inherent magnitude but can be either major or minor, depending on external circumstances or on chance. Of all the responses offered by our sample group to the question of magnitude, 57% indicated that an illness was regarded as major, 41% identified minor illnesses, and less than 1% indicated that any of the terms fell in intermediate categories.

Curability. A related, but somewhat different, attribute of illness is curability, in particular the availability of an herbal remedy or curing ceremony. The possible classes advanced by informants are: (a) there is an herbal remedy; (b) there is no herbal remedy or curing ceremony; (c) there is a curing ceremony but no herbal remedy; (d) there are two varieties of the illness, one with an herbal remedy and the other without. A question that probed this dimension for each of the 76 illness terms elicited acknowledgement of an herbal remedy on 76% of the responses; 14% of the responses indicated that only a ceremony could cure the illness, and 10% said that no cure was available.

Curing personnel. The appropriate person to seek for a cure is another distinguishing attribute of illnesses. The classes offered by informants are: (a) illness for which it is imperative to find a h'ilol; (b) illness for which it is imperative to find a Ladino doctor; (c) illness for which no practitioner need be sought because the illness cures itself; (d) illness for which no practitioner need be sought because the illness is incurable; (e) illness for which either a h'ilol or a Ladino doctor should be sought, or both.

The last option may seem somewhat strange, but it was offered by a number of subjects. A few subjects tend to see Ladino physicians as necessary in some of the 76 illnesses, and the physician option was named frequently (i.e. more than 30%) for six illnesses. For all 76 illnesses, the need for a h'ilol was indicated in 61% of the answers. Approximately 20% of the responses said that the illness "cures itself"; 10% reflected the need for a physician; and 6% said there was no cure.

The blood. The distinction between temperature conditions of the blood is an important attribute of illness in Zinacantan. The condition of the blood implies the nature of the remedy, which always involves producing an opposing effect (for cold blood one eats hot foods, and vice versa). A classification, therefore, could be made either in terms of the blood itself or in terms of the appropriate remedy. The possibilities are normal blood, hot blood, cold blood, and "mixed" blood that alternates between hot and cold. When we asked about the condition of the blood in the 76 named illnesses, only 7% of the total responses mentioned normal blood. By contrast, 40% named hot blood, and 36% named cold blood. Some responses (7%) indicated that the blood could be either hot or cold in a particular illness; and a condition where the blood fluctuated between hot and cold was elicited in 9% of the responses.

Ceremony. Another distinguishing characteristic of illnesses can be the nature of the appropriate curative procedure. We asked about the use of candles in each illness and received three kinds of response: (a) candles are used; (b) candles are not used; (c) the use of candles depends entirely on the results of the h'ilol's pulsing. Sixty percent of the responses indicated that candles were used, 26% that no candles were used, and 1% that the decision rested with the h'ilol. The remaining 13% said the h'ilol was not employed to cure the illness, and thus candles were not used.

Another ceremonial feature that can distinguish illnesses is the number of mountains to be visited. This dimension touches on the magnitude of the curing ceremony. Sixty-three percent of the responses to this question indicated no need for a curing ceremony large enough to visit any mountains. In the remaining responses, as many as nine mountains were mentioned as part of the cure for a few illness terms; but two, three, four, and six mountains were the most common responses (7%, 6%, 12%, and 6%, respectively, for 2, 3, 4, and 6 mountains).

Applicability. Illnesses can be classed according to their applicability to adults and children or men and women. By age: the illness can be contracted only by adults (11% of responses); contracted only by children (6%), contracted by both children and adults (83%). By sex, almost all responses (98%) indicated that an illness affected both men and women.

Contagion. Some informants make a simple distinction between contagious and noncontagious illnesses.

Fatality. Illnesses may be classed into those that are necessarily fatal and those that are not. This dimension overlaps significantly with the dimensions of magnitude.

Duration. One kind of illness passes quickly; another persists for a somewhat longer time.

Repetition in life. One kind of illness attacks a person once in his life and never returns. The other kind can recur frequently.

Occurrence in the world. One kind of illness is always abroad in the community, and at any given time someone is likely to be suffering from it. Another kind of illness enters the municipio infrequently and remains only a limited period of time (usually appearing as an epidemic once in every several generations).

Degree of contagion. Among contagious illnesses, there is one class that is highly contagious, assuming epidemic proportions, and another that is only slightly contagious, communicating itself to only a few people at a time.

Some of these distinctions, especially the last six, seem relatively minor, and for this reason were not incorporated in the questionnaire we used to study the various illness terms. Other dimensions, notably those of curability, curing personnel, and blood condition, are of crucial importance in determining the kind of therapeutic procedure that is appropriate to a given illness.

Zinacanteco Illness Terms

THE LIST OF ILLNESS TERMS presented here is not exhaustive, but it can fairly be said to include the most common ones, and probably all those that are of any importance in Zinacantan. The list was obtained through formal and informal interviews with informants associated with the Harvard Chiapas Project. We initially discussed the terms informally with about fifteen informants, and eleven of these were also interviewed with a questionnaire composed of the various illness dimensions (see Appendix A.) The frames in the questionnaire, refined by this pretest, were then used to interview a larger number (total 69) of h'iloletik and laymen regarding the dimensions associated with each illness. This body of information served as the basis of the controlled study reported in Chapter 7.

In the following presentation, we have attempted to preserve native conceptions when reviewing the manifestations and characteristics of the illnesses. Some illness terms elicited much information about bodily manifestations or symptoms. For other terms, although their implications and characteristics (i.e. their illness dimensions) were known, we received vague and ambiguous information regarding manifestations. These were terms that labeled illnesses the informants had heard of but had no personal experience with. Whenever it was not possible to get a consistent body of data, our presentation of the illness involved is necessarily abbreviated. Quite frequently, for comparative purposes, we have results of a similar study conducted by Holland (1963) in San Larrainzar. When we use the word "informants," we refer to the interviews we conducted regarding details of the *manifestations* of the illness. In citing the *dimensions* associated with each term, we use the word "subjects" or "respondents" to indicate that the information was obtained by the questionnaire mentioned earlier.

1. *Simal ʻobal.* This term appears to refer to the common cold. It is believed to stem from Kahvaltik ta Vinahel (29% of the respondents, however, attributed it to naturalistic causes) and is a minor illness that one can catch repeatedly and that everyone contracts. It does not last long and is not fatal unless a

victim exposes himself to inclement weather, in which case he may die suddenly. Simal 'obal can be cured with an "injection" or with Mejoral (an aspirin-caffein nostrum sold everywhere in Mexico). If one has a strong cough, one can also take *mentolato*, a commercial menthol preparation. The native herbal remedy consists of *flor de difunto* ("corpse's flower," possibly a kind of nard) and *chihil te'* (elderberry) boiled together. Another remedy is ash mixed with salt.

2. *Sik k'ok'*. This term denotes a high fever with chills (the name literally means "hot-cold"), and the illness is a major one. It is sent by Kahvaltik ta Vinahel and circulates through the entire world (i.e., it is inflicted on mankind at large rather than being sent to punish any given individual). If the illness is sik k'ok' alone, it can be cured with injections or medicines. The traditional remedy is an herb called *poshil k'ok'* ("medicine for fever") and/or the ground seeds of a melon taken in warm water. If the illness is mixed with soul-loss or witchcraft, or if someone has sold the victim's soul to the earth, the cure requires a ceremony and may be costly and difficult. A "good" ceremony, one where large candles are lit to the Totilme'iletik, will be of no avail when a Yahval Balamil or a witch is at work. It will be necessary to light only small candles in order to throw the illness back on its sender. In the case of selling to the earth, the h'ilol—if he is very powerful—will have to go down into a cave and perform a ceremony to reclaim the soul.

3. *Komel ta balamil*. This is the famous *espanto*, or soul-loss, which is found throughout Middle America (see Gillin, 1948; Rubel, 1964). Part or all of the victim's soul (*ch'ulel*) is lost or damaged through shock or fright. The term denotes a major illness.

One or more of the ch'ulel's 13 parts may remain in the earth at a point where the victim has fallen or been frightened. At times the ch'ulel may encounter some danger or fall in a dream; and this, too, can result in komel ta balamil. When one is suffering from the illness, he may dream about his soul under the earth: there are only Ladinos and Ladinas there, and he is in their house working for them. A victim of komel may feel headaches, chills, and great fatigue. Often the whole body gradually seems to get colder, and swelling develops; if this continues the victim will die.

To be cured of this illness it is necessary to find a h'ilol who can reclaim the soul from the earth. Alternatively, one can bury ground tobacco and garlic in the ground at the place where the soul was lost and then rub oneself with garlic. This may free the soul by making the Yahval Balamil disgusted with it. The victim can also rub powdered tobacco and garlic on himself for six or nine nights before going to sleep, presumably for the same purpose. As an alternative, he can rub himself with a patent oil called *agua de espíritu* ("spirit water"); this is applied along the lines of the veins, and is sometimes combined with camphor.

4. *Mah sik*. This term appears to mean a localized pain brought on by cold weather. The manifestations our respondents mentioned were ambiguous. *Mah* is a root meaning "strike" or "hit"; and *sik* means "cold." This is said to

be a minor illness, and it comes purely through exposure to the cold or wind. One can cure oneself without seeking a h'ilol or a doctor. Before going to bed a sufferer should rub himself with white salt and lemon; if these are lacking, he can use white salt and rum. If he rubs himself with strong rum before going to sleep, he will sweat during the night and the chill will pass. Mejoral, taken before bed, may also help.

5. *Sim nak'al*. This term refers to an illness characterized by diarrhea. It is said to be a major illness that must be cured by a h'ilol. We also encountered the term *ch'ich' sim nak'al* (bloody diarrhea); some informants say this is the same illness, but others treat it as distinct. The affliction can come either from Kahvaltik ta Vinahel or from witchcraft. The herbal remedy is an infusion of the *nantsi* plant and/or the seeds of the *zapote* (a tropical fruit).

6. *Sarampio*. This term obviously derives from the Spanish *sarampion*, "measles." It denotes a serious illness that requires a h'ilol and a ceremony to cure. Some (41%) say it affects children only; the rest state that all ages are subject to it. The illness comes gradually. First there are chills, fever, and headache, but the patient can still get about. After three days the skin breaks out in small pimples. If these do not appear, the illness is involved with witchcraft, mahbenal (direct "blows" from the gods), or soul-loss. When they do, the illness is a good one—i.e., it comes from Heaven. However, one must still protect himself from cold for three days. If the pimples do not appear one can force them out by drinking water in which a squash has been cooked. If the illness is associated with mahbenal, one must pray or perform a ceremony in order to cure it; and if it is due to soul-loss, one must perform a Lok'esel ta Balamil sequence. In any case, the victim will die if the illness deteriorates, and especially if the pimples do not appear.

7. *Hik'ik'ul 'obal*. This term, "choking cough," labels a major illness and may be related to clinical infection with *Hemophillus pertussis* (whooping cough). The illness is said to affect mainly children, although 35% of the respondents said that adults could be affected. It can produce headache and fever, but its main symptom is coughing, which begins mildly but after two or three days becomes noisy and choking. A victim without a high fever tends to sleep a great deal. One should not eat much during the illness, and should especially avoid fish, which is called "the mother of choking cough."

This illness is believed to come from Kahvaltik ta Vinahel; and 57% of the respondents said that a h'ilol must cure it, although there are medicines that can be taken. One can drink a boiled infusion of *tsonte al krus* (a grass that grows on or near crosses), zapote seeds, *tsonte al toh* ("pine grass"), or *tutsis chon* ("stinky animal," a small lizard that lives at the bottom of walls). Another remedy is honey. If the illness does not get worse, one will recover with these things or with a small ceremony; but if it does deteriorate, then one dies.

8. *Skuyel hch'ul me'yik*. This is one of three varieties of *kuyel* (pox) recognized in Zinacantan. Holland (1963) says it is similar to chicken pox. First come chills, fever, and headache. Then, after three days, the skin breaks out in liquid-filled pimples that look like blisters and are most numerous under

the arms and around the throat. A h'ilol is needed for a cure, although remedies are available. One must light candles to the Totilme'iletik and to Kahvaltik ta Vinahel. Sixty-one percent of the respondents said that this term denoted a major illness.

9. *Muk'ta kuyel.* According to Holland, this possibly corresponds to small-pox. At any rate, 97% of the respondents classified it as a major illness. It is believed to come from Kahvaltik ta Vinahel (64%), but it occurs very infrequently and has not yet been experienced in the present generation. When it comes, it spreads everywhere in epidemic form. There is said to be an herbal remedy available, but 29% of the respondents said that only a ceremonial cure is efficacious. Some respondents stated that the whole municipio gets money together to pay for the ceremony.

First there are chills and fever, and then the body becomes covered with large, discrete lesions. The body of each lesion decomposes at once. If the eye is affected it is said to decompose; and if the inside of the eye is affected it may burst.

10. *Bik'it kuyel.* A milder form of kuyel (75% of the respondents said it was a minor illness). Holland equates it to German measles. Most respondents (78%) attributed this illness to punishment by Kahvaltik ta Vinahel.

11. *Muk'ta k'ok'.* This illness is also termed *bats'i k'ok'*, both terms meaning "big fever." Holland (1963) describes the same term in nearby San Larrainzar as referring to high fevers that possibly result in paralysis, without specifying a more definite translation.

The illness is sent as a strong punishment by Kahvaltik ta Vinahel; but it is rare and has not been seen in this generation. It is said to be a major illness, and it spreads to the entire population when it comes. Respondents were divided on whether an herbal remedy was available, 44% stating that only a ceremony could be used to cure the illness. When it is learned that muk'ta k'ok' is coming (its appearance is heralded in the curers' visions), money will be gathered from the entire municipio, and all the h'iloletik will join in conducting a ceremony on behalf of the entire population. Only prayer can avert the illness before it starts, since there is no preventive remedy. In the past, it is said, many people died from this illness. A high temperature, general debility, and generalized aches and pains are said to be prominent symptoms.

12. *Shenel ch'utel.* This illness involves persistent vomiting and diarrhea. It can come as a punishment from Kahvaltik ta Vinahel, or as mahbenal from the Totilme'iletik or from demons. If it comes from Kahvaltik ta Vinahel, it will spread throughout the world; but if it comes from the Totilme'iletik or from demons, it will afflict only one victim. The illness can also result from selling the soul to the earth. Sometimes shenel ch'utel can be cured, and at other times it is fatal; this depends on its origin. If it comes from demons or from the Totilme'iletik, it is sent because the victim has never had a curing ceremony. If he performs one, the Totilme'iletik will protect him, and he will recover. Sometimes a physician may also be able to treat the illness. But if

the sickness comes too suddenly, nothing can save one, no matter how many doctors or h'iloletik try to treat it. The vomiting and diarrhea are not accompanied by much fever, but the victim sweats heavily while resting.

13. *K'ak'al sik.* This is one of two terms referring to illnesses that may be equivalent to malaria. The illness is only contracted in hot country, where a Zinacanteco body is not accustomed to the environment. Respondents stated that one contracts this illness while bathing in the river: one encounters hairs in the water, and these are the "mother of k'ak'al sik." Others say that it is contracted by drinking the water in a strange town.

At first one feels a great chill and severe headache, and then come chills and fever. The victim suffers sudden attacks of gasping, and if he is struck on the trail, he may collapse. He is confused and disoriented all day, feeling as though he were drunk.

The illness can be cured with the patent remedies Paludrina and Aralen. Otherwise, there are medicinal plants that grow both in hot and cold country. One is called *poshil 'obal,* "cough medicine," but it is also good for k'ak'al sik; another is willow bark. Both of these should be boiled and the water consumed. Curing ceremonies are useless; only the medicines have any effect, and the herbal remedies are better than those sold in the drugstore.

14. *Pasmo.* This is another illness condition that resembles malaria. It is similar to k'ak'al sik but has a different set of associated causes. It is also said to be harder to cure. (Some informants say that in attacks of k'ak'al sik the victim trembles, whereas with pasmo he does not.) Pasmo does not pass quickly. The symptoms are very similar to those of k'ak'al sik; and the illness can be treated with the same medicines, although they will be less effective in this case.

15. *Sikil 'ik'.* This illness is also called *sikil koloal 'il'*; both terms can roughly be translated as "cold wind." The symptoms are chills and fever, and most respondents stated that this was a major illness.

Sikil 'ik' is a severe chill that strikes one on the trail. It can come from demons or from witchcraft (either direct witchcraft or selling the soul to the earth. There are various remedies: a plant called *kurarina,* one called *soro te'* ("fox plant"), and one called *tentsun posh* ("witch's medicine"). All these grow in hot country and are "hot" plants. Each of them must be taken separately. It is necessary to guard the patient from cold for fifteen days; otherwise he will die at once. At the end of this time, during which he cannot drink cold water, the patient takes a steam bath and is ready to start going outdoors again.

16. *Makel.* This term denotes a serious illness having constipation as a prominent symptom, usually accompanied by other symptoms, such as fever. This illness is attributed to many different sources by the respondents. It is said that one can survive for three days and will then die suddenly. Formerly there were no medicines or doctors; but now constipation is curable, although it is said to be quite rare. There is said to be an herbal remedy, but a h'ilol is still needed.

17. *K'ush holol.* This refers to a pain in the head and appears to include protracted headaches. It is said to come as a punishment from the Kahvaltik, although naturalistic sources were also reported. It may be cured with Mejoral bought in the drugstore, although 51% of the respondents said that correct treatment really requires a h'ilol. Others (44%) felt that the illness would disappear by itself.

18. *Sak 'obal.* This is translated as tuberculosis by some informants, but there is of course no certainty that the term is always used to label persons with that disease. The literal meaning is "white cough." A variant is called *ikal sak 'obal*, "black tuberculosis"; it is regarded as a major, protracted illness.

Sak 'obal comes directly through witchcraft, that is, it is inflicted on the victim personally by the witch, with no supernatural intervention. According to other informants, the infective mechanisms include putting a spell on a glass of liquor to be drunk by the victim, or placing small objects, such as worms, into his food and drink. It is extremely difficult to cure, and if it gets worse, the patient will die. One must find a particularly knowledgeable h'ilol who knows what medicines to give. One remedy consists of swallowing cigar tobacco that has been beaten up in warm water; this may induce vomiting and expel the sak 'obal. This may cure "white cough." "Black tuberculosis" cannot be cured, since it is lodged below the throat. The victim gets progressively weaker and dies.

19. *Situbel.* This refers to swelling and is regarded as a major illness that must be cured by a h'ilol. Pathological swelling of the body (especially the limbs) is said to stem from fright or from the soul's being sold to the earth. Most informants say that an herbal remedy is available. One remedy named is *posh nibak* ("Ixtapa medicine"), a bitter plant that is very "hot." One boils it and drinks the liquid. It is very dangerous to be exposed to the cold after taking this medicine. Another remedy is to dry the heart of a vulture and then boil it in a very small jug; the liquid is then drunk. This cure is also hot, and the patient must stay in bed for a month to avoid exposure to the cold.

20. *Sep'.* This term, a major illness, denotes a severe rash or lesion that breaks out over a section of the victim's body and leaves it looking like a vulture's skin. When it begins it covers only a small area, but it may spread. The illness may be contracted in water, but originates from demons and witchcraft. One can get it while bathing or, in the case of women, while washing clothes. It often strikes the hands or feet, and in women it frequently affects the breasts and nipples. If it is not cured, the flesh rots away. Most respondents stated that an herbal remedy was available to treat this illness, and that a h'ilol was also needed for a cure. One way to counteract the torments produced by demons is to torment them in turn with offensive medicines; and some respondents stated that one way to treat sep' is to rub oneself with garlic, tobacco, and urine.

21. *Poslom.* This term denotes a major illness that consists of a discrete lesion developed in some part of the body, usually the arm or leg. First something like a blister appears. The surface of the blister is said to burst, and

what is left looks like a burn. Soon pus appears, and the infected spot develops into an open sore.

Relatively few respondents attributed this illness to a punishment from Heaven. Most said that one encounters it on the trail, through misfortune, and close to 70% of the respondents traced the illness to demons. Some say that the illness comes from an object like a falling star that enters into the flesh or into the stomach. It is also said that after some time the illness changes into another, called *mos*.

Poslom can sometimes be cured if one treats it right at the beginning, before it has had time to become accustomed to the body. If demons are believed to be the source, one can rub the infection with tobacco, garlic, and urine, wrapping it in part of an old skirt. Sometimes this will cure the sore immediately; but if one waits several days before applying the medicine, the cure will take a long time. It may appear that the illness is cured, but after a while another sore opens and it begins again; some say this is because the illness has changed itself into another form inside the body. If poslom enters the stomach, it is supposedly incurable.

22. *Tseluel.* This term refers to a cramp that interferes with locomotion, presumably a cramp of the skeletal muscle. Respondents stated that tseluel can be caused by the cold, by Heaven, or by demons. One can contract tseluel from the cold, especially when there is a *norte* (a three-day storm from the north, characterized by a penetrating damp chill). The chill enters gradually, until the body is chilled and the cramps begin.

Many said that an herbal remedy was available. If the patient is rubbed with alcohol or with a warm rag, the cramps will pass more quickly, but they may hide themselves in the body and return another time. If the patient ties a woman's hair that has been pulled out during combing around his wrists and ankles, the cramps will not spread to the rest of the body. Thread used for weaving can be employed in the same fashion.

23. *Tup' 'ik'.* This can be translated as "attack" and appears to refer to loss of consciousness. Many informants included convulsions as an integral part of the illness. More than half the respondents regarded this as a serious illness, and many stated that no cure was available.

Tup' 'ik' can come either from the Totilme'iletik or from demons. If it comes from the Totilme'iletik there will be only three major attacks. These are a sign that the victim is chosen to be a h'ilol, and during them his soul leaves the body and goes to receive instructions from the Totilme'iletik. He will previously have had dreams in which he received instructions, and the attacks are in part a test of his strength. A h'ilol will pulse to see if the attacks are good or if they come from demons. If they are good, the patient should go on a curing ceremony to all four mountains and will then be ready to make his debut as a h'ilol.

If the attacks come from demons, they can be treated in several ways. One method is to lay the victim's head on the middle of a doorsill. Someone then gives him three blows with a new rope or with yarn used for weaving. Another remedy is to rub the patient's head with willow branches. One can also use a flower called *pom ts'unun* ("sparrow's honey"). At times the demons can be discouraged if the patient is rubbed with an old skirt, but this only works when it is done at the first attack. Otherwise, the illness becomes accustomed to the body, and the patient will suffer from daily attacks for the rest of his life. A similar remedy is to wash the patient's head with urine.

24. *Hak'ob 'ik'*. This is an itchy rash, and is described as a minor illness that will frequently cure itself. It is said to come from a chill. Small, itchy pimples break out on the skin. Since it is a minor ailment, it may be cured with Mejoral. The patient can also rub himself with *unguento de aldea* (some sort of patent preparation) before going to sleep.

25. *Satil*. This term refers to a disturbance of the eye. A sticky liquid is extruded, the eye becomes red and itchy, and vision is blurred. These symptoms sound like a form of conjunctivitis. Satil is classified as a minor illness that comes from punishment by Heaven. It can be treated with a medicine bought at the drugstore, although many respondents also said that it can cure itself.

26. *K'elel*. The term literally means "seeing." An alternative term is *k'ak'al sat*, "hot eye." The meaning of both terms is vague. To some informants they denote an illness suffered by infants as the result of being damaged by someone else's "strong" or "evil" eye. The damage may not be intended, and the person with the evil eye may be unaware of his power. The symptoms described for the victims are various, including diarrhea, stomach ache, and fever. Other informants say that the term *k'elel* refers to an illness that stems from embarrassment, as when a person walks by a large crowd of people or has to speak at a public meeting. There is said to be an herbal remedy, but a h'ilol is also required.

27. *Chlok' hch'ul me'tik ta sat*. "The moon sticks in the eye." A whitish spot or disk similar in appearance to the moon emerges in the eye. The descriptions offered sound like those of a cataract, corneal opacity, or abrasion. If one who already has satil goes outside at night and looks at the moon, it may enter his eye and remain there, manifesting itself as a round, white disk; this is due to the actions of the earth or the moon alone. Many other causes, however, were also reported to bring on the same condition. One remedy consists of mixing Ixtapa salt in a cup of water. Into this one puts 13 black beans and 13 five-centavo pieces. The cup is left outside the house every night for three nights until dew falls in the morning. Each morning, the mixture is brought inside, and one of the coins is held against the eye until the heat of the body has warmed it, then replaced with a cool one. Eventually a few beans are also placed in the eye. Some say that the illness may slowly improve and be cured after the three days.

28. *Nuk'ul*. This is a swelling of the throat and is called a minor illness by most respondents. Many causes were mentioned. Several remedies are available. One is to squeeze a raw *tomato de cáscara* (a small, husk-covered, tomatolike fruit) onto the affected spot and press on it the cold edge of a machete. This is said to reduce the swelling.

29. *Makal ta 'ik'*. This is a confusing term. Several informants identify it with makel, or constipation. Others describe it as a separate illness characterized by general pains throughout the body and inability to walk. The term literally means "closed up by wind," and refers to a major illness caused by witchcraft and demons. Some say it can be cured by drinking water in which powdered tobacco has been mixed; or one can suck on a piece of tobacco and/or rub it over the stomach. Interestingly, close to 15% of the respondents stated that adults, especially females, were most vulnerable.

30. *Mahbenal*. This term, meaning "blows," refers to an illness that is characterized by aches and pains, a sensation that one is being violently struck, weakness, and fever, all of which are caused by the victim's being directly attacked by blows from the Totilme'iletik. All respondents said a h'ilol was required for a cure, and that candles and visits to mountains were an integral part of the ceremony.

31. *E'al*. This is a minor illness, in which white spots appear on the tongue and the interior of the mouth. Holland (1963) reports that in San Larrainzar the illness is said to mainly affect children. The great majority (93%) of our respondents said that both adults and children are affected. This illness may be sent by the Totilme'iletik or may be the result of the heat. It can be treated by putting lemon and white sugar on the tongue.

32. *Ch'ich' sim nak'al*. This term refers to bloody diarrhea and is regarded as a serious illness. It is said to come from Kahvaltik ta Vinahel or from the Totilme'iletik. One does not feel it at the moment it attacks, but only when the stomach and anus begin to hurt. First comes white diarrhea, and then blood. Ch'ich' sim nak'al is more painful than other illnesses. The patient cannot eat beef or pork that still contains blood, since this is "cold" food and will make the illness worse. Nor can he eat rooster, although hen is a hot food and can be eaten in small quantities. Only vegetables and pinole (a maize drink) can be eaten. A curing ceremony may be necessary if the sickness comes from the Totilme'iletik. There are also medicines. The most effective treatment is to boil zapote seeds and the bark of the nantsi together and drink the liquid; this will stop the diarrhea quickly. Somewhat less effective is *refresco de panela* (raw brown sugar in cold water).

33. *K'ush k'abil*. This illness is characterized by pain while urinating and is described as minor. The cause may be witchcraft, although other sources were acknowledged. There is an herbal remedy available.

34. *Taki' chamel*. Several informants consider this the same as ti'ol (No. 67), but we have included it separately because many informants distinguish between the terms. The main clue that we have to the meaning is the word *takih*, which means "to dry up" and perhaps should replace the term taki'. This would produce "drying-up illness," which accords well with informants' descriptions of the affliction as a chronic state of weakness and lassitude. Both this illness and ti'ol are characterized by loss of appetite, loss of interest in life, general malaise, and a gradual wasting away. According to some in-

formants, taki' chamel is due merely to sadness; others attribute it to a variety of causes. It must be cured by a h'ilol, using a curing ceremony.

35. *Chuvah.* This term can be translated as "madness." Some informants attribute it to witchcraft, which works by introducing worms into the victim's ears and nose; others say that demons are the cause. The major symptom is erratic, drunken behavior—shouting, screaming, raucous singing, etc. It is regarded as a major illness by 90% of the respondents.

This illness is frequently caused by demons or witchcraft. It can be cured with medicine. One remedy is a plant called *poshil chuvah* that grows flat on the ground. This is ground up raw, and the juice is drunk; it is also beaten up with cold water, and some is put in the ears and in the nostrils. Another remedy is made by boiling certain large insects that live in hot country and drinking the water. A curing ceremony is said to be useful in many cases.

The use of this term in Zinacantan and in other Maya communities of the area (see Fabrega, Metzger, and Williams, 1970) is instructive from the standpoint of folk medicine. It clearly denotes irregularity in a person's social behavior, and as such may be regarded as a "folk-psychiatric illness." The term may be applied to symptoms that resemble those seen in various psychoses (with delusions and hallucinations prominent), though some respondents report that headaches and temperature are associated with the condition. Apparently the term labels symptoms that in Western medicine have diverse etiological sources.

36. *Ta skuenta (ta hkuentatik).* Roughly, "for his sake" or "for our sake." This idiomatically refers to the infliction of illness by Kahvaltik ta Vinahel or the Totilme'iletik in order to procure proper respect and attention from the victim. It is usually the result of not maintaining a proper relationship with the deities through curing ceremonies. The symptoms can be of any kind, but are said to be incapacitating, with weakness and generalized malaise prominent. The illness must be cured with candles and a ceremony.

37. *Mahben k'ak'al.* This appears to refer to a condition in which heat and prostration are salient features. Some describe it as sunstroke. A few informants identify it with mahbenal (No. 30), but most see it as a separate illness attributable purely to sun and heat. It is regarded as minor. There is said to be an herbal cure, but 29% of the respondents say the illness cures itself.

38. *'Ik'.* Literally, "wind." The symptoms include painful swelling of the extremities, which are made worse by movement. This illness is traced to malevolent sources, and most respondents describe it as major. The remedies may be bought in a drugstore.

39. *Lukum.* This is "worms in the stomach" and is described as stemming largely from naturalistic sources. Twenty-five percent of the respondents said it affects only children. The remedy is made by boiling the skins of peaches. When they have boiled, the water is allowed to cool and then mixed with raw sugar; the patient drinks this. There is also a commercial remedy.

40. *Pumel.* The term literally means "swelling up"—in this case a swelling

of the abdomen, although some informants stated that difficulty in breathing is also a symptom. It is described as a minor illness that frequently cures itself. Most respondents attribute it to naturalistic sources, some saying that it occurs when too much air enters the stomach. It appears to resemble makal ta 'ik' (No. 29), but it is distinguished by a number of informants. The remedy is to suck on powdered tobacco and drink the juice. Another remedy, which one buys at the drugstore, is 20 centavos' worth of bicarbonate, which one drinks with strong rum.

41. *Me'vinik*. This condition is characterized by an accelerated pulse, "pounding of the heart," pains in the chest, and fatigue. The condition may come from overwork or excessive exercise, but is frequently attributed to Kahvaltik ta Vinahel or to the heat. There are remedies sold in the drugstore, such as soda. Another remedy is to drink sugar and lemon juice beaten in cold water. If one cannot obtain these things, he can put three willow branch tips in his belt and produce the same effect.

42. *Shu'it (shuvit)*. Holland (1963) describes the illness labeled by this term as characterized by small dark worms in the intestinal tract. In Zinacantan, "worms" were also involved, as well as pain, weakness, and loss of appetite. Shu'it appears to be very similar to lukum, but was regarded as a distinct illness by many informants. It was described as a major illness, with witchcraft as a prominent cause. Twenty percent said it affected only adults.

43. *K'ush o'onil*. This refers to pain in the chest. It is said to be accompanied by difficulty in breathing and sometimes difficulty in swallowing. Most respondents described it as a major illness sent from Heaven, although witches and demons are also implicated. Some say that it can be cured with a decoction of boiled manzanilla, corn silk, and three tips of red pine.

44. *K'ush ch'util*. This can be translated as "stomach ache" and is associated with abdominal pain and loss of appetite. More than half the respondents stated that it is brought on by naturalistic causes, such as cold, wind, or bad food. It is described as a minor illness.

45. *Makem schikin*. This literally means "his ears [are] closed" and refers to deafness. The condition is caused by the gods, by witches and demons, or by naturalistic events. It is described as a major illness. One remedy is to grind up certain odiferous plants that grow in the hills and put the juice in the victim's ears. If this is done many times, his hearing will gradually improve. One can also obtain a kind of shell that is found on river shores, fill it with hot water, and pour the water in the ears; this will open them up.

46. *Pak chikin*. According to several informants, this is the same as *mak chikin*. It seems to denote a less severe deafness, possibly congenital. Most informants, however, consider it a separate illness and we have maintained the two terms in this list for that reason. Most respondents described it as a minor condition for which no remedy is available.

47. *K'ush chikinin*. This term appears to refer to an earache. It is regarded as a major illness. Forty-nine percent of the subjects attributed it to punishment from the deities, although naturalistic events were frequently cited.

48. *Tup'em sat.* Literally, "extinguished eye," a type of blindness. This is described as a major illness. Some respondents (38%) said that it only affects adults. The condition can come from demons or as punishment from Heaven.

49. *'Unen k'obol.* This terms literally means "little slug" and is a minor affliction of the hand that one contracts from a slug. The slug damages its victim from afar; and he does not feel the illness immediately, but only when a growth begins on the fingers or at the base of the thumb. First there appears a blister, as if from a burn; this fills with liquid and is very painful. There is no fever or other symptom, just pain.

50. *Shok.* This is a dermatological eruption like itch or mange. Holland describes it as warts and moles. It is considered a minor illness by most respondents. Seventy-three percent of the subjects state that a physician is needed for a cure, although an herbal remedy is also said to be useful.

Some respondents stated that this illness is contracted through sexual relations with someone who is infected. It can also come when one is visited in his dreams by a woman, usually old, who comes to frighten him. Sometimes this dream figure is very mangy, in which case the illness is sent by demons.

The illness may appear as white mange or black mange (*'ikal shok*). For the black mange there is no remedy, and the eruption spreads to everyone in the house. It is contagious if one is afraid, but if one is fearless he will not catch it. Also, if one drinks the water in which someone with shok has washed, he will be immune. Black mange produces much itching and cannot be cured rapidly. White mange is not as bad, and the itching is less severe. Neither variety is fatal; one only suffers from the itching. Curing ceremonies are useless, and there is no medicine.

51. *Bate' chamel.* According to some informants, the symptoms of this illness are those of sik k'ok' (No. 2), and this is only a special kind of cause rather than a distinct type of illness. Other informants consider it distinct. The illness is described as a fatal epidemic whose outstanding characteristic is its extreme contagion. It is said that it will kill everyone in any household it touches, even wiping out entire villages.

Some informants stated that bate' chamel can only come through witchcraft performed by the inhabitants of Totolapa and Simojovel (two widely separated Ladino towns in Chiapas). If one has enemies, they may go to one of these towns to procure the illness; or it may befall anyone who directly offends an inhabitant of Totolapa or Simojovel. The illness does not occur in Zinacantan very often because the Totilme'iletik will defend the municipio if a public ceremony is performed. Otherwise there is no remedy.

52. *Sat pukuh.* This could be translated "ugly face" and appears to be a minor facial eruption. Others refer to it as a scarring of the face. It is regarded as a minor condition, but a number of the respondents described it as not really an illness (chamel).

53. *K'ush benchon.* This term refers to toothache or jaw ache and is described as a major illness that only affects adults. It is usually caused by Heaven. There is an herbal remedy called *poshil k'ush benchon.*

54. *P'otbenal.* This term appears to refer to sores in the mouth, or sometimes in the body. It is a major illness that requires a h'ilol. Many informants say that the illness is sent by Heaven or the Totilme'iletik as a punishment for lying. The remedy is a plant, *nichim pimil anal,* which is ground up and applied externally.

55. *Lots'om chih.* This term refers to pain in the muscles or joints of the hand and there is said to be much limitation of activity. It was attributed to naturalistic sources and was described as a minor illness. Thirty-eight percent of the respondents stated that it affected only adults.

56. *Makal snuk' ta sik.* This can be translated to mean "his neck is closed from cold." It refers to an obstruction of the throat associated with hoarseness, pain, and difficulty in speaking. It is described as a minor illness, which can be cured by drinking an infusion of *flor de difunto.*

57. *'Ip hsekubtik.* Literally, "liver illness." This is described as a major illness caused by witchcraft (28%) or excessive drinking (29%). Few informants volunteered specific symptoms associated with this condition. Close to 40% of the subjects stated that it only affected adults, and many said that a physician was needed for a cure.

58. *Empachal.* This term appears to be derived from the Spanish *empacho,* meaning roughly "indigestion." The condition is said to be minor and to come largely from naturalistic sources. Many informants attribute it to food, and a few to hunger and/or excessive drinking. The remedy is to have someone rub the patient with lard, using a hot rag, every night before bed.

59. *Ch'avan sbakel.* The illness so labeled includes chills and bodily pain, often accompanied by feverishness. It is described as a minor illness that requires the services of a h'ilol. It is said to be a punishment from the gods, although 25% of the subjects said it comes from exposure to cold.

60. *Vo'an.* This appears to refer to a growth or tumor of some sort, which is associated with much weakness and tiredness. It is described as a major illness by 80% of the respondents, and is said to stem from malevolent sources. Most subjects indicated that a h'ilol was needed for a cure.

61. *Tashk'a srinyon.* This literally means "the kidney rots" and may actually refer to a kidney ailment. The term appears to be derived from contact with Ladino physicians or druggists. Many informants attribute the illness to an excessive consumption of rum. Over 60% of the subjects said that a physician was needed for a cure, and close to 50% stated that only adults were affected. There is said to be a remedy that can be purchased at the drugstore.

62. *Chakal.* Informants' descriptions of this term can be translated as "tumor," although boils or carbuncles would also be accurate. It is viewed as a major illness by 59% of the subjects. It is said to be a saclike tumor that grows in the body and fills with liquid. It hurts less after it has discharged its contents. If it has not, one can take medicine to make it do so; then it will gradually heal. The illness also causes chills, fever, and pain. The remedy is not taken internally. Instead, one grinds up either squash or matazana seeds and

applies them to the head of the growth to make it burst; the affected area is then washed with a boiled solution of *pak chak*.

63. *Ma'a sat*. This term refers to blindness and is said to be a major illness. Some informants identify this with *tup'em sat* (No. 48), but others describe it as a distinct illness. The difference may be that ma'a sat is supposedly incurable. It was attributed by a large proportion of the subjects to naturalistic sources, and 44% stated that it did not have a cure.

64. *Sal tsil*. This term denotes a skin ailment, and some informants localize it in the face, especially the eyes. Holland (1963) describes it as a discoloration that forms spots and is accompanied by a slight itching. It is viewed as a minor illness that comes largely from naturalistic sources. There is an herbal remedy called *poshil sal tsi'*; one rubs this flower on the affected spot.

65. *Chin* (or *ch'inin chin*). "Pimple" or "itching pimple." This was referred to as a major illness by a large proportion of the respondents, and was attributed to diverse causes. It can be treated with a drugstore ointment called *unguento antiséptico*; however, most respondents state that a h'ilol must be consulted.

66. *Yahba*. Holland (1963) identifies this as adolescent acne, and most of our respondents included skin eruptions as prominent features of the illness. Thirty-six percent of the subjects stated that yahba should not be viewed as an illness. It was attributed to naturalistic sources.

67. *Ti'ol*. This term denotes weakness or tiredness, and is often used to describe a person who is unwilling or unable to work because of laziness. The symptoms are loss of appetite, lassitude, fatigue, and so on. The causes are variously given as sadness and divine punishment. Close to 70% of the respondents described it as a major illness requiring the services of a h'ilol.

68. *Ch'ich' kabnel*. This refers to blood in the urine and is described as a major illness. It is frequently attributed to witchcraft and demons, although naturalistic causes are also cited. One-fourth of the respondents stated that only adults could develop this illness.

69. *Vevech*. This is a gross swelling in the region of the neck, perhaps an enlargement of the thyroid. Some respondents stated that it was associated with pain and difficulty in swallowing. It is said to be caused by demons.

70. *K'ael*. "Rotting." This appears to be venereal disease, or some similar irritation of the genital region. It was frequently attributed to malevolent agents. The condition is said to be a major illness, and more than half the respondents stated that a physician was needed for treatment.

71. *K'asel ta hch'uleltik*. "Breaking a bone in our dreams." The victim dreams of some encounter in which he suffers an injury and then wakes up with symptoms of that injury, such as pain and generalized body aches. This is attributed to punishment by the gods and is a major illness. It is necessary to procure a h'ilol and perform a curing ceremony.

72. *Nelish*. This term refers to crossed eyes. Many informants stated that the term should not properly be regarded as denoting chamel. Most respon-

dents attributed it to Kahvaltik ta Vinahel, and 46% said it affected mainly children.

73. *P'us pat.* Holland (1963) identifies this as a hunched back, and several of our informants gave a similar designation. It was described as a minor illness by 49% of our subjects, and 36% said it affects only adults.

74. *Solem kat.* Possibly equivalent to a rupture or hernia. Some informants indicated that it denoted problems associated with the male genital organs, and that it could cause difficulty in urination. Malevolent sources were frequently cited as causes, and the illness was said to be major.

75. *K'ush sat.* This appears to mean "eye ache." Some informants identify this with satil (No. 25), but others describe it as a separate illness. It is said to produce faulty vision and is viewed as a minor illness stemming from the deities and from naturalistic sources. Many respondents stated that it cures itself.

76. *'Umaꞌ.* This term refers to muteness, and 48% of the respondents stated that it was not really chamel. Punishment by Heaven was most frequently invoked as the cause of this condition. Most respondents stated that the condition is most frequently seen in children, and that no cure is available.

Mathematical Procedures Followed in the Study of Skin Lesions

Modal classification scheme. A 25 × 25 square matrix was formed, with one row and one column for each of the 25 photographs of skin lesions employed in our tests. Each time a subject judged two lesions (e.g., 17 and 24) to be similar a "1" was entered in the corresponding cell of the matrix $(M_{17} N_{24})$. If the subject formed a group of four lesions (e.g., 8, 12, 17, and 24), six similarity entries resulted $(M_8 N_{12}, M_8 N_{17}, M_8 N_{24}, M_{12} N_{17}, M_{12} N_{24}, M_{17} N_{24})$. In general, a group of M items resulted in $M!/2! (M-2)!$ pairings. Each subject's groupings were analyzed in this fashion, and the results were entered in the matrix. The units entered in each cell of the matrix were then totaled and converted to proportions, using 35 (the total number of h'iloletik tested) as the denominator. The resulting matrix can be labeled a "similarity matrix," since each cell records the proportion of the group that joined any two lesions together on the basis of judged similarity. The chi-square test was then applied to each of the 25 rows to evaluate whether the h'iloletik's manner of grouping the lesions differed from that of chance. In 18 instances the test yielded a value that was statistically significant. This far exceeds what could be anticipated on a chance basis, indicating that the h'iloletik had linked the various lesions in a nonrandom fashion.

Each row of the matrix was systematically compared to each remaining row, and two rows (representing two skin lesions) that were similar in terms of their entries were assumed to be conceptually linked by the group. That is, the lesions represented, in addition to being paired together frequently, were also judged to be relatively similar or dissimilar to the remaining 23 lesions. By systematic comparison we were able to identify groups of lesions that tended to show relatively similar entries across the various columns. These groups can be viewed as the subjects' modal categories of skin lesions (i.e., the lesions composing a particular group or cluster were regarded by the subjects as both highly interrelated and noticeably different from the lesions in other groups). The components and boundaries of groups were defined on the basis of the patterning of the similarity scores.

This analytic procedure yielded four groups of lesions, each comprising afflictions that were judged similar by the 35 subjects. This initial categorization or group partition can be viewed as the most abstract and general grouping of skin lesions recognized by h'iloletik. Each discrete group was then arranged in its own matrix, and the lesions within it were once again systematically compared with one another. Again, highly similar lesions were joined together and separated from others, and subgroups were formed from the original group. In essence, four new similarity matrices were formed from the four initial groups of skin lesions, and each matrix was again partitioned on the basis of similarity. The groups formed from this partitioning were separated, and their units were again rearranged and repartitioned by a similar process. This branching procedure was continued until all 25 lesions had been separated and distinguished from one another.

Individual differences of h'iloletik. It will be recalled that each subject, in classifying the lesions, was allowed to form as few as one or as many as 25 groups of photographs, and that the number within each group varied from subject to subject. Thus subject A's first group might contain six lesions; but these same six lesions could be distributed among several of subject B's groups. A measure comparing the different subjects' groupings was computed as follows. First, B was assigned a score to reflect how closely he had approximated A's manner of classifying the lesions. This was computed by the formula

$$S_{ab} = \frac{1}{N_a} \sum_{i=1}^{N_a} \left[\frac{1}{M_i} \sum_{j=1}^{M_i} \left(\frac{X_{ij}}{X_{it}} \right) \left(\frac{X_{ij}}{Y_{jt}} \right) \right]$$

where

S_{ab} = a score reflecting the extent to which B's manner of classifying resembles A's manner of classifying

N_a = number of groups formed by subject A

M_i = number of groups in B's classification that contain lesions of A's group i

X_{ij} = number of lesions in A's group i that are included in B's group j

X_{it} = total number of lesions in A's group i

Y_{jt} = total number of lesions in B's group j

We then computed a score for A to reflect how closely he had approximated B's manner of classifying the lesions. The same formula was used, with the identity of A and B reversed. The two scores were averaged, and the resulting measure was the X_{AB} entry in a 35 × 35 matrix (rows and columns representing subjects); it reflected how closely the two subjects resembled one another in their manner of classifying the lesions. This procedure was followed for every pair of subjects, and the results entered in the matrix. These entries are termed intersubject similarity scores in the text and are used as measures of agreement between the h'iloletik.

Conformance with Western scientific classification. It will be recalled that each subject grouped the 25 lesions in a varying number of categories, and that a particular category might include several different "scientific" types of skin lesions. For example, a subject's group containing five lesions might include two neoplastic lesions and three infectious lesions. Conversely, the lesions included in a given scientific type were often grouped into one or several of the subject's own categories. The extent to which the lesions of each Western scientific type were grouped together or separated in a subject's own classifying scheme was computed by the following formula, which yielded five scores for each subject, one for each Western type of skin lesion.

$$P_i = \frac{1}{M_i} \sum_{j=1}^{M_i} \left(\frac{X_{ij}}{X_{it}} \right) \left(\frac{X_{ij}}{Y_{jt}} \right)$$

where

P_i = the precision with which a subject judges the lesions constituting scientific category i

M_i = the number of categories of the subject which include lesions from scientific category i

X_{ij} = the number of lesions of scientific category i in a particular grouping (j) of the subject

X_{it} = the total number of lesions constituting scientific category i

Y_{jt} = the number of lesions in the subject's category j

Components of Curing Rituals

THIS DISCUSSION will fill out the picture of Zinacanteco curing ritual with more detailed descriptions of some of the basic materials, localities, and ritual sequences that were mentioned in Chapter 11. Included among these are several behavior sequences—e.g., drinking ritual, ritual meals, and pulsing— that are common to virtually all curing ceremonies.

Places

The ritual localities important in Zinacanteco curing start with two features found in every house: the patio cross (*krus ta tiʿ na*) and the fire (*k'ok'*). The typical Zinacanteco house is a one-room, rectangular structure with a steep hip roof of thatch and walls of wattle and daub; but newer types often have adobe walls and a tile roof. (See Warfield, 1963, and Vogt, 1969, for other types and details of construction.) The floor is of hard-packed mud. The house is set in a sitio, an area of land surrounded by a fence and containing the dwellings and outbuildings belonging to one or more members of a patrilinear extended family. These may include various kinds of sheds and possibly a *push*, or sweat bath. This is a small, shedlike structure (often an opening cut into an earth embankment and faced with boards) that is provided with a place to put hot stones, over which water is poured to make steam.

A part of the sitio adjacent to the house constitutes the patio. This is basically nothing more than a cleared area, more or less level and usually immediately in front of the door to the house. Some houses are provided with two doors, one of which gives entry to a second completely or partially enclosed patio at the rear or side of the house. The major feature of the patio is the patio cross, made of wood and usually about one meter high (Vogt, 1969).

Inside the house the major permanent feature of ritual importance is the fire. This is near the center of the room, beneath a smoke hole in the peak of the roof. The fire is permanently located in an area defined by three hearth-stones (*ʿoshyoket*), sometimes broken pots, on which the *comal*, or clay griddle, is rested for making tortillas.

The furnishings of the house that enter into a curing ritual are bed, tables, and chairs. A typical Zinacanteco home has one or more platform beds, consisting of wooden planks laid across a timber framework about two feet above the floor. For an 'Och ta Svolim type of ceremony, the patient's bed may be enclosed with a fence of rough planks, attached to the framework of the platform and running from the floor to about five feet in height. Every house also contains one or more tables and several chairs. These are crude wooden items manufactured in Chamula, and in size they resemble nursery furniture in the United States; i.e., the table stands about a foot high, with the chairs of corresponding size. The table is the most important item for ritual purposes, since it constitutes the principal item used in setting the scene for a ritual situation and is an indispensable part of the ritual meal.

Localities in the hamlets. The sacred localities of Zinacanteco shamanistic ritual are crosses, waterholes, caves, mountains, and churches. All these features exist in and around Hteklum, where they are the focus of the ritual pilgrimages made by h'iloletik while curing and in connection with the public ceremonies. The sacred localities in Hteklum have their counterparts in the hamlets, and these enter in some cases into shamanistic practice. Every waterhole group and hamlet (and some snas) has its own set of sacred places to visit during the K'in Krus ceremony; and Navenchauk, 'Apas, Sekemtik, and possibly other hamlets contain sacred mountains and *kalvarios* that can reportedly be used by curing parties in lieu of or in addition to the major localities in Hteklum. We have no information on the frequency of such ceremonies or on the forms they take.

Localities in Hteklum. By far the most important localities for private curing ceremonies are those in and around Hteklum. These include five sacred mountains, churches, waterholes, crosses, and various topographical features. It is useful to group some of these under the Tzotzil rubric *ch'ul vinahel*, or "holy heaven," which designates places where one can talk with the Totilme'iletik, or ancestral spirits. Each of the sacred mountains, as well as several other localities described below, is a ch'ul vinahel. The term seems to apply only to the established sites where large crosses, with special arrangements for lighting candles, have been set up to facilitate communication with the Totilme'iletik; the churches are in a separate category, and waterholes or other sites serve still another function. In the case of waterholes, many are used only for drawing water for the patient's ritual bath. Their water is a ritual material, but the waterholes themselves usually do not figure in the physical progress of the ceremonial circuit. A few waterholes, however, may be visited briefly, and that at Ni Nab Chilo' can even serve as a ch'ul vinahel.

There are also many crosses marking intersections of trails, minor waterholes, etc., at which the curing party may perform some minor ritual act in passing, such as genuflection, but which are of no further significance to curing ritual.

The locations of the important ritual localities are shown in Figure 5. It seems useful, however, to provide here some brief description of the outstanding features of the sacred localities in Hteklum.

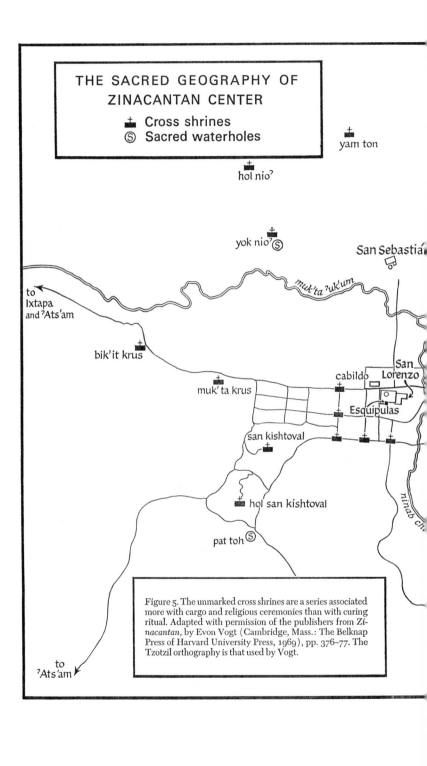

THE SACRED GEOGRAPHY OF
ZINACANTAN CENTER

⚰ Cross shrines
Ⓢ Sacred waterholes

yam ton

hol nioʔ

yok nioʔ Ⓢ

San Sebastiaᵢ

mukʼta ʔukʼum

to
Ixtapa
and ʔAtsʼam

bikʼit krus

cabildo

San
Lorenzo

mukʼ ta krus

Esquipulas

san kishtoval

hol san kishtoval

ninab chʼ

pat toh Ⓢ

to
ʔAtsʼam

Figure 5. The unmarked cross shrines are a series associated
more with cargo and religious ceremonies than with curing
ritual. Adapted with permission of the publishers from *Zinacantan*, by Evon Vogt (Cambridge, Mass.: The Belknap
Press of Harvard University Press, 1969), pp. 376–77. The
Tzotzil orthography is that used by Vogt.

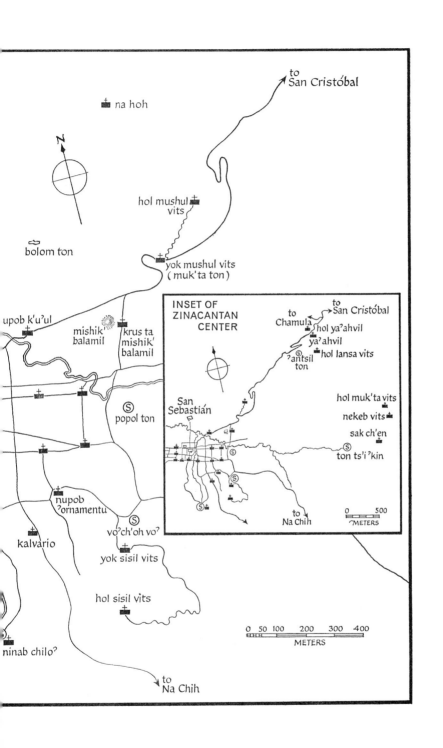

na hoh

to
San Cristóbal

hol mushul
vits

bolom ton

yok mushul vits
(muk'ta ton)

upob k'u'ul

mishik'
balamil

krus ta
mishik'
balamil

INSET OF
ZINACANTAN
CENTER

to
Chamula

to
San Cristóbal

hol ya'ahvil

ya'ahvil

'antsil
ton

hol lansa vits

popol ton

San
Sebastián

hol muk'ta vits

nekeb vits

sak ch'en

ton ts'i'kin

nupob
'ornamentu

vo'ch'oh vo'

to
Na Chih

0   500
METERS

kalvario

yok sisil vits

hol sisil vits

0 50 100   200   300   400
METERS

ninab chilo'

to
Na Chih

Mountains

Bankilal Muk'ta Vits ("older brother big mountain"). This imposing peak at the head of the valley of Hteklum is of great significance because it is the site of the corrals in which the *chanuletik* (animal souls) of the Zinacantecos are kept under the guardianship of the Totilme'iletik. Informants disagree on whether the seat of the Totilme'iletik is also within the mountain. Some state that the assembly of the Totilme'iletik, modeled on that of the officials in the local cabildo, occurs within Kalvario. Despite the conceptual importance of this mountain, it has little importance in curing ritual. Vogt (1969) mentions that it is occasionally visited by curing parties in cases of extreme gravity; but no such cases appear in our own data, although Vogt reports having seen a curing party there.

Mushul Vits. This is a low but distinctly formed round hill that stands out from the range of mountains forming the northern wall of the valley of Hteklum. There is a set of crosses at the top of the mountain and a smaller set at the lowest point of its base in front of a large boulder, Muk'ta Ton ("big rock"). These crosses are typical of those found at the ch'ul vinaheletik—one or more heavy wooden crosses, perhaps six feet high, set in altar-like rock or concrete bases. At the foot of the base there are several stall-shaped enclosures for candles. The construction and maintenance of these crosses is a public function supervised by the authorities at the cabildo.

Kishtoval Vits. ("San Cristóbal mountain"). This is a projecting knoll in the southwest mountain wall of the valley. The major crosses are at the foot, at the edge of a sharp, wooded drop into the valley; there are others, rarely used, higher up.

Sisil Vits. The full name, Ch'ul Me'tik Sisil Vits, means "mountain of our lady St. Cecilia." This is the most pronounced geographical feature of the valley, a precipitous, pyramid-shaped mountain that rises in towering splendor from a point about halfway up the southern wall of the valley, projecting out at a slight angle so that it gives the appearance of being an independent addition to the basic structure of the valley wall. There are two sets of crosses on Sisil Vits. One, at the very top of the mountain, is infrequently used by curing parties, though occasionally a k'esholil may be left there. The other set of crosses is at Yok Sisil Vits ("foot of Sisil Vits"); this is still some distance above the valley floor, just above the waterhole of Vo'ch'ohvo' on the slope of the mountain that faces into the valley. The crosses themselves are in front of a large boulder that protrudes from the mountainside. On some occasions the k'esholil may be left here rather than at Kalvario; if so, it is buried in the narrow space between the base of the crosses and the boulder.

Kalvario. The associations of the Spanish "Calvario," from which this is an obvious borrowing, seem to have little significance in Zinacanteco mythology, despite the striking correspondence between Christian imagery and the Zinacanteco Kalvario, with its row of wooden crosses on a barren hillside. Kalvario is, rather, the preeminent location of the tribal Totilme'iletik. It is here that a curing ceremony typically reaches its climax with the deposit of a k'esholil, a substitute for the patient's soul. And it is here that the Totilme'iletik are believed (at least by some informants) to have their major seat of office.

Kalvario consists of a leveled platform that projects like a rostrum from the hillside between Sisil Vits and Kishtoval Vits at a slightly lower elevation than Yok Sisil Vits. The platform, probably developed from a natural ledge, has been artificially extended and built up with rock walls on the edge and sides overlooking the valley. The crosses are near the precipitous edge of the level area, and the open area behind them (i.e. on the uphill side) is used for the ritual picnic that follows a curing party's prayers at the shrine. On the western side of the platform, about 10–15 feet below its top, is the niche for the deposit of the k'esholil. This is a small chamber in the rock wall of the hillside, whose original form—if any—has been considerably augmented by masonry construction.

According to informants, the Totilme'iletik have their seat of office some distance above the actual crosses, at the very top of the knoll. The crosses merely serve as a doorway to the Totilme'iletik, who are summoned by the curer's prayers and arrive on the scene to partake of the food, liquor, and candles offered to them.

Its'inal Muk'ta Vits ("little brother big mountain"). This mountain, though not in the valley of Hteklum, deserves mention because of its special importance as the site of rainmaking ceremonies, which are conducted by a specialized group of h'iloletik, with permission of the authorities, when drought threatens. The mountain is located to the south of the town of Teopisca, above a Ladino ranch called Chenekultik (see Vogt, 1969), well outside the territory of Zinacantan. Its origin and significance as part of the ritual landscape are obscure.

Waterholes

The seven waterholes from which the water for the patient's ritual bath can be drawn are Ni Nab Chilo', Pat Toh, Popol Ton, Ton Ts'ikin, Ni'o, Vo'ch'ohvo', and Ya'ahvil (see Figure 4). Of these, Ni Nab Chilo' is of special significance. There an underground stream issues forth from the side of a gorge facing on the western slope of Kalvario. The stream is used for washing the patient's clothes. Immediately above the spring itself is a small ledge, overshadowed by the rocky cliff to form a shallow cave or rock shelter; and a set of crosses like those found on the mountains stands against the cliff wall of the cave. Ni Nab Chilo' is used by some h'iloletik in the course of the ceremonial circuit in the same fashion as the mountains, even to the point of burying a k'esholil in front of the crosses.

Caves

There are a number of caves in Hteklum and throughout the municipio that have ritual significance because of their use in witchcraft. Caves and swamps are believed to give access to the world of the Yahval Balamiletik, just as crosses and mountains lead to the Totilme'iletik and churches to the saints. Much witchcraft, then, is believed to take place deep within these caves, where witches go to sell their victims' souls to the earth. The recovery of the souls by a h'ilol involves entering these same caves and swamps to make contact with the Yahval Balamiletik. This procedure is highly reprobated (see Chapter 6), and informants will furnish few details.

Churches

There are three churches in Hteklum; the hamlets of 'Apas, Navenchauk, and 'Ats'am each have a chapel, but these are of little importance in curing ritual. The major church in Hteklum is the Muk'ta Ekleshya ("big church"), the church of San Lorenzo. This faces on a walled plaza, on one side of which is the small chapel of Iskipula (el señor de Esquipulas). Directly across the valley, against the northern wall of mountains, is the church of San Sebastian. (The layout of the altars and images of saints in these three buildings is sketched in Vogt, 1969: 354–55.) Outside San Sebastian and in the plaza between San Lorenzo and Esquipulas are sets of crosses whose function seems analogous to that of the patio cross of a Zinacanteco dwelling.

Directional Orientations

Directional orientations, important generally in the Maya area, are significant in Zinacanteco ritual but curiously underdefined. The terms for east and west in Tzotzil are *lok'eb k'ak'al*, ("place where the sun rises") and *maleb k'ak'al* ("place where the sun sets"). The remaining points of the compass fall under the vague rubric *shokon balamil* ("sides of the earth") with no terminological distinction made between north and south. Directional orientation appears to depend on the path of the sun rather than on a compass, and thus changes somewhat during the year. The expressed ideal is to have ceremonial tables and other ritual elements oriented east-west, but the actual orientation is likely to vary greatly from the compass points. The main altars in the three Hteklum churches are all placed so that a worshiper looks east as he faces them; and each building has a door opposite the altar, that is, facing west. So far, this conforms to Maya patterns observed elsewhere. The crosses at the four major mountain shrines, however, are oriented at right angles to the church altars. At Kalvario the worshipers face south as they pray; at Kishtoval approximately southwest; at Yok Sisil Vits, south; and at Mushul Vits, north. The crosses outside the churches again face east-west.

Ritual Materials

Crosses. The symbolic value of the cross in Zinacantan seems only minimally related to Christianity. It is clear, from informants' statements and from the way they are used, that the crosses in patios and sacred localities are symbolic of doorways where communication can be had with the supernatural world. Most crosses used in curing ritual are permanent constructions. On occasion, however, small temporary crosses may be erected, as when a small cross is placed at the exact site of a soul-loss for use in the Lok'esel ta Balamil sequence.

It is noteworthy that the cross itself is inoperative for ritual purposes without the three pine boughs that are always attached to it during a ceremony. So indispensable are these boughs that Vogt (1969) has been led to suggest that the function of the cross may be primarily to provide a support for them (Vogt, 1969). Crosses are often triple, but even where only one cross is provided (e.g., the patio cross) it is made triple with the pine boughs; and where no cross is available, three pine boughs planted in the ground will suffice.

Pine. The class of plant materials falling under the Tzotzil rubric *toh*, which may be translated as "pine," is one of the basic ritual materials. Two kinds of pine tree grow in great profusion in the region: *bats'i toh*, "true pine," and *'ahan toh*, "corn-ear pine." The first is a variety of white pine (Vogt, 1969) whose wood contains a great deal of pitch and is widely used for kindling, torches, etc. Bats'i toh yields three kinds of ritual materials: *tek'el toh*, the long branches that are attached to the crosses at a shrine; *ni'toh* ("pine nose"), small boughs cut from the growing end of the tree, used for *mak kantela* (also reported for this purpose is *ni' 'ahan toh*); *shak toh*, pine needles used on the floors of the churches and in front of crosses where candles are to be lit.

The second variety of pine, *'ahan toh*, provides the pine boughs used by the *h'ilol* to beat or stroke away the patient's sins and illness at a shrine and to call the soul in a Lok'esel ta Balamil sequence. These boughs are called *ni' 'ahan toh*.

Other "flowers." The principal flower of ritual importance is *tsahal nichim* ("red flower"), the geranium. This is grown in Zinacanteco sitios for commercial sale and is simply purchased for the curing ceremony. The other plants (with the possible exception of *k'os*) are found in the mountains. They include laurel (*tsis' 'uch*), various kinds of *'ech'* (bromeliads, or air plants), and others. The symbolic function of all the flower and plant materials seems to be to represent life forces (Laughlin, 1962).

Incense. There are two kinds of incense (*pom*). One is *bek'tal pom* ("flesh of the incense"), a solidified resin or copal; this also doubles as rosin for the native violinists' bows. The other is *te'el pom* ("incense wood"), which consists of chips of wood from the incense tree (species unknown). These are burned together in the censer, or *yav ak'al* ("place for burning coals"), a crude footed cup of pottery. The censer is filled with glowing coals from the hearth, and chips of incense wood or resin are placed on top.

Candles. These are made by Ladinos and mostly sold in small shops in San Cristóbal (some are available in the few small shops in Hteklum). They are made by a cumbersome method in which the wax is poured over the wicks, collected in a basin below, and poured again and again until a candle is formed. Candles are sold by size, ranging from $1 (about 20 inches tall) to two for 5 ct. (about 3–5 inches tall). The larger candles used in curing are all made of white wax. In the smallest sizes the candles come in tallow and several colors of wax. The seven colors used in witchcraft ceremonies are white, yellow, green, red, black, gold, and tallow.

The number of candles used in a given ceremony is expected to vary among h'iloletik. Some used three at every cross, others two. Some use the 50 ct. size, others the $1 size; and some use only small candles. The candles used by the h'ilol Mariano Anselmo Pérez during a Muk'ta 'Ilel ceremony, for example, are: $12 worth of 50 ct. candles (24 candles); $5 worth of 20 ct. candles (25 candles); 10 ct. worth of each of the seven colors of small candles, at two for 5 ct. (28 candles). In addition, Mariano used $1 worth of incense.

Rum (posh, or "medicine"). Rum is the preeminent medium of exchange and communication in Zinacanteco culture, whether between men or between men and gods. Among the symbolic values of rum in curing are the following:

1. Rum helps the h'ilol to "see"; i.e., intoxication aids his divinatory powers;

2. Rum consumed by the participants in a curing ceremony is simultaneously received by the deities, especially the Totilme'iletik, to whom it serves as a sign of respect and propitiation;

3. The offering of a bottle of rum, as on a ritual table or at a cross, impels the presence of the Totilme'iletik and the Kahvaltik ta Vinahel;

4. The process of drinking rum opens up communication between men and softens their hearts toward each other.

5. Gifts of rum given to the h'ilol, like that consumed during a ceremony, are received as offerings by the deities;

6. Offering rum to another person is a visible sign of respect.

The Zinacanteco *posh* is a clear rum (officially known in Spanish as *aguardiente,* more commonly as *trago*) manufactured from raw, ungranulated sugar. It is sold legally by Ladinos in San Cristóbal and illegally, at a considerably lower price, by the neighboring Chamulas. The Ladino manufacturers, through coercion and bribery, are continually attempting to suppress the sale of Chamula rum, to little effect. Most Zinacantecos, despite occasional confiscations by the native authorities, continue to buy the Chamula product.

Rum is sold and transported in containers of many sizes. When first distilled it is usually stored in large jugs or drums holding 5–20 liters (Ladino trago is often sold in 5-gallon gasoline cans); and for public rites and large private ceremonies Zinacantecos will sometimes purchase it in these containers. For most ceremonial and social purposes, however, the rum is transferred to smaller containers, generally in one of four common sizes: the *cuarta,* a small beer or Coca-Cola bottle; the *media,* a larger beer bottle containing two cuartas; the *limete* of four cuartas, about the size of an American fifth; and the *litro* of five cuartas, equal to one metric liter. Most of the calculations for payment to h'iloletik, gifts, rum to be left at sacred places, and the like are expressed in these measures.

Other foods. Foods of ritual importance include chicken, coffee, *atole* (sweet corn gruel), and Ladino bread. The last, *kashlan vah,* is served with "ceremonial coffee" as part of the ritual meal. It consists of round, flat rolls of wheat bread, sweetened and sometimes garnished with sesame seeds. This is made and sold in San Cristóbal. Coffee, too, is usually purchased in San Cristóbal, although some Zinacantecos, especially in 'Apas, have their own coffee plants. Chiapas is a coffee-growing state, but the price of coffee is not low, and the grade bought by Indians consists mainly of charred corn husks.

Atole is sometimes substituted for coffee as the ceremonial drink in a ritual meal. Atole, or *'ul*, is a thick, viscous liquid made from ground corn and raw sugar. For K'in Krus ceremonies, a special *pahal 'ul*, "sour atole," is made. This is spiced differently, and it is served with *botil* (broad red beans).

Ritual Behavior

Several patterned behavioral sequences are common to many different kinds of curing ceremony, and are "replicated" on different levels of ritual activity throughout the system (Vogt, 1965b). These include many basic elements of formal courtesy that apply to interactions of all sorts: the drinking ritual that pervades every aspect of ceremonial activity from curing to cargo ceremonies; the ritual meal; and such basic elements of curing ritual as pulsing, fetching the h'ilol, and presenting the h'ilol's gift.

Drinking Ritual. The basic materials of drinking ritual are a bottle of rum and a shot glass. In every situation where ritual drinking is required (almost all organized activity in Zinacantan), one person, usually the most junior male present, is designated *hpis vo'*, or drink-pourer.

The hpis vo' first takes the bottle and pours a shot glass full, or nearly so. Ideally, his pouring should be calculated to ensure that the entire bottle will be consumed in a given number of rounds and in equal portions. The pourer hands the glass to the senior male present, or, in the case of a curing ceremony, to the h'ilol; he bows as he does so and is released by a touch from the recipient. In a curing situation, if the h'ilol is praying when this happens, he will pray over the rum, exchange toasts with the others (often omitted), and drink. Otherwise, the recipient engages in toasting, bowing, and releasing with everyone present. The person holding the glass addresses each of the other men in turn, saying *kichban* ("I am going to drink"). Each man comes forward and, depending on whether he is older or younger, either releases the drinker's bow or bows to him, saying *'icho'* ("drink!"). Men of approximately equal age shake hands rather than bowing. After toasting all the men in this fashion, and possibly exchanging toasts with some or all of the women present, the recipient drinks the glassful of liquor in one gulp, grimaces to demonstrate his appreciation of its strength, spits on the floor, and returns the glass to the pourer.

This entire process is repeated down the line of seniority; and after the men are served, the women may drink, also in order of seniority. When everyone has been served, the pourer serves himself and returns the empty bottle. Some variant patterns often occur in curing ceremonies. For example, when three rounds of rum are required at some point in the ceremony, the pourer may serve each person three shots at a time instead of making three rounds.

And at certain places in the ceremony (e.g., when the patient is bathed), the *muk'ta pis* ("big glass") is used. This contains approximately three times the volume of the usual glass.

In the leather shoulder bag that is an invariant feature of their attire Zinacanteco men typically carry an empty bottle and a funnel. These, under certain conditions, can be used for "pouring off." The man accepts a drink and goes through all the motions of toasting, but he takes only a small sip and pours the rest into his bottle. Pouring off usually does not occur until the h'ilol or the senior male gives the signal, and a younger man cannot properly begin to pour off while his elders continue to drink. Pouring off is not likely to begin until everyone has reached a sufficient degree of inebriation, and even then not all drinks will necessarily be poured off; rounds that are part of the ceremonial pattern are more likely to be poured off than those taken for pleasure or tendered as a gesture of courtesy or friendship (for example, drinks exchanged when one curing party meets another on the trail). Women do not pour off into bottles, but often keep a cup or basin for this purpose near them as they work.

The ideal patterns tend to be modified considerably during an actual curing ceremony. When the curing party is large, there is a tendency for the formal toasting and bowing behaviors to slough off as the drinking reaches the tail end of the seniority rank. The most junior men may merely make a perfunctory toasting gesture in the direction of the h'ilol, shake hands among themselves, and drink. The women may be left out of the drinking entirely. And an inexperienced or drunken pourer may fail to distribute the rum properly and remedy the situation by drinking the excess himself.

The ritual meal (Ve'el ta Mesha). The ritual meal requires a small table like that used for the altar. This is oriented with its long axis east-west. The following ritual steps were listed by our informant Domingo.

1. The participants wash their hands and mouths. [They are given a flat gourd bowl of water for washing the hands. This is wrapped in a ceremonial towel (*mantresh*), which is white with red stripes. The bowl is set on the table in front of the h'ilol. He initiates the washing and is followed in order of seniority by the other participants. The bowl is then returned to the women, who hand up a towel-wrapped gourd cup of water for washing the mouth. Starting with the h'ilol, each participant takes a mouthful of water, rinses his mouth, and spits on the floor.]

2. When they finish washing, salt and rum are placed on the table. [A bottle of rum is set at the east end of the table. No one sits at this end of the table, where, according to some informants, the Totilme'iletik appear during the meal. The participants are arranged down the sides and at the west end in order of seniority, alternating from side to side, as in Figure 5. A small dish of salt is set west of the rum.]

3. They place the food on the table. [A clay bowl containing chicken or meat in broth is placed before each participant.]

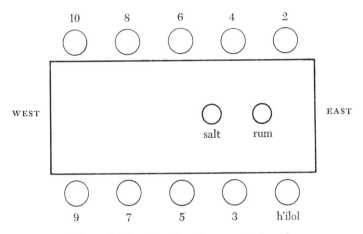

Figure 6. The order of seating at a ritual meal.

4. The h'ilol blesses the meal and prays to the Totilme'iletik.

5. Then they eat. [A stack of tortillas has been placed on the table during the prayer. The h'ilol initiates each stage of the meal. First he takes a tortilla, places salt on it, and eats a bite or two. Everyone follows suit. He then eats the broth by dipping the tortilla into it. Finally, he takes some of the chicken or meat onto the tortilla and eats it. No one precedes the h'ilol at any of these stages. Ideally, the participants should finish eating before the h'ilol. If they do not, and if anything is left in their bowls, they may wrap the meat in a tortilla and place it in their shoulder bags.]

6. After eating, they drink the ceremonial coffee. [Each participant is handed a gourd of coffee (*vo' 'uch'el*), on top of which are two or three kashlan vah; both coffee and bread are wrapped in a ceremonial towel. Again, the h'ilol initiates the eating and drinking. In a variant pattern occasionally observed, the ceremonial coffee and bread are handed to each participant at the beginning of the meal and blessed by the h'ilol. They are consumed first, followed by the chicken or meat. Atole occasionally substitutes for coffee.]

7. After coffee, the h'ilol blesses the bottle of rum, which is then poured out and drunk. This rum is called *ya'lel mesha* ["the water of the table"].

8. Then the dishes are taken away and the participants wash their hands and mouths.

[The table is covered with a mantresh before the rum and salt are set out at the beginning of the meal. The cloth is rolled up to the head of the table while the participants are washing, and after the water has been removed it is rolled down again. Rounds of drinks from a second bottle may be served with the meal—usually one after the washing, another after the chicken is eaten and before the coffee is served, and a third at the very end of the meal, after the rinsing of the mouth. See Vogt (1965b) for a more detailed description of the ritual meal.]

Pulsing (pik ch'ich'). Listening to the blood is the basic diagnostic procedure used by h'iloletik. The patient may come to the curer's house and, after polite conversation, ask for a pulsing; or the diagnosis may take place in the patient's house. The h'ilol seats himself, spits on his fingers, and applies them to the patient's arms inside each wrist and elbow. As he pulses, or immediately afterward, he tells the patient what the blood is saying. It has so far been impossible for us to obtain any statement from a h'ilol regarding how the blood actually communicates. The rate and strength of the pulse undoubtedly have some effect on what the curer says; but we do not know if any regular association is made between different kinds of pulse rate, for example, and particular illnesses.

Courtesy. The curing ceremony is full of ritualized activities that are matters of formal Zinacanteco courtesy rather than special features of the ceremony itself. Formal patterns for approaching a house and greeting its occupants, for example, are followed at all appropriate points in the ceremony. There are similar formalized patterns for asking the curer's service, presenting gifts, and so on.

General Notes

It might be well to briefly review some of the major symbolic and conceptual features of the ceremonies. One interesting aspect of Zinacanteco curing is the use of markers to set off the sacred from the profane—especially when a sacred background has to be established in what is ordinarily a profane setting, such as a private home. The most important sacred marker in a house is the table: simply by orienting an ordinary wooden table east-west and placing on it candles with their wicks pointing east, one converts the house from a profane to a sacred location. An even more definitive marker, when used, is the mantresh, which unequivocally marks a ritual occasion when placed on the table.

Pine boughs and needles play a similar role. Pine boughs are the indispensable accompaniment of sacred ritual at crosses, as are pine needles freshly sprinkled before a cross to prepare it for ritual use. The incense burner, too, invariably accompanies prayer either before crosses or at the table.

The proper use of ritual materials converts them into offerings for the gods, which in part accounts for the lavish expenditure of these materials during a curing ceremony. Flowers, candles, food, rum, and gifts are all received by the gods—but only after they are transformed by their prescribed use in the ceremony. We can see the ceremony, then, as a transaction in which the participants offer the gods not only the ritual sacrifices themselves but the ceremonial labor needed to convert them to divine use.

The Totilme'iletik and Kahvaltik ta Vinahel are believed to be present at various stages of a ceremony, summoned by the curer's prayers and by the ritual placement of rum on the table, in the hearth, and before crosses. Rum is the outstanding avenue of communication between the individual, other men, and the gods. All situations of ritual drinking in Zinacantan, curing ceremonies included, also symbolize the existing seniority relationships of the participants. In a curing ceremony the patient tends to move to the head of the seniority arrangement (drinking right after the h'ilol and marching directly in front of him), whatever his actual standing. This may express the extraordinary position in which his illness temporarily places him, as the center of the supportive activities of all participants.

Examples of Curing Prayers

SPACE DOES NOT PERMIT the presentation of anything like a complete range of curing prayers or an analysis of their content. It is hoped that these will appear in a later publication. The following samples of prayers used in different kinds of curing situations were collected from the h'ilol Telesh Komis Rodrigo of Paste'. The translations are very rough. The Tzotzil of Zinacanteco prayers is in large part antiquated and obscure, and it is difficult to translate it adequately. Nonetheless, our examples should at least give some idea of the ideas and symbols used in curing ritual.

1. *Prayer for Calling the Soul in a Lok'esel ta Balamil Sequence*
(for a patient named Juan)

Come now, Juan, come from where you have stayed in the earth.
You are not only seated there, you are not only huddled there.
From where you were frightened, from where you were affrighted,
Your feet were frightened, your hands were frightened.
Near you, in front of you,
The divine heaven, the divine earth,
The divine father accompanies you,
The divine mother accompanies you,
The six divine mayoles,
The six divine assistants [the mayoletik of the Totilme'iletik],
Six divine feet, six divine hands.
Come now, Juan; not only may you be lying there face down,
Not only may you be lying there on your side;
The extent to which you were frightened in such a place,
That you were affrighted in such a place,
In whatever place, in whatever direction,
Be it a place below or above,
Remember your house, remember your dwelling place,
Your father, your lord,
Your mother, your mother-in-law.

Get up so you may come,
Get ready to come;
You come accompanied by the holy father,
You come accompanied by the holy mother,
Six divine mayoles, six divine assistants.
Come now, Juan, come.

2. *Prayer for Saluting the Candles*
(*by the mother of a child patient*)

God, Jesus Christ, my lord.
How much my father, how much my lord,
If you are going to support, if you are going to protect
The back, the side (i.e. the body)
Of my beloved gift (soul),
Which is in your protection, which is of your suffering
In the afternoons, in the mornings,
Which does not feel well now,
Which now is not in a state of well-being.
Each flower of your vision, each flower of your face [these refer
    to days, because, it is said, the face of the Sun is like a flower],
Which has an illness, which has pain.
If you are going to support, if you are going to protect,
Divine fathers, divine mothers,
May you take your suffering.
Support him, protect him,
Do not let him weep, do not let him howl.
May you take his back, his side;
Give it your holy protection, give it your holy support.
My divine great father, my holy great lord,
Take your suffering,
Support, protect, watch, guard
The back, the side of my precious gift
Let not my back, my sides, remain abandoned;
In the afternoons, in the mornings,
For this I ask divine pardon, divine permission;
For this my beloved father, my beloved mother [the h'ilol]
Speaks for me, defends me—
He accepted my words, he accepted my task,
His head did not say no, his heart did not say no.
My beloved father, my beloved mother,
Protect him, support him;
My fathers, my mothers,
Support, protect,
That he may still have time to pass,
That he may still have his road to travel.

An illness, a pain, a sickness, an ending
How he is already suffering,
My beloved son, my beloved child,
My beloved gift.

3. *Prayer of the H'ilol to Kahvaltik ta Vinahel
and to the Totilme'iletik*

In the holy name of god, Jesus Christ, my lord,
As much as my father, as much as my lord,
Coming young, coming high,
The flower of your sight, the flower of your visage [i.e. every day].
It is for this that I ask divine pardon,
It is for this that I ask divine permission,
Because perhaps it is an illness, perhaps it could be an ending [death],
Because perhaps it is a sickness, perhaps a pain;
Where did it come from, where did it start?
Perhaps it was sent by one of his fathers,
Perhaps it was sent by one of his mothers,
Perhaps it was sent by someone young,
Perhaps it was sent by someone older.
Look how he is suffering, how he suffers.
You have him in your sight, you have him in your vision.
May you seize, holy father, may you seize, holy mother,
Holy Kalvario, holy father, holy Kalvario, holy mother;
How much I am going to put together, how much I am going to
    prepare;
I reach to speak to you, I reach to move my lips to you;
With a little incense, with a little smoke,
I ask divine pardon, divine license;
Take his labors, take his sufferings,
If they are going to stop, if you are going to protect him,
His back, his sides;
Your beloved sons, your beloved children,
Your beloved flowers, your beloved sprouts [possibly = people].
He is suffering, he is suffering,
He is like a rag, he is like an old board,
He does not feel well, he is not in good health,
Every flower of your sight, every flower of your face;
Seize, holy father, seize, holy mother.
What is thought, what is measured,
If there is healing, if there is reviving,
If there is grace, if there is blessing,
Of his back, of his side,
Your beloved son, your beloved child;
If you are going to fix him up for me,

If you are going to secure him for me
With the thirteen holy servants [the flowers, in thirteen bunches,
   used in the curing ceremony].
Take the thirteen holy flowers, thirteen holy leaves,
Which he is going to receive, which he is going to possess,
With which he is going to bathe,
With which he is going to wash his head.
Now comes young, now comes high [the sun],
The flower of your sight, the flower of your visage;
For this I am going to speak to you,
For this I am going to move my lips to you,
If there is healing, if there is reviving,
If he still has time to travel,
If he still has time to walk,
The flower of your vision, the flower of your faces;
If he does not die until later,
If he does not become cold until later;
His sin, his perdition [possibly reference to witchcraft],
Perhaps it is his sin,
Perhaps it is perdition of his father, his mother;
For this I ask divine pardon, divine permission;
In the flower of your sight, in the flower of your face,
In the place where his heart is content [his house],
In the place where he wakes up [his house],
I am going to speak to you, I am going to move my lips to you;
The flower of your vision, the flower of your visages [the sun]
Comes young, comes high;
Seize, holy fathers, holy mothers,
All holy fathers, all holy mothers,
All holy gods, all holy saints;
I reach to move your noses, to move your ears [the prayers intrude
   on the senses of the gods],
I reach to speak to you, to move my lips to you,
Around [i.e. around the ceremonial circuit]
Your holy vision, your holy faces,
Holy fathers, holy mothers, my lord.

Bibliography

Ackerknecht, Erwin H. 1942a. Problems of primitive medicine. *Bull. Hist. Med.* 11: 503–21.
——1942b. Primitive medicine and culture pattern. *Bull. Hist. Med.* 12: 545–74.
——1943. Psychopathology, primitive medicine, and primitive culture. *Bull. Hist. Med.* 14: 30–67.
——1945a. On the collecting of data concerning primitive medicine. *Amer. Anthrop.* 47: 427–32.
——1945b. Primitive medicine, *New York Acad. Sci. Trans.* II, 8: 26–37.
——1946a. Natural diseases and rational treatment in primitive medicine. *Bull. Hist. Med.* 19: 467–97.
——1946b. Contradictions in primitive surgery. *Bull. Hist. Med.* 20: 184–87.
——1947. Primitive surgery. *Amer. Anthrop.* 49: 25–45.
——1955. Primitive medicine, pp. 10–17, in A short history of medicine, Erwin H. Ackerknecht, ed. New York: Ronald.
Alland, Alexander, Jr. 1970. Adaptation in cultural evolution: An approach to medical anthropology. New York: Columbia University Press.
Attneave, F. 1959. Applications of information theory to psychology. New York: Holt, Rinehart, & Winston.
Becker, W. C. 1959. A genetic approach to the interpretation and evaluation of process reactive distinction in schizophrenia. *J. Abnor. & Soc. Psychol.* 53: 229–36.
Berlin, B., D. E. Breedlove, and P. H. Raven. 1968. Covert categories and folk taxonomies. *Amer. Anthrop.* 70: 290–99.
Boyer, L. B. 1962. Remarks on the personality of shamans, with special reference to the Apache of the Mescalero Indian Reservation. In W. Muensterberger and S. Axelrad, eds., The psychoanalytic study of society, II, 233–54. New York: International Universities Press.
——1964. Further remarks concerning shamans and shamanism, *Israel Ann. Psychiat.* 2: 235–57.

Boyer, L. B., et al. 1964. Comparisons of the shamans and pseudoshamans of the Apaches of the Mescalero Indian Reservation: A Rorschach study. *J. Proj. Tech.* 28: 173–80.

———1967. Apache "learners" and "nonlearners." *J. Proj. Tech.* 31: 22–29.

Broom, L., et al. 1967. Acculturation: An exploratory formulation. In P. Bohannan and F. Plog, eds., Beyond the frontier: Social process and cultural change, pp. 255–86. Garden City, N.Y.: Natural History Press.

Bruner, Jerome. 1968. Processes of cognitive growth in infancy. Heinz Werner Lecture, presented at Heinz Werner Institute in Developmental Psychology, Clark University, February 8–9.

Bruner, Jerome, and Mary Potter. 1964. Interference in visual recognition. *Science* 144: 424–25.

Bunzel, Ruth. 1952. Chichicastenango. Locust Valley, N.Y.: American Ethnological Society.

Cancian, Francesca M. 1966. Patrones de interacción en las familias Zinacantecas. In E. Z. Vogt, ed., Los Zinacantecos, pp. 251–74. Mexico, D.F.: Instituto Nacional Indigenista.

Cancian, Frank. 1963. Informant error and native prestige ranking in Zinacantan. *Amer. Anthrop.* 65: 1068–75.

———1965. Economics and prestige in a Maya community: The religious cargo system in Zinacantan. Stanford, Calif.: Stanford University Press.

———1972. Change and uncertainty in a peasant economy: The Maya corn farmers of Zinacantan. Stanford, Calif.: Stanford University Press.

Chance, N. A. 1965. Acculturation, self-identification, and personality adjustment. *Amer. Anthrop.* 67: 372–93.

Clements, F. E. 1932. Primitive concepts of disease. *Univ. Calif. Publ. Amer. Archeol. & Ethnol.* 32: 185–252.

Cockburn, T. Aidan. 1971. Infectious diseases in ancient populations. *Curr. Anthrop.* 12: 45–62.

Colby, B. N., and Pierre L. Van den Berghe. 1961. Ethnic relations in southeastern Mexico. *Amer. Anthrop.* 63: 772–92.

Colby, Lore. 1960. Tzotzil Dictionary. Unpublished ms., Harvard Chiapas Project.

Collier, Jane F. 1966. El noviazgo Zinacanteco como transacción económica. In E. Z. Vogt, ed., Los Zinacantecos, pp. 235–50. Mexico, D.F.: Instituto Nacional Indigenista.

———1973. Law and social change in Zinacantan. Stanford, Calif.: Stanford University Press.

Conklin, Harold C. 1954. The relation of Hanunoo culture to the plant world. Unpublished Ph.D. dissertation, Yale University.

———1955. Hanunoo color categories. *Southwest. J. Anthrop.* 11: 339–44.

Devereux, G. 1956. Normal and abnormal: The key problem of psychiatric anthropology. In J. B. Casagrande and T. Gladwin, eds., Some uses of anthropology: Theoretical and applied. Washington, D.C.: Anthropological Society of Washington.

Donabedian, Avedis. 1966. Evaluating the quality of medical care. *Milbank Mem. Fund Quart.* 44: 166–206.

Doob, L. W. 1960. Becoming more civilized: A psychological exploration. New Haven: Yale University Press.

Dunn, Fredrick L. 1968. Epidemiological factors: Health and disease in hunter-gatherers. In R. B. Lee and I. Devore, eds., Man the hunter, pp. 221–28. Chicago: Aldine.

Early, John D. 1965. The sons of San Lorenzo in Zinacantan. Ph.D. dissertation, Harvard University.

Edel, Matthew D. 1962. Zinacantan's ejido: The effects of Mexican land reform on an Indian community in Chiapas. Unpublished ms., Harvard University.

Ekman, Paul. 1969. Pan-cultural elements in facial displays of emotion. *Science* 164: 86–88.

Engel, George L. 1960. A unified concept of health and disease. *Persp. Biol. & Med.* 3: 459–85.

Erasmus, C. J. 1952. Changing folk beliefs and the relativity of empirical knowledge. *Southwest. J. Anthrop.* 8: 411–28.

Evans-Pritchard, E. E. 1937. Witchcraft, oracles, and magic among the Azandes. Oxford: Clarendon Press.

Fabrega, Horacio, Jr. 1971. The study of medical problems in preliterate settings. *Yale J. Biol. & Med.* 43: 385–407.

———1972. Medical anthropology. In Bernard Siegel, ed., Biennial review of anthropology, 1971. Stanford, Calif.: Stanford University Press.

———1973. Disease and social behavior: An elementary exposition. M.I.T. Press. Scheduled for November 1973.

Fabrega, Horacio, and Duane Metzger. 1968. Psychiatric illness in a small Ladino community. *Psychiatry*, 31: 339–51.

Fabrega, Horacio, Duane Metzger, and Gerald Williams. 1970. Psychiatric implications of health and illness in a Maya Indian group: A preliminary statement. *Soc. Sci. & Med.* 3: 609–26.

Fabrega, Horacio, and J. D. Swartz. 1967. Correlates of personality organization in schizophrenic patients: An analysis of means of genetic level scores on the Holtzman Inkblot Techniques. *J. Nerv. & Ment. Dis.* 146: 127–35.

Feinstein, Alvan R. 1967. Clinical judgment. Baltimore: Williams & Wilkins.

Foster, George M. 1953. Relationships between Spanish and Spanish-American folk medicine. *J. Amer. Folkl.* 66: 201–17.

Frake, Charles O. 1961. The diagnosis of disease among the Subanun of Mindanao. *Amer. Anthrop.* 63: 113–32.

Frank, Jerome D. 1961. Persuasion and healing. Baltimore: Johns Hopkins.

Gajdusek, D. Carleton. 1964. Factors governing the genetics of primitive human populations. *Cold Spr. Harbor Symp. Quant. Biol.* 29: 121–35.

Gardner, Riley W., D. N. Jackson, and S. J. Messick. 1960. Personality organization in cognitive controls and intellectual abilities. *Psychological Issues*, II, No. 4, Monogr. 8. New York: International Universities Press.

Gardner, Riley W., and Alice Moriarty. 1968. Personality development at pre-adolescence: Explorations of structure formation. Seattle: University of Washington Press.

Garner, W. R. 1962. Uncertainty and structure as psychological concepts. New York: Wiley.

Geertz, Clifford. 1966. Religion as a cultural system. In M. Banton, ed., Anthropological approaches to the study of religion, pp. 1–46. London: Tavistock.

Gillin, John. 1948. Magical fright. *Psychiatry* 11: 387–400.

Goldberg, Harvey E. 1961. The coheteros of San Cristóbal. Unpublished ms., Harvard Chiapas Project.

Goodenough, Ward H. 1957. Cultural anthropology and linguistics. In P. L. Garvin, ed., Report of the 7th annual round table meeting of linguistics and language study, *Monog. Ser. Lang. & Ling.* 9: 167–73. Washington, D.C.: Georgetown University Press.

Gouldner, Alvin W. 1960. The norm of reciprocity: A preliminary statement. *Amer. Sociol. Rev.* 25: 161–78.

Graves, T. D. 1967. Acculturation, access, and alcohol in a tri-ethnic community. *Amer. Anthrop.* 69: 306–21.

Guiteras-Holmes, Calixta. 1961. Perils of the soul: The world view of a Tzotzil Indian. New York: Free Press.

Handelman, Don. 1967. The development of a Washo shaman. *Ethnology* 6: 444–64.

———1968. Shamanizing on an empty stomach. *Amer. Anthrop.* 70: 353–56.

Holland, William R. 1963. Medicina Maya en los Altos de Chiapas. Mexico: Instituto Nacional Indigenista.

Holland, William R., and Roland G. Tharp. 1964. Highland Maya psychotherapy. *Amer. Anthrop.* 66: 41–52.

Hughes, Charles C. 1963. Public health in nonliterate societies. In I. Galdston, ed., Man's image in medicine and anthropology, pp. 157–233. New York: International Universities Press.

Kerr, M., and D. G. Trantow. 1968. Perspectives—and a suggested framework—for defining, measuring, and assessing the quality of health services. In Health services and mental health administration, pp. 38–76. Washington, D.C.: U.S. Public Health Service.

Kiev, Ari, ed. 1964. Magic, faith, and healing. New York: Free Press.

Last, John M. 1965. Evaluation of medical care. *Med. J. Austral.* 2: 781–85.

Laughlin, Robert. 1962. El símbolo de la flor en la religión de Zinacantan. *Estud. Cult. Maya*, II, 123–39. Mexico, D.F.: Seminario de Cultura Maya, Universidad Nacional Autonoma de Mexico.

Lévi-Strauss, Claude. 1963a. The effectiveness of symbols. In C. Lévi-Strauss, ed., Structural anthropology, pp. 186–205. New York: Basic Books.

———1963b. The sorcerer and his magic. In C. Lévi-Strauss, ed., Structural anthropology, pp. 167–85. New York: Basic Books.

———1966. The savage mind. Chicago: University of Chicago Press.

Livingstone, F. B. 1958. Anthropological implications of sickle-cell gene distribution in West Africa. *Amer. Anthrop.* 60: 533–62.

Lounsbury, Floyd G. 1956. A semantic analysis of the Pawnee kinship usage. *Language*, 32: 158–94.

McNemar, Q. 1955. Psychological statistics. 2d ed. New York: Wiley.

Madsen, William. 1955. Shamanism in Mexico. *Southwest. J. Anthrop.* 11: 48–57.

Meadow, Richard H. 1965. Modern and ancient Maya settlement patterns. Unpublished ms., Harvard University.

Mechanic, David. 1962. The concept of illness behavior. *J. Chron. Dis.* 15: 189–94.

Metzger, Barbara. 1959. An ethnographic history of Zinacantan. Unpublished ms., Harvard Chiapas Project.

————1960. Notes on the history of Indian-Ladino relations in Chiapas. Unpublished ms., Harvard Chiapas Project.

Metzger, Duane, and Gerald Williams. 1963. Tenejapa medicine: The curer. *Southwest. J. Anthrop.* 19: 216–34.

————1966. Some procedures and results in the study of native categories: Tzeltal "firewood." *Amer. Anthrop.* 68: 389–407.

Nash, June. 1967. Death as a way of life: The increasing resort to homicide in a Maya Indian community. *Amer. Anthrop.* 69: 455–70.

Neel, James V. 1970. Lessons from a "primitive" people. *Science*, 170: 815–22.

O'Nell, C. W., and H. A. Selby. 1968. Sex differences in the incidence of *susto* in two Zapotec pueblos: An analysis of the relationships between sex role expectations and a folk illness. *Ethnology*, 7: 95–105.

Parsons, Talcott. 1951. Illness and the role of the physician. *Amer. J. Orthopsychiatry.* 21: 452–60.

Pike, Kenneth. 1954. Language in relation to a unified theory of the structure of human behavior. Glendale, Calif.: Summer Institute of Linguistics.

Pozas, Ricardo A. 1959. Chamula: Un pueblo Indio de los Altos de Chiapas. Mexico, D.F.: Instituto Nacional Indigenista.

Rassmussen, Knud. 1929. Intellectual culture of the Iglulik Eskimo: Report of the Fifth Thule Expedition, 1921–24, Vol. III, No. 7. Copenhagen: Gyldendalske Boghandel, Nordisk Forlag.

Rivers, W. H. R. 1924. Medicine, magic, and religion. London: Kegan Paul, Trench, Trubner.

Romano V., Octavio Ignacio. 1965. Charismatic medicine, folk healing, and folk-sainthood. *Amer. Anthrop.* 67: 1151–73.

Rubel, Arthur. 1960. Concepts of disease in Mexican-American culture. *Amer. Anthrop.* 62: 795–814.

————1964. The epidemiology of a folk illness: *Susto* in Hispanic America. *Ethnology* 3: 268–83.

Sakoda, J. M., B. M. Cohen, and G. Beall. 1954. Test significance for a series of statistical tests. *Psychol. Bull.* 51: 172–75.

Shweder, Richard Allan. 1968. Cognitive aspects of shamanism: Experimental results. Unpublished ms., Harvard Chiapas Project.

Siegel, Sidney. 1956. Nonparametric statistics for the behavioral sciences. New York: McGraw-Hill.

Silverman, Julian. 1967. Shamans and acute schizophrenia. *Amer. Anthrop.* 69: 21–31.

Simmons, O. G. 1955. Popular and modern medicine in Mestizo communities of coastal Peru and Chile. *J. Amer. Folkl.* 68: 37–71.

Stauder, Jack. 1961. Zinacantecos in hot country. Unpublished ms., Harvard Chiapas Project.

Steffy, R. A., and W. C. Becker. 1961. Measurement of the severity of disorder in schizophrenia by means of the Holtzman Inkblot Test. *J. Consult. Psychol.* 25: 555.

Van den Berghe, Pierre L., and Benjamin N. Colby. 1961. Ladino-Indian relations in the highlands of Chiapas, Mexico. *Social Forces*, 40: 63–71.

Vayda, Andrew P., and Roy A. Rappaport. 1968. Ecology, cultural and noncultural. In J. A. Clifton, ed., Introduction to cultural anthropology, pp. 476–97. Boston: Houghton Mifflin.

Vogt, Evon Z. 1961. Some aspects of Zinacantan settlement patterns and ceremonial organization. *Estud. Cult. Maya*, I, 131–46. Mexico, D.F.: Seminario de Cultura Maya, Universidad Nacional Autonoma de Mexico.

———1964. Some implications of Zinacantan social structure for the study of the ancient Maya. *Actas y Memorias del XXXV Congreso Internacional de Americanistas, 1962, Mexico* 1: 307–19.

———1965a. Ceremonial organization in Zinacantan. *Ethnology*, 4: 39–52.

———1965b. Structural and conceptual replication in Zinacantan culture. *Amer. Anthrop.* 67: 342–53.

———1969. Zinacantan: A Maya community in the highlands of Chiapas. Cambridge, Mass.: Harvard University Press.

Wallace, Anthony F. C. 1961. Culture and personality. New York: Random House.

Warfield, James P. 1963. House architecture in Zinacantan. Unpublished ms., Harvard Chiapas Project.

Weathers, Nadine. 1947. Tzotzil phonemes, with special reference to allophones of B. *Int. J. Amer. Ling.* 13: 108–11.

———1950. Morphological analysis of a Tzotzil (Mayan) text. *Int. J. Amer. Ling.* 16: 91–98.

Weinerman, E. Richard. 1966. Research into the organization of medical practice. *Milbank Mem. Fund Quart.* 44: 104–45.

Werner, H. 1948. The comparative psychology of mental development. Rev. ed. Chicago: Follett.

Wiesenfeld, Stephen L. 1967. Sickle-cell trait in human biological and cultural evolution. *Science* 157: 1134–40.

Wilson, George Carter. 1963. Drinking and drinking customs in a Mayan community. Unpublished ms., Harvard Chiapas Project.

Index